Medical Applications of Intelligent Data Analysis:

Research Advancements

Rafael Magdalena–Benedito
University of Valencia, Spain

Emilio Soria
University of Valencia, Spain

Juan Guerrero Martínez
University of Valencia, Spain

Juan Gómez–Sanchis
University of Valencia, Spain

Antonio Jose Serrano–López
University of Valencia, Spain

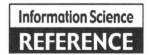

Managing Director:	Lindsay Johnston
Senior Editorial Director:	Heather A. Probst
Book Production Manager:	Sean Woznicki
Development Manager:	Joel Gamon
Acquisitions Editor:	Erika Gallagher
Typesetter:	Nicole Sparano
Cover Design:	Nick Newcomer, Lisandro Gonzalez

Published in the United States of America by
Information Science Reference (an imprint of IGI Global)
701 E. Chocolate Avenue
Hershey PA 17033
Tel: 717-533-8845
Fax: 717-533-8661
E-mail: cust@igi-global.com
Web site: http://www.igi-global.com

Library of Congress Cataloging-in-Publication Data

Medical applications of intelligent data analysis: research advancements / Rafael Magdalena-Benedito ... [et al.], editors.
     p. ; cm.
  Includes bibliographical references and index.
  Summary: "This book explores the potential of utilizing medical data through the implementation of developed models in practical applications"--Provided by publisher.
  ISBN 978-1-4666-1803-9 (hardcover) -- ISBN 978-1-4666-1804-6 (ebook) -- ISBN 978-1-4666-1805-3 (print & perpetual access)
  I. Magdalena Benedito, Rafael, 1968-
  [DNLM: 1. Decision Support Systems, Clinical. 2. Knowledge Bases. W 26.55.D2]
  610.285--dc22
                              2012002868

British Cataloguing in Publication Data
A Cataloguing in Publication record for this book is available from the British Library.

Table of Contents

Foreword..xvi

Preface...xviii

Chapter 1
Intelligent Management of Sepsis in the Intensive Care Unit 1
  Vicent J. Ribas, Universitat Politècnica de Catalunya, Spain
  Juan Carlos Ruiz-Rodríguez, Servei de Medicina Intensiva, Grup de Recerca en Shock, Disfunció
    Orgánica i Ressuscitació, Hospital Universitari Vall d'Hebron, Institut de Recerca Vall d'Hebron,
    Universitat Autònoma de Barcelona, Spain
  Alfredo Vellido, Universitat Politècnica de Catalunya, Spain

Chapter 2
Statistical Pattern Recognition Techniques for Early Diagnosis of Diabetic Neuropathy by
Posturographic Data 17
  Claudia Diamantini, Università Politecnica delle Marche, Italy
  Sandro Fioretti, Università Politecnica delle Marche, Italy
  Domenico Potena, Università Politecnica delle Marche, Italy

Chapter 3
Preprocessing MRS Information for Classification of Human Brain Tumours 29
  C. J. Arizmendi, Universitat Politècnica de Catalunya, Spain & Universidad Autonoma
    de Bucaramanga, Colombia
  A. Vellido, Universitat Politècnica de Catalunya, Spain
  E. Romero, Universitat Politècnica de Catalunya, Spain

Chapter 4
Semi-Supervised Clustering for the Identification of Different Cancer Types
Using the Gene Expression Profiles.. 50
  Manuel Martín-Merino, University Pontificia of Salamanca, Spain

Chapter 5
Real-Time Robust Heart Rate Estimation Based on Bayesian Framework and Grid Filters 67
    Radoslav Bortel, Czech Technical University in Prague, Czech Republic
    Pavel Sovka, Czech Technical University in Prague, Czech Republic

Chapter 6
Automated Diagnostics of Coronary Artery Disease: Long-Term Results and
Recent Advancements 91
    Matjaž Kukar, University of Ljubljana, Slovenia
    Igor Kononenko, University of Ljubljana, Slovenia
    Ciril Grošelj, University Medical Centre Ljubljana, Slovenia

Chapter 7
The Use of Prediction Reliability Estimates on Imbalanced Datasets:
A Case Study of Wall Shear Stress in the Human Carotid Artery Bifurcation 113
    Domen Košir, University of Ljubljana, Slovenia & Httpool Ltd., Slovenia
    Zoran Bosnić, University of Ljubljana, Slovenia
    Igor Kononenko, University of Ljubljana, Slovenia

Chapter 8
Pattern Mining for Outbreak Discovery Preparedness 125
    Zalizah Awang Long, Malaysia Institute Information Technology, Universiti Kuala Lumpur, Malaysia
    Abdul Razak Hamdan, Universiti Kebengsaan Malaysia, Malaysia
    Azuraliza Abu Bakar, Universiti Kebengsaan Malaysia, Malaysia
    Mazrura Sahani, Universiti Kebengsaan Malaysia, Malaysia

Chapter 9
Development of Surrogate Models of Orthopedic Screws to Improve Biomechanical Performance:
Comparisons of Artificial Neural Networks and Multiple Linear Regressions 138
    Ching-Chi Hsu, Graduate Institute of Applied Science and Technology, National Taiwan University
        of Science and Technology, Taiwan

Chapter 10
Dashboard to Support the Decision-Making within a Chronic Disease: A Framework for Automatic
Generation of Alerts and KPIs 160
    Leonor Teixeira, University of Aveiro / GOVCOPP / IEETA, Portugal
    Vasco Saavedra, University of Aveiro, Portugal
    João Pedro Simões, Accenture, Portugal

Chapter 11
Identification of Motor Functions Based on an EEG Analysis 172
    Aleš Belič, University of Ljubljana, Slovenia
    Vito Logar, University of Ljubljana, Slovenia

Chapter 12
Visual Data Mining in Physiotherapy Using Self-Organizing Maps: A New Approximation
to the Data Analysis 187
Yasser Alakhdar, University of Valencia, Spain
José M. Martínez-Martínez, University of Valencia, Spain
Josep Guimerà-Tomás, University of Valencia, Spain
Pablo Escandell-Montero, University of Valencia, Spain
Josep Benitez, University of Valencia, Spain
Emilio Soria-Olivas, University of Valencia, Spain

Chapter 13
Kernel Generative Topographic Mapping of Protein Sequences 195
Martha-Ivón Cárdenas, Universitat Politècnica de Catalunya, Spain
Alfredo Vellido, Universitat Politècnica de Catalunya, Spain
Iván Olier, The University of Manchester, UK
Xavier Rovira, Institut de Neurociències, Universitat Autònoma de Barcelona, Spain
Jesús Giraldo, Institut de Neurociències and Unitat de Bioestadística, Universitat Autònoma
*   de Barcelona, Spain*

Chapter 14
Medical Critiquing Systems 209
Ian Douglas, Florida State University, USA

Chapter 15
Learning Probabilistic Graphical Models: A Review of Techniques and
Applications in Medicine 223
Juan I. Alonso-Barba, University of Castilla-La Mancha, Spain
Jens D. Nielsen University of Castilla-La Mancha, Spain
Luis de la Ossa, University of Castilla-La Mancha, Spain
Jose M. Puerta, University of Castilla-La Mancha, Spain

Chapter 16
Natural Language Processing and Machine Learning Techniques
Help Achieve a Better Medical Practice 237
Oana Frunza, University of Ottawa, Canada
Diana Inkpen, University of Ottawa, Canada

Chapter 17
Modeling Interpretable Fuzzy Rule-Based Classifiers for Medical Decision Support 255
Jose M. Alonso, University of Alcala, Spain
Ciro Castiello, University of Bari, Italy
Marco Lucarelli, University of Bari, Italy
Corrado Mencar, University of Bari, Italy

Chapter 18
Extraction of Medical Pathways from Electronic Patient Records..273
    Dario Antonelli, Politecnico di Torino, Italy
    Elena Baralis, Politecnico di Torino, Italy
    Giulia Bruno, Politecnico di Torino, Italy
    Silvia Chiusano, Politecnico di Torino, Italy
    Naeem A. Mahoto, Politecnico di Torino, Italy
    Caterina Petrigni, Politecnico di Torino, Italy

Chapter 19
Building a Lazy Domain Theory for Characterizing Malignant Melanoma 290
    Eva Armengol, Artificial Intelligence Research Institute (IIIA-CSIC), Spain
    Susana Puig, Hospital Clínic i Provincial de Barcelona, Spain

Compilation of References 309

About the Contributors 334

Index...345

Detailed Table of Contents

Foreword.. xvi

Preface.. xviii

Chapter 1
Intelligent Management of Sepsis in the Intensive Care Unit 1

    Vicent J. Ribas, Universitat Politècnica de Catalunya, Spain
    Juan Carlos Ruiz-Rodríguez, Servei de Medicina Intensiva, Grup de Recerca en Shock, Disfunció
      Orgánica i Ressuscitació, Hospital Universitari Vall d'Hebron, Institut de Recerca Vall d'Hebron,
      Universitat Autònoma de Barcelona, Spain
    Alfredo Vellido, Universitat Politècnica de Catalunya, Spain

Sepsis is a transversal pathology and one of the main causes of death in the Intensive Care Unit (ICU). It has in fact become the tenth most common cause of death in western societies. Its mortality rates can reach up to 60% for Septic Shock, its most acute manifestation. For these reasons, the prediction of the mortality caused by Sepsis is an open and relevant medical research challenge. This problem requires prediction methods that are robust and accurate, but also readily interpretable. This is paramount if they are to be used in the demanding context of real-time decision making at the ICU. In this brief contribution, three different methods are presented. One is based on a variant of the well-known support vector machine (SVM) model and provides and automated ranking of relevance of the mortality predictors while the other two are based on logistic-regression and logistic regression over latent factors. The reported results show that the methods presented outperform in terms of accuracy alternative techniques currently in use in clinical settings, while simultaneously assessing the relative impact of individual pathology indicators.

Chapter 2
Statistical Pattern Recognition Techniques for Early Diagnosis of Diabetic Neuropathy by
Posturographic Data 17

    Claudia Diamantini, Università Politecnica delle Marche, Italy
    Sandro Fioretti, Università Politecnica delle Marche, Italy
    Domenico Potena, Università Politecnica delle Marche, Italy

The goal of this chapter is to describe the use of statistical pattern recognition techniques in order to build a classification model for the early diagnosis of peripheral diabetic neuropathy. In particular, the authors present two experimental methodologies, based on linear discriminant analysis and Bayes vector quantizer algorithms respectively. The former algorithm has demonstrated the best performance in distinguish between non-neuropathic and neuropathic patients, while the latter is able to build models that recognize the severity of the neuropathy.

Chapter 3

Preprocessing MRS Information for Classification of Human Brain Tumours 29

C. J. Arizmendi, Universitat Politècnica de Catalunya, Spain & Universidad Autonoma de Bucaramanga, Colombia

A. Vellido, Universitat Politècnica de Catalunya, Spain

E. Romero, Universitat Politècnica de Catalunya, Spain

Brain tumours show a low prevalence as compared to other cancer pathologies. Their impact, both in individual and social terms, far outweighs such low prevalence. Their anatomical specificity also makes them difficult to explore and treat. The use of biopsies is limited to extreme cases due to the risks involved in the surgical procedure, and non-invasive measurements are the standard for diagnostic exploration. The usual measurement techniques come in the modalities of imaging and spectroscopy. In this chapter, the authors analyze magnetic resonance spectroscopy (MRS) data from an international database and illustrate the importance of data preprocessing prior to diagnostic classification.

Chapter 4

Semi-Supervised Clustering for the Identification of Different Cancer Types
Using the Gene Expression Profiles.. 50

Manuel Martín-Merino, University Pontificia of Salamanca, Spain

DNA Microarrays allow for monitoring the expression level of thousands of genes simultaneously across a collection of related samples. Supervised learning algorithms such as k-NN or SVM (Support Vector Machines) have been applied to the classification of cancer samples with encouraging results. However, the classification algorithms are not able to discover new subtypes of diseases considering the gene expression profiles. In this chapter, the author reviews several supervised clustering algorithms suitable to discover new subtypes of cancer. Next, he introduces a semi-supervised clustering algorithm that learns a linear combination of dissimilarities from the a priori knowledge provided by human experts. A priori knowledge is formulated in the form of equivalence constraints. The minimization of the error function is based on a quadratic optimization algorithm. A L2 norm regularizer is included that penalizes the complexity of the family of distances and avoids overfitting. The method proposed has been applied to several benchmark data sets and to human complex cancer problems using the gene expression profiles. The experimental results suggest that considering a linear combination of heterogeneous dissimilarities helps to improve both classification and clustering algorithms based on a single similarity.

Chapter 5

Real-Time Robust Heart Rate Estimation Based on Bayesian Framework and Grid Filters 67

Radoslav Bortel, Czech Technical University in Prague, Czech Republic

Pavel Sovka, Czech Technical University in Prague, Czech Republic

In this chapter, the authors discuss derivation, implementation, and testing of a robust real-time algorithm for the estimation of heart rate (HR) from electrocardiograms recorded on subjects performing vigorous physical activity. They formulate the problem of HR estimation as a problem of inference in a Bayesian network, which utilizes prior information about the probability distribution of HR changes. From this formulation they derive an inference procedure, which can be implemented as a grid filter. The resulting algorithm can then follow even a rapidly changing HR, whilst withstanding a series of missed or false QRS detections. Also, the HR estimate is complete with confidence intervals to allow the identification of the moments, where the precision of HR estimation is lowered. Additionally, the computational complexity of this algorithm is acceptable for battery powered portable devices.

Chapter 6

Automated Diagnostics of Coronary Artery Disease: Long-Term Results and
Recent Advancements 91

Matjaž Kukar, University of Ljubljana, Slovenia
Igor Kononenko, University of Ljubljana, Slovenia
Ciril Grošelj, University Medical Centre Ljubljana, Slovenia

The authors present results and the latest advancement in their long-term study on using image processing and data mining methods in medical image analysis in general, and in clinical diagnostics of coronary artery disease in particular. Since the evaluation of modern medical images is often difficult and time-consuming, authors integrate advanced analytical and decision support tools in diagnostic process. Partial diagnostic results, frequently obtained from tests with substantial imperfections, can be thus integrated in ultimate diagnostic conclusion about the probability of disease for a given patient. Authors study various topics, such as improving the predictive power of clinical tests by utilizing pre-test and post-test probabilities, texture representation, multi-resolution feature extraction, feature construction and data mining algorithms that significantly outperform the medical practice. During their long-term study (1995-2011) authors achieved, among other minor results, two really significant milestones. The first was achieved by using machine learning to significantly increase post-test diagnostic probabilities with respect to expert physicians. The second, even more significant result utilizes various advanced data analysis techniques, such as automatic multi-resolution image parameterization combined with feature extraction and machine learning methods to significantly improve on all aspects of diagnostic performance. With the proposed approach clinical results are significantly as well as fully automatically, improved throughout the study. Overall, the most significant result of the work is an improvement in the diagnostic power of the whole diagnostic process. The approach supports, but does not replace, physicians' diagnostic process, and can assist in decisions on the cost-effectiveness of diagnostic tests.

Chapter 7

The Use of Prediction Reliability Estimates on Imbalanced Datasets:
A Case Study of Wall Shear Stress in the Human Carotid Artery Bifurcation 113

Domen Košir, University of Ljubljana, Slovenia & Httpool Ltd., Slovenia
Zoran Bosnić, University of Ljubljana, Slovenia
Igor Kononenko, University of Ljubljana, Slovenia

Data mining techniques are extensively used on medical data, which is typically composed of many normal examples and few interesting ones. When presented with highly imbalanced data, some standard classifiers tend to ignore the minority class which leads to poor performance. Various solutions have been proposed to counter this problem. Random undersampling, random oversampling, and SMOTE (Synthetic Minority Oversampling Technique) are the most well-known approaches. In recent years several approaches to evaluate the reliability of single predictions have been developed. Most recently a simple and efficient approach, based on the classifier's class probability estimates was shown to outperform the other reliability estimates. The authors propose to use this reliability estimate to improve the SMOTE algorithm. In this study, they demonstrate the positive effects of using the proposed algorithms on artificial datasets. The authors then apply the developed methodology on the problem of predicting the maximal wall shear stress (MWSS) in the human carotid artery bifurcation. The results indicate that it is feasible to improve the classifier's performance by balancing the data with their versions of the SMOTE algorithm.

Chapter 8

Pattern Mining for Outbreak Discovery Preparedness 125

Zalizah Awang Long, Malaysia Institute Information Technology, Universiti Kuala Lumpur, Malaysia

Abdul Razak Hamdan, Universiti Kebengsaan Malaysia, Malaysia

Azuraliza Abu Bakar, Universiti Kebengsaan Malaysia, Malaysia

Mazrura Sahani, Universiti Kebengsaan Malaysia, Malaysia

Today, the objective of public health surveillance system is to reduce the impact of outbreaks by enabling appropriate intervention. Commonly used techniques are based on the changes or aberration in health events when compared with normal history to detect an outbreak. The main problem encountered in outbreaks is high rates of false alarm. High false alarm rates can lead to unnecessary interventions, and falsely detected outbreaks will lead to costly investigation. In this chapter, the authors review data mining techniques focusing on frequent and outlier mining to develop generic outbreak detection process model, named as "Frequent-outlier" model. The process model was tested against the real dengue dataset obtained from FSK, UKM, and also tested on the synthetic respiratory dataset obtained from AUTON LAB. The ROC was run to analyze the overall performance of "frequent-outlier" with CUSUM and Moving Average (MA). The results were promising and were evaluated using detection rate, false positive rate, and overall performance. An important outcome of this study is the knowledge rules derived from the notification of the outbreak cases to be used in counter measure assessment for outbreak preparedness.

Chapter 9

Development of Surrogate Models of Orthopedic Screws to Improve Biomechanical Performance: Comparisons of Artificial Neural Networks and Multiple Linear Regressions 138

Ching-Chi Hsu, Graduate Institute of Applied Science and Technology, National Taiwan University of Science and Technology, Taiwan

An optimization approach was applied to improve the design of the lag screws used in double screw nails. However, finite element analyses with an optimal algorithm may take a long time to find the best design. Thus, surrogate methods, either artificial neural networks or multiple linear regressions, were used to substitute for the finite element models. The results showed that an artificial neural network method can accurately develop the objective functions of the lag screws for both the bending strength and the pullout strength. A multiple linear regression method can successfully develop the objective function of the lag screws for the pullout strength, but it failed to construct the objective function for the bending strength. The optimal design of the lag screws could be obtained using the artificial neural network method and genetic algorithms.

Chapter 10

Dashboard to Support the Decision-Making within a Chronic Disease: A Framework for Automatic Generation of Alerts and KPIs 160

Leonor Teixeira, University of Aveiro / GOVCOPP / IEETA, Portugal

Vasco Saavedra, University of Aveiro, Portugal

João Pedro Simões, Accenture, Portugal

This chapter describes a monitoring system based on alerts and Key Performance Indicators (KPIs), applied in clinical context, within a chronic disease (haemophilia). This kind of disease follows the patient through his/her life, and its treatment requires an almost permanent exchange of data/information with healthcare professional (HCPs), with the information and communications technologies (ICTs) a key contribution in this process. However, most applications based on those ICTs do not allow the analysis of heterogeneous data in real time, requiring the availability of clinicians to check the data and analyze the information to support the clinical decision process. Since time is a scarce resource in the context of healthcare providers, and information a crucial resource in the decision support process, real-time monitoring systems can help finding the right balance between those two resources, presenting the key information in an appropriate format, through alerts and KPIs. The system described in this chapter, named hemo@care_dashboard, aims to support clinical decision-making of healthcare professionals of a specific chronic disease, providing real time information in a push logic through alerts and KPIs, displayed on a dashboard.

Chapter 11

Identification of Motor Functions Based on an EEG Analysis 172
Aleš Belič, University of Ljubljana, Slovenia
Vito Logar, University of Ljubljana, Slovenia

A combination of several techniques is necessary for a reliable identification of activities based on EEG signals. A separation of the overlapping patterns in the EEG signals is often performed first. These separated patterns are then analysed by some artificial intelligence methods in order to identify the activity. As pattern separation and activity identification are often linked, the two processes must be tuned to a specific problem, thus losing some generality of the procedure. The complexity of the patterns in EEG signals is often too great for completely automated pattern recognition. In this case, phase demodulation was introduced as a procedure for the extraction of the phase properties of the EEG signals. These phase shifts are known to correlate with the brain activity; therefore, phase-demodulated EEG signals were used to predict the motor activity. Three studies with off-line identification of the motor activities have been performed so far. In the first study, a continuous gripping force was predicted. In the second study, index- and middle-finger activation was predicted, and in the final study, wrist movements were analysed. The presented procedure can be used for designing a continuous brain-computer interface.

Chapter 12

Visual Data Mining in Physiotherapy Using Self-Organizing Maps: A New Approximation
to the Data Analysis 187
Yasser Alakhdar, University of Valencia, Spain
José M. Martínez-Martínez, University of Valencia, Spain
Josep Guimerà-Tomás, University of Valencia, Spain
Pablo Escandell-Montero, University of Valencia, Spain
Josep Benitez, University of Valencia, Spain
Emilio Soria-Olivas, University of Valencia, Spain

The basis of all clinical science developments is the analysis of the data obtained from a particular problem. In recent decades, however, the capacity of computers to process data has been increasing exponentially, which has created the possibility of applying more powerful methods of data analysis. Among these methods, the multidimensional visual data mining methods are outstanding. These methods show all the variables of one particular problem on the whole allowing to the clinical specialist to extract his own conclusions. In this chapter, a neural approximation to this kind of data mining is shown by means of the valuation analysis of the knee in athletes in the pre- and post-surgery of the anterior cruciate ligament, studying variables of force and measurements at different distances of the knee.

Chapter 13

Kernel Generative Topographic Mapping of Protein Sequences 195

Martha-Ivón Cárdenas, Universitat Politècnica de Catalunya, Spain
Alfredo Vellido, Universitat Politècnica de Catalunya, Spain
Iván Olier, The University of Manchester, UK
Xavier Rovira, Institut de Neurociències, Universitat Autònoma de Barcelona, Spain
Jesús Giraldo, Institut de Neurociències and Unitat de Bioestadística, Universitat Autònoma
*   de Barcelona, Spain*

The world of pharmacology is becoming increasingly dependent on the advances in the fields of genomics and proteomics. The –omics sciences bring about the challenge of how to deal with the large amounts of complex data they generate from an intelligence data analysis perspective. In this chapter, the authors focus on the analysis of a specific type of proteins, the G protein-couple receptors, which are the target for over 15% of current drugs. They describe a kernel method of the manifold learning family for the analysis of protein amino acid symbolic sequences. This method sheds light on the structure of protein subfamilies, while providing an intuitive visualization of such structure.

Chapter 14

Medical Critiquing Systems 209

Ian Douglas, Florida State University, USA

Computer Science has traditionally focused on the functional aspects of design, underemphasizing the human element in the success of any technology. The failure of technologies and the accidents that happen during use require the consideration of the user and the technologies as symbiotic parts of a whole systems approach to improving diagnosis and treatment. This chapter provides an overview of the history of the critiquing approach to knowledge systems that illustrates a more human-centered approach. It is an approach that, unlike traditional knowledge-based systems, aims to provide a check on human reasoning, rather than a replacement for it. The chapter will also discuss future possibilities for research, in particular the use of social networking and recommender systems, as a means to enhance the approach.

Chapter 15

Learning Probabilistic Graphical Models: A Review of Techniques and
Applications in Medicine 223

Juan I. Alonso-Barba, University of Castilla-La Mancha, Spain
Jens D. Nielsen University of Castilla-La Mancha, Spain
Luis de la Ossa, University of Castilla-La Mancha, Spain
Jose M. Puerta, University of Castilla-La Mancha, Spain

Probabilistic Graphical Models (PGM) are a class of statistical models that use a graph structure over a set of variables to encode independence relations between those variables. By augmenting the graph by local parameters, a PGM allows for a compact representation of a joint probability distribution over the variables of the graph, which then allows for efficient inference algorithms. PGMs are often used for modeling physical and biological systems, and such models are then in turn used to both answer probabilistic queries concerning the variables and to represent certain causal and/or statistical relations in the domain. In this chapter, the authors give an overview of common techniques used for automatic construction of such models from a dataset of observations (usually referred to as learning), and they also review some important applications. The chapter guides the reader to the relevant literature for further study.

Chapter 16
Natural Language Processing and Machine Learning Techniques
Help Achieve a Better Medical Practice 237
Oana Frunza, University of Ottawa, Canada
Diana Inkpen, University of Ottawa, Canada

This book chapter presents several natural language processing (NLP) and machine learning (ML) techniques that can help achieve a better medical practice by means of extracting relevant medical information from the wealth of textual data. The chapter describes three major tasks: building intelligent tools that can help in the clinical decision making, tools that can automatically identify relevant medical information from the life-science literature, and tools that can extract semantic relations between medical concepts. Besides introducing and describing these tasks, methodological settings accompanied by representative results obtained on real-life data sets are presented.

Chapter 17
Modeling Interpretable Fuzzy Rule-Based Classifiers for Medical Decision Support 255
Jose M. Alonso, University of Alcala, Spain
Ciro Castiello, University of Bari, Italy
Marco Lucarelli, University of Bari, Italy
Corrado Mencar, University of Bari, Italy

Decision support systems in Medicine must be easily comprehensible, both for physicians and patients. In this chapter, the authors describe how the fuzzy modeling methodology called HILK (Highly Interpretable Linguistic Knowledge) can be applied for building highly interpretable fuzzy rule-based classifiers (FRBCs) able to provide medical decision support. As a proof of concept, they describe the case study of a real-world scenario concerning the development of an interpretable FRBC that can be used to predict the evolution of the end-stage renal disease (ESRD) in subjects affected by Immunoglobin A Nephropathy (IgAN). The designed classifier provides users with a number of rules which are easy to read and understand. The rules classify the prognosis of ESRD evolution in IgAN-affected subjects by distinguishing three classes (short, medium, long). Experimental results show that the fuzzy classifier is capable of satisfactory accuracy results – in comparison with Multi-Layer Perceptron (MLP) neural networks – and high interpretability of the knowledge base.

Chapter 18
Extraction of Medical Pathways from Electronic Patient Records 273
Dario Antonelli, Politecnico di Torino, Italy
Elena Baralis, Politecnico di Torino, Italy
Giulia Bruno, Politecnico di Torino, Italy
Silvia Chiusano, Politecnico di Torino, Italy
Naeem A. Mahoto, Politecnico di Torino, Italy
Caterina Petrigni, Politecnico di Torino, Italy

With the introduction of electronic medical records, a large amount of patients' medical data has been available. An actual problem in this domain is to perform reverse engineering of the medical treatment process to highlight medical pathways typically adopted for specific health conditions. This chapter addresses the ability of sequential data mining techniques to reconstruct the actual medical pathways followed by patients. Detected medical pathways are in the form of sets of exams frequently done together, sequences of exam sets frequently followed by patients and frequent correlations between exam sets. The analysis shows that the majority of the extracted pathways are consistent with the medical guidelines, but also reveals some unexpected results, which can be useful both to enrich existing guidelines and to improve the public sanitary service.

Chapter 19
Building a Lazy Domain Theory for Characterizing Malignant Melanoma 290
Eva Armengol, Artificial Intelligence Research Institute (IIIA-CSIC), Spain
Susana Puig, Hospital Clínic i Provincial de Barcelona, Spain

In this chapter, the authors propose an approach for building a model characterizing malignant melanomas. A common way to build a domain model is using an inductive learning method. Such resulting model is a generalization of the known examples. However, in some domains where there is not a clear difference among the classes, the inductive model could be too general. The approach taken in this chapter consists of using lazy learning methods for building what the authors call a lazy domain theory. The main difference between both inductive and lazy theories is that the former is complete whereas the latter is not. This means that the lazy domain theory may not cover all the space of known examples. The authors' experiments have shown that, despite of this, the lazy domain theory has better performance than the inductive theory.

Compilation of References 309

About the Contributors 334

Index 345

Foreword

"All models are wrong but some are useful"

George E.P. Box

The first sentence of this foreword includes the philosophy of the day–to-day clinical data analysis. The human body is one of the most complex systems to analyze, so to establish an exact model of any of its parts is an extremely difficult task, and very often the proposed model does not contain all the peculiarities of the phenomenon under study.

The analysis of clinical data is not new; its history lasts more than 100 years. In the early stages, techniques used were mainly contrast hypothesis, linear models, factorial analysis. Those days nor the capacity nor the computational power of current computers were available, but, although, from a present point of view, models used were very primitive, and results obtained showed their usefulness.

Terms like soft computing, data mining, machine learning, intelligent data analysis, extracting knowledge of massive data sets, are all equivalent to refer to the process of extracting knowledge from datasets. Applications of those techniques are wide in almost all fields of knowledge with multiple benefits. Clinical problems are the perfect target for those methods: big amount of data with many different types of variables, that many times contain errors or are incomplete. Moreover, data are, very often, related to difficult predictions or complex diagnostics.

The authors of the different chapters in this handbook show the applications of those techniques to different clinical problems. Chapters include problems of prediction, pattern classification (diagnostic) and multidimensional visualization that allow the specialist to extract conclusions about data. All of them are practical applications than emphasize the validity and wide use of those techniques. Many different kinds of models like, neural models (Multilayer perceptron and Self organizing Maps), support vector machines, Bayesian networks, and fuzzy models have been applied to different kinds of data; i.e. genetic, from UCI, dermatological, electroencephalographical, et cetera.

Summarizing, the reader hold between his/her hands a complete exposition of the state of the art of the applications of those techniques in clinical practice. Bearing in mind the evolution in this field we could complete professor's Cox sentence and say:

"In clinic, all models are wrong but some are very useful"

Josep Redón
European Society of Hypertension, & University of Valencia, Spain

Josep Redón I Mas *was born in Valencia in 1950. He earned his Master's degree in Medicine completed at the Medical School of the University of Valencia (1968-1974) with 12 A+ grades and with an A grade on the Master's final examination. His PhD was earned at the University of Valencia. He was Specialist in Internal Medicine from the Medical Postgraduate Training Program (MIR) done at the Jiménez Diaz Foundation, Madrid, and at the University Hospital La Fe in Valencia. Editorial Activity of his includes: a) Member of the Editorial Board of indexed journals in the field of Hypertension: Journal of Hypertension, Blood Pressure Monitoring; b) Reviewer of both Cardiovascular and Internal Medicine journals: Circulation, Hypertension, Journal of Hypertension, American Journal of Hypertension, American Journal of Medicine, American Journal of Kidney Disease, European Heart Journal, and Nephrology Dialysis and Transplantation; c) Author of numerous editorials and review articles by invitation.*

Preface

What is Intelligent Data Analysis? And furthermore, what can Intelligent Data Analysis bring to Health Sciences? These questions are well grounded, because the name "Intelligent Data Analysis" itself is very ambiguous. The main idea underlying this concept is extracting knowledge from data.

Man now lives in the Age of Information. Health Sciences are fully embedded in Information Technologies. Technology is ubiquitous; technology is cheap. Technology is everything nowadays. Moore's Law has brought the world to the Technology Information Society, and even the furthest away corner in the world is today covered by telecommunications technology. A high-end technology cellular phone exhibits more computing power that the computer that drove man to the moon 30 years ago, and we use it for playing bird-killing online games!

It is easy and cheap to acquire, monitor, and measure any set of variables, digitize the data, and store in a hard disk or in the Cloud. Because it is easy and cheap, the society and management boards are prone to do it. But to whom much has been given, much will be expected, or this should be the right way. The cheap, powerful computing capabilities of nearly every appliance, the fast data highways that plough and fly through the Earth, and the nearly unlimited storage resources available everywhere, at any time, are flooding us with digital data. The Age of Information could also be defined as the Curse of Data, because it is quite cheap and easy to gather and store data. But people need information, so they chase knowledge. They have the haystack, but they want the needle.

Biology and Health Sciences are very complex fields. These sciences have made a long walk from the ancient times, but processes involved in biology, medicine and physiology are much too intricate to be faithfully modeled. It is not easy to extract knowledge starting from raw data, and it is also not cheap. The curse of cheap hardware, cheap bandwidth, and a cheap processor is an extraordinary large amount of data, a very large number of variables, and very little knowledge about what is cooking inside this data.

During the recent past, scientists and technologists have relied on traditional statistics to cope with the task of extracting information from data. Statistics building has been deeply rooted in the ground of Mathematics since the seventeenth century, but during the last few decades, this enormous amount of data and variables has overwhelmed the capabilities of classical statistics. There is no way for classical methods to deal with such amount of data. It's impossible to visualize even the lesser information, and man is unable to extract knowledge from these radiant, brand-new gathered datasets.

Mathematics is also now coming to help, going back to classical statistics and bringing tools that enable us to extract some information from these huge datasets. These new tools are called "Intelligent Data Analysis." But Mathematics is not the only discipline involved in Data Analysis. Engineering, computing sciences, database science, machine learning, and even artificial intelligence are bringing their powers to this newly born data analysis discipline.

So Intelligent Data Analysis is defined as the tools that enable for extracting the information under lying a very large amount of data, with a very large amount of variables, data that represents very complex, non-linear, real-life problems, which are intractable with the old tools people were used to. People must be able to cope with high dimensionality, sparse data, very complex and unknown relationships, biased, wrong or incomplete data, and mathematics algorithms or methods that lie in the foggy frontier of Mathematics, Engineering, Physics, Computer Science, Statistics, Biology or even Philosophy.

Moreover, Intelligent Data Analysis can help starting from the raw data, coping with prediction tasks without knowing the theoretical description of the underlying process, classification tasks of new events based off of past ones, or modeling the aforementioned unknown process. Classification, prediction, and modeling are the cornerstones that Intelligent Data Analysis can bring to us.

And in this brave New Information World, information is the key. It is the key, the power, and the engine that moves the economy. The world is moving with markets data, medical epidemiologic sets, Internet browsing records, geological surveys data, complex engineering models, and so on. Nearly every man activity nowadays is generating a big amount of data that can be easily gathered and stored, and the greatest value of that data is the information that lies behind it.

This book approaches Intelligent Data Analysis from a very practical point of view. There are many theoretical, academic books about theory on data mining and analysis, but the approach in this book comes from a real health-world view: solving common life problems with data analysis tools. It is an "engineering" point of view, in the sense that the book presents a real problem, usually defined by complex, non-linear and unknown processes, and then offers a Data Analysis based solution that enables for solving the problem or even to infer the process underlying the raw data. The book gives practical experiences with intelligent data analysis.

So this book is aimed to medicine and biology scientists and engineers carrying out research in very complex, non linear areas, such as medicine, genetics, biology, and data processing, with large amounts of data that need to extract some knowledge starting from the data, knowledge that can take the flavor of prediction, classification, or modeling. But this book also brings a valuable point of view to engineers and businessmen that work in companies, trying to solve practical, economical, or technical problems in the field of their company activities or expertise. The pure practical approach helps to transmit the idea and the aim of the author to communicate the way to approach and to cope with problems that would be intractable in any other way. And at last, final courses of academic degrees in Engineering, Mathematics, Medicine, or Biology can use this book to provide students with a new point of view for approaching and solving real, practical problems when underlying processes are not clear.

Obviously a prior knowledge of statistics, discrete mathematics, and machine learning is desirable, although authors provide several references to help engineers and scientists use the experience and the know-how described in every chapter to their own benefit. The book is structured as follows.

Chapter 1, "*Intelligent Management of Sepsis in the Intensive Care Unit,*" Ribas, Ruiz, and Vellido is about sepsis. Sepsis is a pathology affecting all people and is one of the main causes of death in the Intensive Care Unit. Indeed, it is the tenth most common cause of death in western countries (death rates up to 60% for its most severe stages). The aim of this chapter is to provide interpretable and actionable indicators for the assessment of the Risk of Death in Severe Sepsis. Three different methods are presented: Relevance Vector Machines (a sub-class of Support Vector Machines) that provides an automated ranking of relevance of the mortality predictors, Logistic-Regression models that are widely used by the medical community, and Logistic-Regression over Latent Factors (i.e. Logistic-Regression combined with Factor Analysis). The new methods are compared against other state-of-the-art methods widely used in clinical practice (APACHE II).

Chapter 2, "*Statistical Pattern Recognition Techniques for Early Diagnosis of Diabetic Neuropathy by Posturographic Data*," by Diamantini, Fioretti, and Potena, describes the use of Statistical Pattern Recognition techniques for the early diagnosis of Peripheral Diabetic Neuropathy, with the twofold aim of distinguishing between non-neuropathic and neuropathic patients and of recognizing the severity of the neuropathy. The chapter presents two experimental methodologies, which are based on Linear Discriminant Analysis and Bayes Vector Quantizer algorithms, respectively.

In Chapter 3, "*Preprocessing MRS Information for Classification of Human Brain Tumours*," Arizmendi, Vellido and Romero analyze Magnetic Resonance Spectroscopy data from Brain Tumors database in order to prove the importance of data preprocessing prior to diagnostic classification.

In Chapter 4, "*Semi-supervised Clustering for the Identification of Different Cancer Types using the Gene Expression Profiles*," Martín-Merino covers the DNA Microarrays, which allow for monitoring the expression level of thousands of genes simultaneously across a collection of related samples. Supervised learning algorithms such as k-NN or SVM (Support Vector Machines) have been applied to the classification of cancer samples using the gene expression profiles. However, they are not able to discover new subtypes of diseases. This chapter studies several supervised clustering algorithms suitable to discover new subtypes of cancer. Next, a semi-supervised clustering algorithm is introduced that allows for incorporating *a priori* knowledge provided by human experts. The performance of the algorithms is illustrated considering several complex human cancer problems.

Chapter 5, "*Real-Time Robust Heart Rate Estimation Based on Bayesian Framework and Grid Filters*," by Bortel and Sovka, describes a robust real-time algorithm for the estimation of heart rate (HR) from strongly corrupted electrocardiogram records. The problem of HR estimation is formulated as a problem of inference in a Bayesian network, which utilizes prior information about the probability distribution of HR changes. From this formulation, an inference procedure is derived and implemented as a grid filter. The resulting algorithm can then follow even a rapidly changing HR, whilst withstanding a series of missed or false QRS detections. Additionally, the computational complexity of this algorithm is acceptable for battery powered portable devices.

In Chapter 6, "*Automated Diagnostics of Coronary Artery Disease: Long-term Results and Recent Advancements*," Kukar, Kononenko, and Groselj analyze the clinical diagnostics of coronary artery disease by using advanced analytical and decision support tools. They study various topics, such as improving the predictive power of clinical tests by utilizing pre-test and post-test probabilities, texture representation, multi-resolution feature extraction, feature construction and data mining algorithms that significantly outperform the medical practice. Finally, they present the results during a long term study.

Chapter 7, "*The Use of Prediction Reliability Estimates on Imbalanced Datasets: A Case Study of Wall Shear Stress in the Human Carotid Artery Bifurcation*," by Kosir, Bosnic, and Kononenko demonstrate the positive effects of using proposed algorithms on artificial datasets. They then apply the developed methodology on the problem of predicting the maximal wall shear stress (MWSS) in the human carotid artery bifurcation. The results indicate that it is feasible to improve the classifier's performance by balancing the data with the authors' versions of the SMOTE algorithm.

In Chapter 8, "*Pattern Mining for Outbreak Discovery Preparedness*," Long, Hamdan, Bakar, and Sahani review data mining techniques focusing on frequent and outlier mining to develop generic outbreak detection process model, named as "Frequent-outlier" model. The process model was tested against the real dengue dataset obtained from FSK, UKM, and also tested on the synthetic respiratory dataset obtained from AUTON LAB. The ROC was run to analyze the overall performance of "frequent-outlier" with CUSUM and Moving Average (MA).

Chapter 9, "*Development of Surrogate Models of Orthopedic Screws to Improve Biomechanical Performance: Comparisons of Artificial Neural Networks and Multiple Linear Regressions*," Hsu evaluates the strengths and limitations of the surrogate methods in developing the objective functions of the lag screws used in double screw nails and investigates the design improvements of this orthopaedic device.

In Chapter 10, "*Dashboard to Support the Decision-making within a Chronic Disease: A Framework for Automatic Generation of Alerts and KPIs*," by Teixeira, Saavedra, and Simoes, given the importance that the real-time information has within the scope of clinical decisions, with increased relevancy in the context of chronic diseases, the present chapter discusses the role of an application for monitoring real-time data in a specific chronic disease, based on alerts and KPIs. Moreover, those concepts are demonstrated by a practical application, developed in collaboration with the Haematology Service of Coimbra Hospital Centre (SH_CHC), in order to provide a quick reading of the relevant information for decision-making through a set of alerts and KPIs, based on a push strategy, displayed on a dashboard.

Chapter 11, "*Identification of Motor Functions Based on an EEG Analysis*," by Belic and Logar, is about phase characteristics of the electroencephalographic (EEG) signals are getting a lot of attention latey as phase-locking seems to be one of the most important mechanisms for binding of brain regions during complex activity. Working memory and motor activity tasks have been extensively used in search for existence of the phase locking activity in the EEG. The area of 2D image compression also showed that when using frequency based methods for image compression, the phase properties of the image carry the most important information of the image composition while amplitude is of secondary importance and does not affect the possibility to recognise the de-compressed image. However, phase properties of signals are relatively difficult to extract from the signals in real-time and are strongly affected by the measurement noise. A phase demodulation method for the analysis of the EEG signals is shown and illustrated in the Chapter Identification of motor functions based on EEG analysis. The method provides promising results with respect to brain-computer interface development.

In Chapter 12, "*Visual Data Mining in Physiotherapy Using Self-Organizing Maps: A New Approximation to the Data Analysis*," by Alakhdar, Martínez, Guimerá, Escandell, Benitez, and Soria, deals with Anterior Cruciate Ligament injury (ACL), which is the most frequent lesion in the knee joint, and the most of torn ligaments occurs during the participation in sports activities. Among the different surgical techniques, most authors consider the intra-articular reconstruction techniques. In this study, the semitendinosus tendon graft was used. After surgery, the subject must undergo a period of rehabilitation. This period is considered as important as the surgery or even more. Thus, in order to facilitate the functional recovery of the affected knee, monitoring, control, and an evaluation of the patient are crucial. For this purpose, a neural approximation based on multidimensional visual data mining methods, the self-organizing maps (SOM), is shown by means of the valuation analysis of the knee in athletes in the pre- and post-surgery of the anterior cruciate ligament, studying variables of force and measurements at different distances of the knee. The goal is to check if the analysis of these variables permits to know if the recovery process has satisfied its final aim. Together with the measurements of the thigh contour and the muscle strength, in the SOM analysis it is also included the age, weight, and height of each patient.

In Chapter 13, "*Kernel Generative Topographic Mapping of Protein Sequences*," Cárdenas, Vellido, Olier, Rovira, and Giraldo work on the world of pharmacology, which is becoming increasingly dependent on the advances in the fields of genomics and proteomics. The —omics sciences bring about the challenge of how to deal with the large amounts of complex data they generate from an intelligent data analysis perspective. In this chapter, the authors focus on the analysis of a specific type of proteins, the G protein-coupled receptors (GPCRs), which regulate the function of most cells in living organisms.

They describe a kernel method of the manifold learning family to analyze the grouping of their amino acid symbolic sequences. This grouping into types and subtypes, based on sequence analysis, may significantly contribute to helping drug design and to a better understanding of the molecular processes involved in receptor signaling both in normal and pathological conditions.

In Chapter 14, "*Medical Critiquing Systems,*" Douglas provide an overview of the history of the critiquing approach to knowledge systems that illustrates a more human-centered approach. It is an approach that unlike traditional knowledge-based systems, aims to provide a check on human reasoning, rather than a replacement for it. The chapter will also discuss future possibilities for research, in particular the use of social networking and recommender systems, as a means to enhance the approach.

In Chapter 15, "*Learning Probabilistic Graphical Models: A Review of Techniques and Applications in Medicine,*" by Alonso, Nielsen, de la Ossa, and Puerta, First a brief introduction to the most important and most commonly used types of probabilistic graphical models is given, besides their specification, parametrization, and interpretation. A special focus on the Bayesian Belief network model is made. Then an overview of the most typical frameworks for learning models from data is studied and the ideas that lie behind the development of these frameworks are discussed. A review of recent and classical applications of probabilistic graphical models and learning in the areas of diagnostic and prognostic reasoning, and automatic discovery of causal relationships and regulatory networks in genetics. The chapter concludes with a brief discussion on the most interesting publicly available software packages for learning and modelling using probabilistic graphical models.

Chapter 16, "*Natural Language Processing and Machine Learning Techniques Help Achieve a Better Medical Practice,*" by Frunza and Inkpen, presents several natural language processing and machine learning techniques that can help the medical practice by means of extracting relevant medical information from the wealth of textual data. The chapter describes three major tasks: building intelligent tools that can help in the clinical decision making, tools that can automatically identify relevant medical information from the life-science literature, and tools that can extract semantic relations between medical concepts. The chapter also presents methodological settings accompanied by representative results obtained on real-life data sets for all three tasks.

Chapter 17, "*Modeling Interpretable Fuzzy Rule-Based Classifiers for Medical Decision Support,*" by Alonso, Castielo, Lucarelli, and Mencar, is about intelligent systems for medical decision support may be of little use if the knowledge at the basis of decisions is not easily comprehensible to physicians (and patients). This chapter describes a methodology for designing fuzzy rule-based classifiers based on linguistic rules that are easy to read and understand. Moreover, it shows a proof of concept based on a real-world case study for predicting the evolution of the end-stage renal disease in subjects affected by Immunoglobin-A Nephropathy.

In Chapter 18, "*Extraction of Medical Pathways from Electronic Patient Records,*" Antonelli, Baralis, Bruno, Chiusano, Mahoto, and Petrigni, a huge amount of medical data storing the medical history of patients has made available in recent years by the introduction of electronic medical records. An actual problem in this domain is to perform reverse engineering of the medical treatment process to highlight medical pathways typically adopted for specific health conditions, as well as discovering deviations with respect to predefined care guidelines. This information can support healthcare organizations in improving the current treatment process or assessing new guidelines. The chapter addresses the ability of sequential data mining techniques to reconstruct the actual medical pathways followed by patients. Detected medical pathways are in the form of sets of exams frequently done together, sequences of exam sets frequently followed by patients and frequent correlations between exam sets. The analysis shows that the majority of the extracted pathways are consistent with the medical guidelines, but also reveals some unexpected results that can be useful both to enrich existing guidelines and to improve the public sanitary service.

Finally, in Chapter 19, "*Building a Lazy Domain Theory for Characterizing Malignant Melanoma*," Armengol and Puig describe an application focused on building a model able to characterize (and distinguish) early malignant melanoma from benignant skin lesions. The procedure followed for constructing such model is using lazy learning methods instead of inductive learning methods that is the most usual approach. Authors experimentally compared the performance of the domain theories generated by two lazy learning methods (k-NN and LID) with the ones generated by decision trees. Results show that lazy learning theories have aspects that allow practitioners to consider them better than the inductive domain theories. In addition, when comparing the predictivity of the theories, the lazy domain theories show to be better than the inductive ones.

The Editors

Rafael Magdalena-Benedito
University of Valencia, Spain

Emilio Soria
University of Valencia, Spain

Juan Guerrero Martínez
University of Valencia, Spain

Juan Gómez-Sanchis
University of Valencia, Spain

Antonio Jose Serrano-López
University of Valencia, Spain

Chapter 1
Intelligent Management of Sepsis in the Intensive Care Unit

Vicent J. Ribas
Universitat Politècnica de Catalunya, Spain

Juan Carlos Ruiz-Rodríguez
*Servei de Medicina Intensiva, Grup de Recerca en Shock, Disfunció Orgánica i Ressuscitació,
Hospital Universitari Vall d'Hebron, Institut de Recerca Vall d'Hebron, Universitat Autònoma de
Barcelona, Spain*

Alfredo Vellido
Universitat Politècnica de Catalunya, Spain

ABSTRACT

*Sepsis is a transversal pathology and one of the main causes of death in the Intensive Care Unit (ICU).
It has in fact become the tenth most common cause of death in western societies. Its mortality rates can
reach up to 60% for Septic Shock, its most acute manifestation. For these reasons, the prediction of the
mortality caused by Sepsis is an open and relevant medical research challenge. This problem requires
prediction methods that are robust and accurate, but also readily interpretable. This is paramount if they
are to be used in the demanding context of real-time decision making at the ICU. In this brief contribution, three different methods are presented. One is based on a variant of the well-known support vector
machine (SVM) model and provides and automated ranking of relevance of the mortality predictors
while the other two are based on logistic-regression and logistic regression over latent Factors. The
reported results show that the methods presented outperform in terms of accuracy alternative techniques
currently in use in clinical settings, while simultaneously assessing the relative impact of individual
pathology indicators.*

DOI: 10.4018/978-1-4666-1803-9.ch001

INTRODUCTION

Sepsis and its associated complications, Septic Shock and Multiorganic Dysfunction Syndrome (MODS) are considered the most frequent causes for morbidity and mortality for patients admitted to the Intensive Care Unit (ICU)(Livingston DH., 1995).

Sepsis is characterized by the systemic response to infection and from a clinical point of view it is recognized by a set of clinical signs and symptoms corresponding to the response of the organism to the presence of microorganisms or their toxic products.

The evolution and prognosis of septic patients is variable and unpredictable. Some patients with Sepsis have a fulminant evolution leading, within hours, to death of a refractory Septic Shock. However, other patients survive the hyperacute phase and develop MODS, which also lead to death. Fortunately, other patients present a favorable evolution and successfully recover from Sepsis.

The diagnosis of a Septic Shock is not trivial and it is usually carried out in challenging clinical emergency situations. Early recognition of signs of decreased perfusion before the onset of hypotension, appropriate therapeutic response, and removal of the center of the infection are the keys to survival of patients with Septic Shock. Given the criticality of this pathology, it is of capital importance to have available an early indication of this condition in order to allow doctors to act rapidly at the onset of Sepsis.

Needless to say, the ICU environment can be unforgiving in terms of decision making tasks. Clinicians in general might benefit from at least partially automated computer-based decision support, but those clinicians making real-time executive decisions at ICUs in particular will require methods that are not only reliable, but also, and this is a key issue, readily interpretable. This work aims to address these needs through the design and development of computer-based decision making tools to assist clinicians at the ICU. These developments will focus on the problem of Sepsis in general and, more specifically, on the problem of survival prediction for patients with Severe Sepsis. The tools at the core of Sepsis data analysis will stem from the fields of multivariate statistics, machine learning and computational intelligence.

BACKGROUND

The incidence of Sepsis and its associated complications: Septic Shock and MODS are difficult to establish and their causes are multiple and varied: longevity, associated pathologies (diabetes mellitus, hepatic cyrrhosis, neoplasias, chronic renal insufficiency, and so on), the increased use of invasive techniques, corticoid administration, chemotherapy and immunosupressants, organ transplants, and so on (Luce J., 1987).

Studies carried out in the eighties probably underestimated the real incidence of Sepsis. In 1990 the US Center for Disease Control (CDC) calculated that between 1979 and 1987 there were 450,000 cases of Sepsis causing the death of 100,000 people. The incidence of Sepsis increased from 73.6 cases/100,000 people patients in 1979 to 175.9 cases/100.000 people in 1989 (CDC, 1990).

Now it is commonly accepted that the incidence of Sepsis is much higher. Angus *et al.* (Angus DC., 2001) describes an incidence of 3 cases / 1000 people, which implies that in the US there may appear 750,000 cases of Sepsis per year out which 51.1% will require ICU admission, with a hospital mortality rate of 28.7% (resulting in more than 215,000 deaths/year). These figures are similar to those of secondary deaths of acute myocardial infarction. It is expected that this incidence will increase 1.5% each year due to increased longevity, more aggressive treatment and the increased number of patients taking immunosuppressants. Therefore, the expected incidence for the years 2010-2020 is 934,000-1,110,000 cases. Besides this study, Martin *et al.* (Martin GS., 2000) studied the incidence of Sepsis during 1979-2000 in the US and found out that the number of Septic patients augmented from 164,072 in 1979 to 659,935 in 2000 (i.e. an increase of 13.7% each year). The reported incidence of Sepsis increased from 82.7 cases / 100,000 people to 240.4 cases / 100,000 people (annual increase of 8.7%).

In Europe, the incidence of Sepsis has been estimated in 450,000 cases out of which 55% evolve to Septic Shock with an associated mortality of 40%. The mortality rates for those patients evolving to MODS range between 70-90%. In Spain, Sepsis is responsible for the death of 150,000 patients each year.

Besides its incidence, Sepsis also supposes a burden to National Health Systems. For example, the average expenditure for each case of Sepsis in the US is 22,100 USD. The total expenditure caused by Sepsis is around 16.7 billion USD (Angus DC., 2001).

Sepsis takes place in 9% of ICU admissions (Brun-Bruisson C., 1995) and constitutes the principal cause of death in critically ill patients as opposed to the general population where it is considered the 13th cause of death (CDC, 1993). The mortality rate for Sepsis is 45%, reaches 60% for Septic Shock and 90% for MODS with three or more organs in failure (Vincent JL., 1998).

From a physiopathologic point of view, Sepsis is the immunologic response of the host against microorganisms or products derived from those, and it is characterized by the systemic inflammatory processes that end up damaging the endothelial cells. This inflammatory response to infection, which initially has defensive properties, by mechanisms yet not very well understood may become uncontrolled and result, in most severe cases, in the death of the patient as a result of refractory shock or MODS.

Clinical Overview

Sepsis and its sequelae, namely Septic Shock and MODS, are presented as a clinical and physio-pathologic continuum. In its initial phase, infection may evolve towards Sepsis and this Sepsis may also evolve towards Severe Sepsis, Septic Shock and MODS. This continuous process presents a higher severity at each stage and clearly influences prognosis. The definitions of Sepsis and its associated processes where established in 1992 (Conference, 1992) and where updated in subsequent conferences (2000 and 2003) and studies (Levy M.M., 2003).

Therefore, Sepsis and its sequelae represent a continuum of clinical and pathophysiologic severity. Of course, the degree of severity independently affects prognosis. Some clinically recognizable stages of Sepsis include the following:

- **Severe Sepsis:** Sepsis associated with organ dysfunction, hypoperfusion abnormality, or Sepsis-induced hypotension. Hypoperfusion abnormalities include lactic acidosis, oliguria, and acute alteration of mental status.
- **Sepsis Induced Hypotension:** Presence of a systolic blood pressure of less than 90 mmHg or its reduction by 40 mmHg or more from the baseline in the absence of other cause for hypotension.
- **Septic Shock:** A subset of Severe Sepsis (i.e. it includes organ dysfunction and is therefore very closely related to MODS, as it shall be seen below), defined as Sepsis-induced hypotension and persisting despite adequate fluid resuscitation (fluid administration), along with the presence of hypoperfusion abnormalities or organ dysfunction. Patients receiving inotropic or vasopressor agents may no longer be hypotensive by the time they manifest hypoperfusion abnormalities or organ dysfunction.

However, they would still be considered to suffer from Septic Shock.

- **Multiple Organ Dysfunction Syndrome:** Defined as the detection of altered organ function in the acutely ill patient. The term *dysfunction* identifies this process as a phenomenon in which organ function is not capable of maintaining homeostasis.

In normal clinical practice, and while treating the syndromes outlined above, clinicians are always trying to catch up with the pathology. In other words, they are treating the more severely ill patients at late stages of evolution. It is also apparent that many of these patients who have more complex illnesses may be suffering from a combination of chronic and acute disease.

The rationale for using scoring systems in a clinical environment is to ensure that the increased complexity of disease in patients currently being treated is consistently represented for all those involved in the form of evaluations and descriptions. A specific goal of severity scoring systems is to use these important patient attributes to describe the relative risks of patients and identify where along the continuum of severity the patient resides. This should reduce the variability due to patient Factors so that the incremental impact of new or existing therapies can be more precisely determined. Also, more precise measurements of patient risk should lead to new insights into disease processes and serve as a tool with which clinicians could more accurately monitor patients and guide the use of new therapies.

In 1994, the ESICM (European Society of Intensive Care Medicine) (Vincent J.L., 1996) organized a consensus meeting in Paris to create a so-called Sequential Organ Failure Assessment (SOFA) Score with the aim of objectively and quantitatively describing the degree of organ dysfunction/failure over time in groups of patients or even individuals. The main two major applications of the SOFA score are:

- Improving the understanding of the natural history of organ dysfunction/failure and the interrelation between the failure of various organs / systems.
- Assessing the effect of new therapies on the course of organ dysfunction/failure. This could be used to characterize patients at admission in the ICU, serve as an ICU entry criterion and evaluate treatment efficacy.

Originally, the SOFA score was not designed to predict outcome but to describe a series of complications on the critically ill. Although any assessment of morbidity is related to mortality to some extent, the SOFA score was not designed just to describe organ dysfunction/failure according to mortality. However, and as investigated in this work, SOFA scores greater than 7 could present important ICU outcome prediction capabilities. Moreover, when combined with additional parameters, it provides a very powerful set of features not only for outcome assessment but also for the study of the evolution of Sepsis into its more severe states. The latter is one of the main design objectives of this particular score.

The SOFA limits the number of organs/systems under study to six, namely: Respiratory (inspiration air pressure), Coagulation (Platelet Count), Liver (Bilirrubine), Cardiovascular (Hypotension), Central Nervous System (Glasgow Coma Score), Renal (Creatinine or Urine Output). Scoring for each system ranges from 0 for *normal function* to 4 for *maximum failure/dysfunction*. The final SOFA score is the addition of the dysfunction indexes for all organs/systems. Therefore, the maximum possible SOFA score is 24, corresponding to maximum failure for all of the six organs/systems considered.

The APACHE II ("Acute Physiology and Chronic Health Evaluation II") is the severity-of-disease classification system (Knaus W.A., 1985) most widely used in clinical practice. After admission of a patient to an ICU, an integer score from 0 to 71 is computed based on several measurements. Higher scores imply a more severe disease and, therefore, a higher risk of death.

APACHE II was designed to measure the severity of disease for adult patients admitted to ICUs. The minimum age is not specified in the original study (Knaus W.A., 1985), but a reasonable limit recommends using APACHE II only for patients older than 15 years. This scoring system is applied in different ways:

- Some procedures are only carried out in, and some drugs are only prescribed to, patients with a given APACHE II score.
- The APACHE II score can be used to describe the morbidity of a patient when comparing his/her outcome with that of other patients.
- Predicted mortalities are averaged for groups of patients in order to specify the group's morbidity.

The score is calculated from 12 routine physiological measurements (such as blood pressure, body temperature, heart rate, etc.) during the first 24 hours after admission, plus information about previous health status and some information obtained at admission (such as age). The resulting score should always be interpreted in relation to the illness of the patient. After the initial score has been determined within 24 hours of admission, no new score can be calculated during the ICU stay. If a patient is discharged from the ICU and readmitted, a new APACHE II score must be calculated. In the proposed work, the APACHE II score will be used to assess patient severity and also as a baseline for comparing risk of death in Severe Sepsis.

SEVERE SEPSIS MORTALITY PREDICTION WITH LOGISTIC REGRESSION OVER LATENT FACTORS AND RELEVANCE VECTOR MACHINES

In this section we propose the use of a latent model-based feature extraction approach to obtain new sets of descriptors, or prognostic Factors for the prediction of mortality due to Sepsis. The experimental results reported in this study are readily interpretable. Interpretability is, needless to say, a sensitive issue in the medical ambit, and one that should not be underestimated: The lack of translation of the prognostic Factors into usable clinical knowledge would risk rendering the proposed approach useless (Martín J.D., 2010).

In this section we propose the use of different prediction models, including logistic regression from a set of latent features extracted from the original data and Relevance Vector Machines. Latent model-based feature extraction is used to obtain new sets of descriptors, or prognostic Factors for the prediction of mortality due to Sepsis. These Factors are used to predict mortality through standard LR, which is a method commonly used in medical applications (Kumar U.A., 2009) (Ture M., 2008) and widely trusted by clinicians. The prediction accuracy results obtained with the extracted Factors improve on those obtained with current standard data descriptors and therefore provide support for the use of these new Factors as risk-of-death predictors in ICU environments. Relevance Vector Machines not only provide accurate predictions, but also an estimation of the relative relevance of individual features in such prediction.

Materials

This work resorts to a prospective study approved by the Clinical Investigation Ethical Committee of the *Hospital Universitari del Vall d'Hebrón* in Barcelona, Spain, and to a database collected by the Research Group on Shock, Organic Dysfunction and Resuscitation of Vall d' Hebron's Intensive Care Unit. The database consisted of data collected in the ICU at this hospital between June 2007 and November 2008. During this period of time, 156 patients were admitted to the ICU (including medical and surgical patients) with Severe Sepsis.

The mean age of the patients in the analyzed database was 57.24 (with standard deviation +-15.25) years, 41.03% of patients were female and the diagnosis on admission was 64.10% *medical* and 35.90% *surgical*. The origin of primary infection for the cases on the database was 49.36% pulmonary, 14.74% abdominal, 10.26% urinary, 7.05% skin/muscle, 2.56% central nervous system (CNS), 1.28% catheter related, 0.64% endovascular, 5.13% biliary, 2.56% mediastinum and 6.41% unknown.

The collected data show the worst values for all variables during the first 24 hours of evolution for Severe Sepsis. Organ dysfunction was evaluated by means of the SOFA score (Vincent J.L., 1996) as shown in the table below. Severity was evaluated by means of the APACHE II score (for further reference, see (Knaus W.A., 1985)).

The population under study, 56.41% received mechanical ventilation with a PaO2/FiO2 of 166 +-100, 73% received vasoactive drugs, the platelet count was $1.84 \cdot 10^5$ +-$1.36 \cdot 10^5$/L, the Lactate Levels were 3.40 +-3.60 mmol/L, and the APACHE II score was 22.73 +-8.53.

In 2004, the Surviving Sepsis Campaign (SSC) defined a set of guidelines for the management of Severe Sepsis and Septic Shock (Masur H., 2004). More specifically, these set of guidelines were proposed for both the first 6 hours of evolution and the first 24 hours. The compliance of the SSC bundles for the first 6 hours was 31.41%, out

of which 77.56% had Haemocultures performed, 85.90% received antibiotics, 57.05% had their lactate monitored, 69.87% received Volume (i.e. Fluid Resuscitation) 18.59% received transfusions and 4.89% received Dobutamine. The SVCO$_2$ values were 45.53+-70.76 and the Hematocrit 26.53+-12.92 for the first 6 hours. The compliance of the first 24 hour SSC bundles was 51.92%, the glycaemia was <150 mg/dL in 62.18% of cases and Plateau Pressure (PPlateau) <30 cm H$_2$O in 44.23% of cases. The mortality rate intra-ICU for our study population was 34% for the period of study.

Feature Extraction Methods

Out of the broad palette of existing feature extraction methods, some of the most widely used are Principal Component Analysis (PCA) (Jolliffe, 2002), Non-Negative Matrix Factorization (NMF) (Seoung S.H., 1999) and Factor Analysis (Thayer D.T., 1982). NMF is also a natural way of obtaining a meaningful base because the observations are all positive, and most are multinomially distributed. Provided that this Factorization does not give a ranking of the elements of the base as in the case of PCA, an arbitrary dimension of the sub-base that spans the observation can be selected. The bases (Factors) that are obtained with both methods span a subspace which reconstructs the original observation with an error.

The covariance matrix can be decomposed into the sum of two terms: the product of the base that we use in order to represent the observed data, plus an error term, in the form $\Sigma = \Lambda\Lambda^T + \Psi$. In PCA and NMF, the covariance of the error term is a full matrix, which means that the Factor base does not account for all the interactions between the observed variables. In other words, the error term still contains information about interactions or relations between these variables in addition to the specific information of each variable (diagonal term of Ψ).

To overcome this limitation, we propose the use of FA, which finds a decomposition of the covariance matrix $\Sigma = \Lambda\Lambda^T + \Psi$ such that Ψ is a diagonal matrix. This method selects the Factors following a criterion based on the correlation between features of the observation vector. In our implementation, the model is estimated using maximum likelihood (ML), which explicitly assumes a Gaussian distribution for x. Nevertheless, and independently of assumptions concerning data distribution, ML searches for a decomposition of Σ so that the error matrix Ψ has a diagonal structure. Therefore, the model generates the observation from a set of latent variables that are independent of the error term, and takes into account all the correlations between variables.

Factor Analysis through ML Estimation

The likelihood function for the sample X and probability distribution f is:

$$L(X,\Theta) = \prod_{i=1}^{n} f(x_i, \Theta)$$

and, as result, the log-likelihood function is defined as

$$l(x,\Theta) = \ln L(X,\Theta) = \sum_{i=1}^{n} \ln f(x_i, \Theta),$$

which has a support function

$$S(\Lambda,\Psi;S) = tr((\Lambda\Lambda^T + \Psi)^{-1}S) - \ln\left|(\Lambda\Lambda^T + \Psi)^{-1}S\right| - p.$$

This support function is a linear function of the log-likelihood $l(X;\Sigma)$. The minimum of $S(\Lambda,\Psi;S)$ corresponds to a maximum of $l(X;\Sigma)$. This minimization can be performed by means of an iterative Newton-Raphson method, which results in an eigen value equation, by minimizing separately for Λ (over a fixed Ψ) and subsequently minimizing over Ψ.

Relevance Vector Machines

A general regression problem can be written as (A. J. Smola., 2002):

$$y = w^T \phi(x),$$

Where $\phi(x)$ is a basis function. In order to estimate the weights w from our support, it is assumed that each target t_i in the training sample (valued 1 for survival and -1 for exitus in this work) represents the true model y_i contaminated with i.i.d Gaussian noise $\varepsilon_i \sim N(0,\sigma^2)$ so that $\forall i$:

$$t_i = w^T \phi(x_i) + \varepsilon_i$$

For N i.i.d training points

$$p(t \mid x_i, w, \sigma^2) =$$

$$\prod_{i=1}^{N} N(w^T \phi(x_i), \sigma^2) = \frac{1}{(2\pi\sigma^2)^{N/2}} e^{\frac{\|t-\Phi w\|}{2\sigma^2}},$$

where t is the vector of training targets t_i, the $N \times M$ Matrix Φ is built so that the ith row represents vector $\phi(x_i)$. The growth of weights w can be constrained by defining an explicit prior probability distribution on w. Assuming a Gaussian distribution on w and defining $S = sI$ as the hyperparameter matrix where I is the $N \times N$ Identity matrix and $s = [s_1 \cdots s_N]$ is a vector where each s_i describes the inverse variance for each w_i. For each weight, the hyperparameter s_i modifies the relevance of the prior.

The posterior probability over the unkown parameters is

$$p(w, s, \sigma^2 \mid t) = p(w \mid t, s, \sigma^2)p(s, \sigma^2 \mid t)$$

$$p(w \mid t, s, \sigma^2) = \frac{|\Sigma|^{1/2}}{(2\pi)^{N/2}} e^{\frac{-1}{2}(w-\mu)^T \Sigma^{-1}(w-\mu)},$$

Here $\Sigma = \left(\dfrac{1}{\sigma^2}\Phi^T\Phi + S\right)^{-1}$ and $\mu = \dfrac{1}{\sigma^2}\Sigma\Phi t$

Assuming uniform hyperpriors, we can calculate the following marginal likelihood function in Box 1, which has to be maximized w.r.t. σ^{-2} and s.

It is important to note that during the iterative process to solve the former optimization some s_i may tend towards infinity, which entails $\lim\limits_{s_i \to \infty} \Sigma = 0$ and $\lim\limits_{s_i \to \infty} \mu = 0$. In this situation, some w_i will take values close to zero, which means that the adaptive effect of the hyperparameters will effectively disable the input features that are deemed to be irrelevant for the prediction. This is, in fact, a form of *soft* feature selection, or, more precisely, a form of *automatic relevance determination*.

Logistic Regression

Logistic regression studies binomially distributed variables of the form $C_i \sim B(n_i, p_i)$ where n_i and p_i correspond to the number of patients and the probability of exitus. In this work C_i is a class label that takes the value 1 for survival and -1 for exitus. The logistic model proposes that, for each patient i, there is a set of explanatory variables that might inform the final probability. Thus, the model takes the form $p_i = E\left(\dfrac{C_i}{n_i} \mid X_i\right)$, for each

Table 1. List of SOFA scores with their corresponding mean and standard deviation values

System	Mean (SD)
Cardiovascular (CV)	2.8 (1.50)
Respiratory (RESP)	2.41 (1.06)
Central Nervous System (CNS)	0.42 (0.86)
Hepatic (HEPA)	0.39 (0.86)
Renal (REN)	0.97 (1.16)
Hematologic (HEMATO)	0.88 (1.16)
Global SOFA Score	7.95 (3.67)
Organs in Dysfunction (SOFA 1-2)	1.73 (1.12)
Organs in Failure (SOFA 3-4)	1.15 (0.89)
Total Organs in Dysfunction	3.20 (1.41)

variable i (be it from the original set of variables in Table 2 or one of the extracted Factors).

Here, the natural logarithms of the odds ratio for the unknown binomial probabilities are modeled as a linear function of X_i:

$$\ln\left(\frac{p_i}{1 - p_i}\right) = \beta_0 + B^T X_i,$$

where β_0 is the intercept and B is the vector of logistic regression coefficients. In our work, the intercept and regression coefficients have been estimated by ML with a generalized linear model.

Box 1.

$$\ln p(t \mid s, \sigma^{-2}) = \frac{1}{2}\sum_{i=1}^{M} \ln s_i - \frac{N}{2}(\ln(\sigma^{-2}) + \ln(2\pi)) + \frac{1}{2}(\sigma^{-2}t^T t - \mu^T \Sigma^{-1}\mu + \ln|\Sigma|),$$

Table 2. List of variables

Variable	Description
V1	Age
V2	Gender
V3	Focus of Sepsis
V4	Germ Class
V5	Polymicrobial Infection
V6	Base Pathology
V7	Cardiovascular SOFA score
V8	Respiratory SOFA score
V9	CNS SOFA score
V10	Hepatic SOFA score
V11	Renal SOFA score
V12	Hematologic SOFA score
V13	Total SOFA score
V14	Organs in Dysfunction for SOFA 1-2
V15	Organs in Dysfunction for SOFA 3-4
V16	Total Number of Organs in Dysfunction
V17	Mechanical Ventilation
V18	Oxygenation Index PaO_2/FiO_2
V19	Vasoactive Drugs
V20	Platelet Count
V21	APACHE II score
V22	Surviving Sepsis Campaign 6h (Resuscitation Bundles)
V23	Hemocultures 6h
V24	Antibiotics 6h
V25	Volume 6h
V26	Central Venous Saturation of O_2 6h
V27	Hematocrit 6h
V28	Transfusions 6h
V29	Dobutamine 6h
V30	Surviving Sepsis Campaign 24 h (Treatment Bundles)
V31	Glycaemia 24h
V32	PPlateau
V33	Worst Lactate Levels
V34	O_2 Central Venous Saturation

RESULTS

Factor Interpretation from a Clinical Point of View

As described in the previous subsections, the application of FA resulted in a consistent 14-Factor model of the original data set. The cumulative proportion of total (standardized) sample variance explained by this model was found to be 79.12%.

The table in Figure 1 summarizes the matrix of loadings corresponding to the original variables listed in Table 2. Taking into consideration the highest Factor loadings (in absolute value) for every given variable, these Factors were mapped into different easily interpretable clinical descriptors, explained as follows:

- **Factor 1:** Related to cardiovascular function and, more specifically, to the cardiovascular SOFA score and vasoactive drugs c.f. Table 1.
- **Factor 2:** Corresponds to haematologic function (haematologic SOFA score measured by platelet count).
- **Factor 3:** Corresponds to the use of Mechanical Ventilation and PPlateau.
- **Factor 4:** Also corresponds to respiratory function, Respiratory SOFA score (PaO_2/FiO_2 relation).
- **Factor 5:** Related to the microorganism producing the Sepsis and whether this Sepsis is polimicrobial or not.
- **Factor 6:** It corresponds to the 24 h. SSC bundles and glycaemic indexes.
- **Factor 7:** It corresponds to renal function measured by the SOFA score and the total SOFA score.
- **Factor 8:** Related to the hepathic function measured by the SOFA score.

Figure 1. Loadings matrix

	F1	F2	F3	F4	F5	F6	F7	F8	F9	F10	F11	F12	F13	F14
v1	.33	-.60	-.05	-.03	-.05	-.11	.58	-.12	.10	.09	.84	-.00	.17	.21
v2	.06	-.02	.18	.06	.12	-.04	.10	-.12	.13	-.02	-.10	.24	.12	.10
v3	.11	.00	-.05	-.28	-.03	.01	.03	.19	-.05	.06	.13	**-.43**	.16	**.26**
v4	-.16	-.06	.00	-.06	**.97**	-.06	-.02	-.01	-.07	-.02	-.06	-.01	-.07	-.08
v5	-.04	.00	.02	-.10	**.76**	-.15	-.07	-.03	-.12	-.03	.02	.06	-.01	.03
v6	-.11	.19	.02	.14	.00	-.05	-.00	-.07	-.01	-.04	.08	**.84**	-.08	.03
v7	**.95**	.06	.15	-.06	-.06	-.00	.08	.13	-.06	.02	-.00	-.07	.12	-.03
v8	.01	-.04	.36	**.89**	-.11	-.00	.01	.11	.03	.02	.11	.04	.02	-.07
v9	.02	.05	.03	-.02	-.03	-.02	.06	.01	.13	.11	**.96**	.01	.09	.13
v10	.08	.12	.03	.10	-.08	.12	.01	**.88**	.05	.22	.07	-.04	.11	.29
v11	.18	.12	.04	-.05	-.09	.02	**.91**	.07	-.06	.11	.04	-.00	.29	-.06
v12	.12	**.93**	.09	-.01	.02	-.02	.03	.16	-.03	.08	-.01	.04	.10	.23
v13	.57	.37	.23	.24	-.08	.06	**.38**	.34	.04	.16	.22	-.01	.21	.20
v14	.00	.27	-.12	.03	-.05	.03	.09	.11	.04	**.92**	.10	-.08	.08	.10
v15	.51	.27	.36	.19	-.14	.02	.30	.31	.08	-.37	.25	.04	.19	.01
v16	.34	.44	.06	.17	-.12	.05	.20	.30	.09	**.49**	.33	-.08	.20	.01
v17	.10	-.03	**.93**	.14	-.00	-.01	.08	.06	.12	-.09	.08	.02	.18	-.15
v18	.10	-.04	.03	**-.76**	.09	.02	.01	-.00	-.09	-.09	.10	-.24	-.15	-.08
v19	**.88**	.10	.13	-.08	-.13	.01	.06	.01	.11	-.01	-.06	-.06	.05	.02
v20	-.10	-.64	.12	.02	.09	.07	-.12	-.12	.01	-.21	-.08	-.17	-.14	.07
v21	.03	.16	.27	.21	-.01	.01	.35	.05	.09	.05	.21	.10	**.66**	.07
v22	.03	.06	.02	.07	.01	.06	-.01	.08	.48	.13	.02	.06	.04	.03
v23	.21	.04	-.02	-.03	-.07	-.03	.03	.04	**.66**	-.09	.09	.06	-.12	.06
v24	.04	-.01	.01	.06	-.14	.05	-.02	.06	**.68**	-.01	.02	-.08	.00	.01
v25	.52	.07	.06	-.06	.03	.11	-.02	.00	.41	-.00	-.04	-.03	.13	-.06
v26	-.00	.08	-.07	.02	.03	-.21	-.02	.18	.11	.14	.08	.06	-.11	-.00
v27	.04	-.15	.06	-.04	-.01	-.05	-.07	.03	.3	-.01	.05	.23	.05	-.22
v28	.01	.10	-.07	-.00	.03	-.06	-.05	.09	.05	.12	.00	.01	.01	**.25**
v29	.09	.14	.21	-.15	.03	.05	.01	.06	.04	.06	-.01	.13	.09	.08
v30	.01	.02	-.05	-.03	-.10	**.73**	-.00	.11	.07	-.02	.02	-.03	-.00	.02
v31	.01	-.05	-.01	.01	-.10	**.98**	.02	.05	.07	.09	-.01	-.01	-.03	-.10
v32	-.22	.06	**-.52**	-.17	-.03	.06	.03	.13	.09	.09	.06	-.04	-.18	.03
v33	.25	.17	.22	.07	-.09	.05	.18	.15	.05	-.03	-.06	.02	**.48**	.08
v34	.09	.11	-.01	-.02	.01	.06	.05	**.40**	.12	-.02	-.03	-.01	.08	-.06

- **Factor 9:** It corresponds to the administration of antibiotics and haemocultures taken during the first 6 h. of evolution.
- **Factor 10:** Relates to the number of dysfunctioning organs for a SOFA 1-2 and the total number of dysfunctioning organs.
- **Factor 11:** It corresponds to the CNS function measured in the SOFA score and the total number of dysfunctioning organs.
- **Factor 12:** Relates to the base pathology and the loci of Sepsis.
- **Factor 13:** Corresponding to the global APACHE II score.
- **Factor 14:** Relates to the focus of Sepsis, transfusions and hepathic SOFA score.

The Factors obtained with this method are coherent with the SOFA score as a description and measure of organ failure and dysfunction (Vincent J.L., 1996), combined with the management guidelines defined by the Surviving Sepsis Campaign (Masur H., 2004). Therefore, it can be safely concluded that they are related to SOFA and the actions taken to mitigate this organ deterioration.

This is a result of particular interest. One of the main challenges in mortality prediction is that of producing flexible models that can robustly fit the observed data without the need for unnecessary contextual assumptions, and in the presence of subtle interactions between covariates. This happens because standard medical indicator-based models typically rely on hand-crafted parametric solutions to get around the problem (Tagliaferri R., 2010). One clear example of this is the categorization of the SOFA score prognostic indicators described in materials section. The obtained FA solution goes beyond this categorization while accounting for covariate interactions.

As mentioned in the introduction to the study, the interpretability of results is paramount in real clinical applications (Martín J.D., 2010). The reported FA not only complies with this requirement: it also provides a parsimonious data representation that can be used as a basis for mortality prediction related to the Sepsis pathology (Figure 1).

Mortality Prediction with RVM

The performance of the model was evaluated by bagging (bootstrap aggregating). One thousand training sets consisting of 104 samples each were generated by sampling uniformly and with replacement.

For each new training set, approximately 52 training instances from the original database were left out and used to evaluate the system performance (i.e. out-of-bag prediction). The model performance was averaged over the 1,000 bagged training sets.

The RVM yielded an accuracy of mortality prediction of 0.75 as measured by the area under the ROC plot (AUC); a prediction error of 0.27; sensitivity (proportion of correctly predicted survivors out of all survivors) of 0.78; and specificity (proportion of correctly predicted exitus out of all exitus) of 0.71.

Beyond classification accuracy, and as described in the previous section, RVM performs soft feature selection through automatic feature relevance determination. The following relevance vector (with the weights associated to each input feature) was obtained:

- Number of organs in dysfunction ($w_1 = -0.19$)
- Mechanical Ventilation ($w_2 = -0.07$)
- **APACHE II** ($w_3 = -0.17$)
- Resuscitation Bundles (6h) ($w_4 = 0.04$)

- **Volume (6h)** ($w_5 = 0.08$)
- Treatment Bundles (24h) ($w_6 = 0.02$)
- **Worst Lactate** ($w_7 = -0.27$)

The coefficients corresponding to the rest of features were set to values close to zero as part of the training process. This effectively reduces the complexity of the prediction procedure (34 features reduced to just 7) and improves its interpretability. Given that a linear basis function was been used to estimate the relevance vector, it becomes apparent that the negative weights (number of organs in dysfunction, mechanical ventilation, APACHE II and worst lactate) are related to a higher mortality risk (note again that we have coded survival as 1 and exitus as -1), whereas the SSC bundles (both for 24 and 6 h) and Volume Resuscitation (during the first 6h of evolution) are associated to a protective effect. The resuscitation bundles (6h) include: antibiotic administration, performance of haemocultures and administration of vasoactive drugs. Volume resuscitation during the first 6h of evolution has been considered as a separate variable. In fact, timely administration of antibiotics and performance of haemocultures are considered critical to improving the prognosis of Septic patients. Equally important is the knowledge of which features are deemed not to be relevant by RVM.

Mortality Prediction Using Logistic Regression over Latent Factors

We now progress to the task of mortality prediction itself, using the obtained 14-Factor FA solution as starting point. The performance of the model was also evaluated by means of bagging (bootstrap aggregating). One thousand new training sets consisting of 104 samples were generated by sampling uniformly and with replacement. For each new training set, approximately 52 training instances from the original database were left out. These left-out instances were used to evaluate the system performance (i.e. out-of-bag prediction). The model performance was averaged over the 1,000 bagged training sets.

Table 3 shows the coefficient estimates β, Z-Scores and p-values resulting from fitting a logistic regression model to the 14 Factors (inputs) and the outcome in the ICU (output). The Z-Scores measure the effect of removing one Factor from the model (R. Tibshirani, 2008). A Z-score greater than 1.96 in absolute value is significant at the 5% level and provides a measure of the relevance for the prediction of a given Factor.

Here, Factor 3, which is related to *Mechanical Ventilation* and *Pplateau*, shows the strongest effect together with Factor 13, which is related to the APACHE II score. Factor 8 (Hepatic Function measured with the SOFA Score) and Factor 10 (related to the number of Dysfunctional Organs) are also found to be relevant.

Table 4 shows the theoretical 95% confidence intervals for the LR coefficients and their corresponding odds-ratio. More specifically, $CI_i = \beta_i \pm 1.96\sigma_i$ and $OR_i = e^{CI_i}$.

It is worth noting at this stage that, with LR, the Factors related to the *Surviving Sepsis Campaign* show no strong effect on mortality prediction. However, it is interesting to note that Factor 9 (antibiotic administration and haemocultures) presents a higher impact than that of Factor 6 (24 h. bundles with glycaemic indexes). For our ICU, 85.90% of patients received antibiotics during the first 6 h of evolution and 77.56% had haemocultures during the same period of time. In fact, timely administration of antibiotics and performance of haemocultures are considered critical to improving the prognosis of Septic patients.

Regression on the 14 Factors together with bagging resulted in an AUC of 0.75, a prediction error over the test data of 0.22, a sensitivity of 0.64, and a specificity of 0.84.

Mortality Prediction Using Logistic Regression over the Original Data

Further experiments aimed to compare the predictive ability of the FA 14-Factor solution with that of the original data attributes were carried out. For that, the most significant clinical attributes were selected in a backward feature selection process (in our case, the backward feature selection removes those variables resulting in non-significant z-scores). The selected attributes were: the total number of organs in dysfunction; the APACHE II score; and the worst lactate levels. The corresponding coefficients, z-scores and p-values for these three variables are presented in Tables 5 and 6.

Regression on the most significant attributes together with bagging yield an AUC of 0.71, a lower result than the one obtained with the FA solution. This experiment also yielded a prediction error over the test data of 0.25 (higher than the FA solution), a sensitivity of 0.72, and a specificity of 0.77.

Mortality Prediction Using the ROD Formula over the APACHE II Score

The Risk-of-Death (ROD) formula based on the APACHE II score can be expressed as (Knaus W.A., 1985):

$$\ln\left(\frac{ROD}{1 - ROD}\right) = -3.517 + 0.146A + \varepsilon$$

Where A is the APACHE II score and ε is a correction Factor depending on clinical traits at admission in the ICU. For instance, if the patient has undergone post-emergency surgery, ε is set to 0.613. The application of this formula with a threshold to the population under study yields an error rate of 0.28 (higher than previous results), a sensitivity of 0.55 (very low) and a specificity of 0.82. The AUC was 0.70.

Table 3. Results for logistic regression over 14 Factors (Z-score>1.96 results in p-values <0.05). Most relevant Factors are presented in bold lettering.

	β Coefficient	Z-Score	p-value
Intercept	**0.95**	**3.52**	**0.008**
F1	-0.39	-1.14	0.27
F2	-0.45	-1.84	0.53
F3	**-1.03**	**-3.72**	**0.005**
F4	-0.16	-0.66	0.45
F5	0.02	0.09	0.8
F6	0.47	0.58	0.18
F7	-0.61	-1.82	0.17
F8	**-0.61**	**-2.55**	**0.04**
F9	0.22	1.07	0.35
F10	**-0.50**	**-2.06**	**0.02**
F11	-0.31	-1.24	0.27
F12	-0.02	-0.09	0.52
F13	**-0.88**	**-3.11**	**<0.001**
F14	0.21	0.91	0.39

Table 4. 95% CI and odds-ratio

	CI-High	CI-Low	OR-High	OR-Low
Intercept	1.47	0.42	4.36	1.52
F3	-0.49	-1.57	0.61	0.21
F8	-0.14	-1.09	0.87	0.34
F10	-0.02	-0.98	0.98	0.37
F13	-0.32	-1.43	0.72	0.24

Table 5. Logistic regression results

	β Coefficient	Z-Score	p-value
Intercept	4.16	4.85	<0.001
Num. Org. Dysf.	-0.57	-2.05	0.03
APACHE II	-0.09	-2.15	0.03
Worst Lactate	-0.30	-2.49	<0.001

Table 6. 95% CI and odds-ratio

	CI-High	CI-Low	OR-High	OR-Low
Intercept	5.78	2.55	12.82	324
Num. Org. Dysf.	-0.04	-1.10	0.33	0.95
APACHE II	-0.01	-0.17	0.85	0.99
Worst Lactate	-0.10	-0.51	0.60	0.91

FUTURE RESEARCH DIRECTIONS

The performance of the proposed method has been evaluated in a single ICU and a limited population sample. From a clinical standpoint, future work should lead towards a multi-centric prospective study, in order to validate its generalizability.

From a Machine Learning point of view, we intend to study the marginal dependence between the different clinical traits involved in Sepsis by means of Algebraic Statistical Models (ASM). The idea behind this approach is that ASM naturally map with graphical models in general and Markov Random Fields and Bayes Neworks in particular. The parameterizations obtained combined with the graphical models naturally give way to the deployment of Kernel Methods that are not only general but also interpretable from a clinical point of view.

CONCLUSION

Sepsis is a prevalent pathology in the clinical ICU environment, and one with relatively high mortality levels associated. Its medical management is therefore both a sensitive issue and a serious challenge to health care systems.

The clinical indicators of Sepsis currently in use are known to be of limited relevance as mortality predictors. In the assessment of ROD for critically ill patients, sensitivity is of paramount importance due to the fact that more aggressive treatment and therapeutic actions may result in better outcomes for high risk patients. As validated by the results reported in Table 7 for APACHE II and similar ones reported in other studies (Gómez M., 1995), the ROD formula presented in (Knaus W.A., 1985) is poor in terms of sensitivity (i.e., it results in a high number of false positive cases). This is despite the fact that it is widely accepted in practice and yields acceptable accuracy results. Its poor sensitivity may be the result of its formula

Table 7. Results summary table for relevance vector machines (RVM), logistic regression (LR), LR over latent Factors (LR-FA) and the APACHE II ROD

Method	AUC	Error	Sens.	Spec.
RVM	0.79	0.27	0.78	0.71
LR	0.75	0.22	0.64	0.84
LR-FA	0.71	0.25	0.72	0.77
APACHE II	0.7	0.28	0.55	0.82

being based on clinical traits and the APACHE II score only.

In this study, we have put forward a new and simple method for the assessment of ROD in Septic patients. It proposes a change of data representation in the form of feature extraction using FA, and uses LR over the resulting latent Factors for the prediction itself. The main advantage of the proposed approach is that it removes collinearities and noisy inputs while keeping the method simple and fully interpretable from a clinical point of view. In other words, the strength of this study lies in the fact that it is possible to derive a prognostic score from a set of physiopathologic and therapeutic variables, which are available at the onset of Severe Sepsis.

The proposed method may be understood as a generalization of the ROD formula introduced in (Knaus W.A., 1985), where the ε corrective Factor, which models clinical traits at admittance in the ICU, is accounted for by the latent-Factor representation. It takes not only the contribution of the APACHE II score into consideration, but also other important clinical traits such as the number of dysfunctioning organs combined with the Sequential Organ Failure Assessment (SOFA), which also impacts on the mortality rates of Septic patients. The reported ROD assessment takes into consideration the Respiratory and Hepatic SOFA scores. It is precisely all the extra parameters considered in our experiments the reason behind the significant improvement on sensitivity. This improvement is achieved while keeping model complexity under control and without compromising the interpretability of the results (given that all the parameters involved are routinely monitored in an ICU).

The proposed RVM method is also a generalization of the ROD formula introduced in (Knaus W.A., 1985), where the ε corrective Factor, which not only takes the contribution of the APACHE II score into consideration, but also other important life-threatening clinical traits such as the number of organs in dysfunction combined with mechanical ventilation, and worst lactate levels, which in turn are also aligned with those traits obtained with the LR and FA methods. The prognosis indicator is also balanced with the most important procedures from the SSC to overcome Sepsis such as the administration of volume, antibiotics, vasoactive drugs and the performance of haemocultures.

ACKNOWLEDGMENT

This research was partially funded by the Spanish MICINN project TIN2009-13895-C02-01.

REFERENCES

Angus, D. C., Linde-Zwirble, W. T., Lidicker, J., Clermont, G., Carcillo, J., & Pinsky, M. R. (2001). Epidemiology of severe sepsis in the United States: Analysis of incidence, outcome and associated costs of care. *Critical Care Medicine, 29*, 1303–1310. doi:10.1097/00003246-200107000-00002

Bone, R. C., Balk, R. A., Cerra, F. B., Dellinger, R. P., Fein, A. M., & Knaus, W. A. (1992). Definitions of sepsis and organ failure and guidelines for the use of innovative therapies in sepsis. *Chest, 101*(6), 1644–1655. doi:10.1378/chest.101.6.1644

Brawnwald, E., Fauci, A. S., Kasper, D. L., Hauser, S. L., Long, D. L., & Jameson, J. L. (2008). *Harrison's principles of internal medicine*. London, UK: McGraw-Hill Medical Publishing Division.

Brun-Buisson, C., Doyan, F., Carlet, J., Dellamonica, P., Gouin, F., & Lepoutre, A. (1995). Incidence, risk Factors, and outcome of severe sepsis and septic shock in adults. *Journal of the American Medical Association, 274*, 968–974. doi:10.1001/jama.1995.03530120060042

Center for Disease Control. (1990). Increase in national hospital discharge survey rates for Septicemia: United States, 1979-1987. *Morbidity and Mortality Weekly Report, 39*, 31–34.

Centers for Disease Control and Prevention. (1993). Mortality patterns-United States, 1990. *Monthly Vital Statistics Report, 41*, 5.

Dellinger, R. P., Carlet, J. M., Masur, H., Gerlach, H., Calanda, T., & Cohen, J. (2004). Surviving sepsis campaign guidelines for management of severe sepsis and septic shock. *Intensive Care Medicine, 30*, 536–555. doi:10.1007/s00134-004-2210-z

Hastie, T., Tibshirani, R., & Friedman, J. H. (2008). *The elements of statistical learning*. Springer.

Jolliffe, I. (2002). *Principal component analysis*. New York, NY: Springer.

Knaus, W. A., Draper, E. A., Wagner, D. P., & Zimmerman, J. E. (1985). APACHE II: A severity of disease classification system. *Critical Care Medicine, 13*, 818–829. doi:10.1097/00003246-198510000-00009

Kurt, I., Ture, M., & Turhan Kurum, A. (2008). Comparing performances of logistic regression classification and regression tree, and neural networks for predicting coronary arterial disease. *Expert Systems with Applications, 34*(1), 366–374. doi:10.1016/j.eswa.2006.09.004

Lee, D. D., & Seung, S. (1999). Learning the parts of objects by non-negative matrix Factorization. *Nature, 6755*(401), 788–791.

Levy, M. M., Fink, M. P., Marshall, J. C., Abraham, E., Angus, D., & Cook, D. … Ramsay, G. (2003). *2001 SSCM/ESICM/ACCP/SIS International Sepsis Definitions Conference* (pp. 530-538).

Lisboa, P. J. G., Vellido, A., Tagliaferri, R., Napolitano, F., Ceccarelli, M., Martin-Guerrero, J. D., & Biganzoli, E. (2010). Data mining for cancer research. *IEEE Computational Intelligence Magazine, 5*(1), 14–18. doi:10.1109/MCI.2009.935311

Livingston, D. H., Mosenthal, A. C., & Deith, E. A. (1995). Sepsis and multiple organ dysfunction syndrome: A clinical-mechanistic overview. *New Horizons (Baltimore, Md.), 3*, 257–266.

Luce, J. (1987). Pathogenesis and management of septic shock. *Chest, 91*, 883–888. doi:10.1378/chest.91.6.883

Martin, G. S., Mannino, D. M., Eaton, S., & Moss, M. (2003). The epidemiology of sepsis in the United States from 1979 to 2000. *The New England Journal of Medicine, 348*, 1546–1554. doi:10.1056/NEJMoa022139

Martín, J. D., & Lisboa, P. J. G. (2010). Computational intelligence in biomedicine: Some contributions. *Proceedings of the 18th European Symposium on Artificial Neural Networks (ESANN)*, (pp. 429-438).

Paliwal, M., & Kumar, U. A. (2009). Neural networks and statistical techniques: A review of applications. *Expert Systems with Applications, 36*(1), 2–17. doi:10.1016/j.eswa.2007.10.005

Scholkopf, B., & Smola, A. J. (2002). *Learning with kernels*. Boston, MA: MIT Press.

Thayer, D. T., &. R. (1982). EM algorithms for ML Factor analysis. *Psychometrica, 47*, 69–76. doi:10.1007/BF02293851

Vincent, J. L. (1996). Definition and pathogenesis of septic shock. *Current Topics in Microbiology and Immunology, 216*, 1–13. doi:10.1007/978-3-642-80186-0_1

Vincent, J. L., de Mendoça, A., Cantraine, F., Moreno, R., Takala, J., & Suter, P. M. (1998). Use of the SOFA score to assess the incidence of organ dysfunction/failure in intensive care units: Results of a multicenter, prospective study. *Critical Care Medicine, 26*, 1793–1800. doi:10.1097/00003246-199811000-00016

Vincent, J. L., Moreno, R., Takala, J., Willats, S., De Mendoca, A., & Burining, H. (1996). The SOFA (Sepsis-related organ failure assessment) score to describe organ dysfunction/failure. *Critical Care Medicine, 22*, 707–710.

Wong, D. T., Crofts, S. L., McGuire, G. P., & Byrick, R. J. (1995). Evaluation of predictive ability of APACHE II system and hospital outcome in Canadian intensive care unit patients. *Critical Care Medicine, 23*(7), 1177–1183. doi:10.1097/00003246-199507000-00005

Chapter 2
Statistical Pattern Recognition Techniques for Early Diagnosis of Diabetic Neuropathy by Posturographic Data

Claudia Diamantini
Università Politecnica delle Marche, Italy

Sandro Fioretti
Università Politecnica delle Marche, Italy

Domenico Potena
Università Politecnica delle Marche, Italy

ABSTRACT

The goal of this chapter is to describe the use of statistical pattern recognition techniques in order to build a classification model for the early diagnosis of peripheral diabetic neuropathy. In particular, the authors present two experimental methodologies, based on linear discriminant analysis and Bayes vector quantizer algorithms respectively. The former algorithm has demonstrated the best performance in distinguish between non-neuropathic and neuropathic patients, while the latter is able to build models that recognize the severity of the neuropathy.

INTRODUCTION

Neuropathy affects up to 50% of diabetic patients showing different clinical features. Peripheral Neuropathy (PN) is one of most prevalent types of diabetic neuropathy. An early diagnosis in asymptomatic patients is useful in order to make the patients aware of their condition and to activate educational programs oriented to encourage some changes in lifestyle. Moreover, effective treatments are available to prevent further complications. Nerve conduction studies are the gold standard for diagnosing PN but these tests can be

DOI: 10.4018/978-1-4666-1803-9.ch002

challenging for both the patient and the testing physician, hence they are typically prescribed in the presence of strong clues for neuropathy. These observations suggest the need of new, easy, and reliable tools for the early diagnosis of PN.

The loss of sensory perception secondary to PN has a markedly detrimental effect on postural stability during stance and gait. Evaluation of postural steadiness is usually based on the interpretation of centre-of-pressure (COP) measures using a dynamometric platform. High correlations have been found in previous works between the severity of neuropathy and the COP measures. Hence it is sensible to assume that posturographic data based on COP measures can be used as input to statistical pattern recognition techniques to automatically build a diagnosis model. An approach using classical Linear Discriminant Analysis (LDA) has been recently proposed in Fioretti, Scocco, and Ladislao (2010).

In this chapter we survey the main features of the cited paper, by discussing the issues related to the application of such parametric technique for PN diagnosis. Next, we compare this approach with a more general, non-parametric methodology. In particular, the use of the supervised learning algorithm called Bayes Vector Quantizer (BVQ) is discussed. BVQ is applied to nearest neighbor types classifiers, resulting in a simple and cheap classification rule. Its roots in statistical pattern recognition, in particular in Bayes decision theory for the minimization of average misclassification risk, guarantee higher robustness and accuracy performance than traditional nearest neighbor, and the ability to deal with asymmetric classification costs and unbalanced data.

In the following Sections we first introduce both the application domain and some Statistical Pattern Recognition concepts and techniques used in this Chapter. Afterwards, the BVQ algorithm is described as well as the experimental methodology we use for designing a 3-class classification model. Results and future research directions are discussed in the remaining of the Chapter.

BACKGROUND

Static Posturography Applied to Diabetic Neuropathic Subjects

The most prevalent type of diabetic neuropathy is distal symmetric, primarily sensory, peripheral polyneuropathy. This can be the result of progressive nerve fiber loss, with a reduction of nerve conduction velocity. The altered proprioception results in abnormal postural control and in an augmented risk of falls for the patients. Improved glycemic control may slow the progress of neuropathy so that an early diagnosis of peripheral neuropathy in asymptomatic patients is very important in order to avoid non-reversible consequences of this disease.

Electromyography and nerve conduction studies are the gold standard for diagnosing peripheral neuropathy. These tests can be grueling for both the patient and the testing physician and so are underused in diagnosing peripheral neuropathy, especially in the elderly. Literature shows a number of screening instruments and methods that have been proposed to detect diabetic neuropathy at a preclinical stage, as alternative diagnostic procedures besides electromyography as those described in Perkins, Olaleye and Zinman (2001). These methods are generally characterized by a low sensitivity when compared with standard diagnostic tests (i.e. nerve conduction velocity) and give rise to qualitative rather than quantitative results. These characteristics of the proposed screening tests do not allow us to obtain reliable information on the degree of severity of the neuropathic impairment. Moreover, only combinations of more than one test allow obtaining acceptable sensitivity in detecting distal symmetric polyneuropathy.

Motor performance of diabetic patients with peripheral neuropathy has been examined in a quantitative manner by means of static posturography. This latter is a quantitative, non-invasive test measuring the amount of oscillatory motions (sway) during quiet standing. The subject is asked to maintain the standing upright position, and the centre-of-pressure (COP) is measured. The centre-of-pressure is the point of application of the resultant force exchanged between feet and floor and can be easily measured by means of a dynamometric platform. The ability to maintain the standing position is usually evaluated both with eyes open and with eyes closed conditions.

The analysis of literature shows that in case of diabetic patients suffering peripheral neuropathy, static posturography has revealed, as expected, a more unstable posture. However, classical static posturography has not been able, until now, to discriminate subjects with subclinical peripheral neuropathy from subjects without this complication. It is worth emphasizing the fact that all the literature concerning the application of static posturography to the study of diabetic peripheral neuropathy based its findings mainly on parameters extracted by a "geometric" analysis of the COP trajectory during a standing balance test. However literature shows that different types of modelling techniques can be applied to the recorded posturographic data in order to infer some information about the characteristics of the motor control deputed to the posture maintenance as for instance the sway density plot analysis proposed in Baratto, Morasso, Re and Spada (2002). The main drawback of the conventional techniques used for the analysis of posturographic signal is that they completely ignore the dynamics governing the time-evolution of the COP signal. On the contrary, the second kind of parameterization is aimed to characterize the COP movement by means of models that try to describe its dynamics.

The background hypothesis of both kinds of parameterizations is that the quiet standing position can be considered as the dynamic stability of a continuously moving body that receives information on the position of its segments and on the changes of the surrounding environment, and consequently adapts itself to maintain balance.

Specific aspects to be taken in consideration when static posturography results are analysed

are the variability of the parameter values i.e. the sensitivity of the results with respect to the test conditions (for instance: sensory status, age, health condition) and the ability of the posturographic method to preserve useful information hidden in the posturographic recording subjected to an unfavourable signal-to-noise-ratio. This implies that attention has to be given to possible spurious sources of variability such as the characteristics of the data acquisition, the influence of the anthropometric characteristics of the subject, and in general the experimental protocol (foot placement, environment conditions, length of data acquisition etc.).

All these aspects were taken into account in Fioretti et al, (2010) that represents the first successful attempt to discriminate the presence or absence of diabetic neuropathy by means of static posturography tests. Their 2-class model was able to classify neuropathic and non-neuropathic diabetic subjects with a 95% level of accuracy in predicting neuropathic subjects and 75% in predicting non-neuropathic ones. However, the same authors did not succeed in discriminating the severity of the disease, i.e., they failed in obtaining a satisfactory 3-class model able to distinguish patients that are at a preclinical (asymptomatic) stage, from those that have a more severe (symptomatic) impairment, and from the diabetic non-neuropathic subjects. The statistical classification technique used in that study was the classical Linear Discriminant Analysis (LDA). LDA is the optimal linear Statistical Pattern Recognition methodology to apply when a-priori classification is available; LDA will be introduced in the following Section. Unfortunately, as stated also in Fioretti et al., LDA requires a proper data preparation and an accurate choice of variables which:

- Must be *linearly independent*;
- Should present *low values of correlation*;
- Must have distributions verifying conditions of *homoschedasticity* and *normality*.

Moreover, the application of LDA to posturographic data introduced the problem of data *reliability*, related to the fact that posturographic parameters are submitted to many sources of variability. Reliability is also connected with the evaluation of correlation between variables. In Fioretti et al. only posturographic parameters with at least a *fair-to-good* level of reliability were taken into account; furthermore some parameters were submitted to *normalization procedure* deemed necessary to eliminate dependence with anthropometric factors, too.

Statistical Pattern Recognition

Statistical Pattern Recognition is the classical discipline where classification problems have been formalized in statistical terms for the first time. For a comprehensive introduction to the discipline, see (Fukunaga, 1990). The pattern recognition problem is formalized by assuming that an object x in a domain of interest can be described by a *pattern*, that is a vector $X = (x_1, x_2...x_n)$ in an n-dimensional space, where the i-th component is the value of a measure performed on x. The n components of the vector are also called features, and the vector space takes the name of feature space consequently. For instance, a person can be characterized by features like age, height, weight, and described by a point in a three dimensional vector space. The recognition problem is then the problem to assign an object to one of a finite, discrete set of classes (say, e.g. hypertension, normal, hypotension) given its pattern. Let us denote by $C = \{c_1, c_2..., c_C\}$ the set of classes. *Statistical Pattern Recognition* assumes that classes can be statistically characterized by a class-conditional probability density function (cpdf) $p_i(X)=p(X \mid c=c_i)$, and an a-priori class probability $P_i =P(c_i)$, $i = 1,..,C$. Hereafter we use boldface characters to denote random vectors/variables when needed, while the lower-case symbol p and the upper-case symbol P are used to denote continuous and discrete distributions respectively.

One of the fundamental results in Statistical Pattern Recognition is that the optimal way to achieve a classification is to follow the Bayes decision rule. For a two-class case, the Bayes rule can be written as:

If $q_1 > q_2$ *Then* c_1 *Else* c_2,

where $q_i=P(c=c_i \mid X = X)$ is the *a posteriori probability* of class c_i given X, and can be derived by the Bayes theorem

$$q_i = \frac{P_i \cdot p_i(X)}{p(X)},$$

where $p(X)$ is the probability density function of X.

It is straightforward to generalize the rule to the case of C classes: given a pattern X simply decide for the class with the maximum a posteriori probability (MAP rule).

The Bayes rule is optimal in that it allows to achieve the minimum error probability. Again, we give the formula for error probability for the two-class case, leaving the reader to generalize to the case of C classes:

$$\varepsilon = P_1 \int_{\Omega_2} p_1(X)dX + P_2 \int_{\Omega_1} p_2(X)dX,$$

where Ω_i is the region of the feature space where X is classified to c_i.

This theoretical framework cannot be applied directly in most practical applications, since class statistics are unknown. Then, in practice Pattern Recognition may be considered a problem of estimating probabilities starting from a set of class samples, called training set. Either parametric or non-parametric approaches can be used to this end: the former assumes a functional form of class-conditional pdf and samples are used to estimate cpdf parameters. Non-parametric approaches do not make any assumption concerning the structure of the cpdf, and rely only on training samples to build the classifier. The quality of such a classifier can be evaluated referring to the *Confusion Matrix*, whose elements represent the number of samples belonging to class c_i that are classified in the class c_j. In 2-class problems, the confusion matrix assumes the form in Table 1. where C_i is the number of correctly classified samples of class c_i, M_{ij} is the number of samples belonging to c_i that are misclassified as class c_j, and N_i is the cardinality of class c_i. Hence, the accuracy can be estimated as the ratio between the sum of elements in the main diagonal and the sum of all elements in the matrix. The error probability is given as 1-accuracy. In two classes case, various measures can also be derived by the confusion matrix like precision, recall, sensitivity and specificity, as follows:

$$precision = \frac{C_1}{C_1 + M_{21}}; \quad recall = \frac{C_1}{C_1 + M_{12}};$$

$$sensitivity = recall; \quad specificity = \frac{C_2}{C_2 + M_{21}};$$

In particular specificity and sensitivity are often used in medical domain, when the classification problem is to recognize a class of interest (presence of disease) with respect to a control class (absence of disease). They measure the accuracy in predicting the control class and the class of interest respectively. In this work we use a domain independent approach to evaluate models by referring to the error probability (or the accuracy) and discussing the confusion matrices.

One example from parametric methods is Linear Discriminant Analysis (LDA). LDA assumes that classes are Normally distributed, with the same covariance matrix. In this case the Bayes rule can be rewritten as

If $\sum^{-1} \cdot (\mu_1 - \mu_2) \cdot X - \alpha > 0$ Then class c_1 else class c_2,

Table 1. Confusion matrix

		Predicted class membership		
		c_1	c_2	
Real class membership	c_1	C_1	M_{12}	$N_1 = C_1 + M_{12}$
	c_2	M_{21}	C_2	$N_2 = C_2 + M_{21}$

where μ_i is the mean vector of class c_i, $\sum$ is the (common) covariance matrix, and α is a constant. In practice, a hyperplane separating the two classes is defined (a linear discriminant), whose parameters can be easily estimated from known samples.

A well known non-parametric method is the k-Nearest Neighbour (kNN). The classification criterion is the following: given a sample X of unknown class, find the k elements of the training set that fall nearest to X, and decide for the class represented by a majority of kNNs. kNN is a simple and intuitive approach; however it is computationally expensive when the training set is large, since the distance of the unknown sample X from any training samples must be computed. Furthermore, its classification performance can be poor, especially in problems with more than two classes. In what follows, we will describe a variant of the Nearest Neighbour method that overcomes some of these limitations.

We conclude this introduction to pattern recognition by observing that a proper selection of the features is critical and strongly affects classification performance: turning to our first example, it is apparent that no effective decision about hypertension can be taken by considering only a person's height! Furthermore low informative features have a deteriorating effect on both parametric and non parametric methods, as they augment the dimension of the feature space without providing significant information. Therefore classification is typically preceded by a feature selection pre-processing step, and the definition of efficient and effective features selection methods is a key problem in pattern recognition. Among the many techniques developed, Fisher's Linear Discriminant Analysis (FLDA) is one of the most known. When the covariance matrices are equals, it correspond to the LDA described above. As a matter of fact, $\sum^{-1}(\mu_1 - \mu_2) \cdot X$ gives a new representation of X, by projecting it on a reduced (i.e. one-dimensional) space, represented by the line normal to the separating hyperplane. However FLDA is a more general method, which can deal also with different covariance matrices. For more details on FLDA we refer the reader to (Fukunaga, 1990 pg. 134). Fisher's method still relies on the Normality assumption. In order to obtain more accurate results for general pdf, a non-parametric version of FLDA (called NDA) based on the kNN principle is presented (Fukunaga, 1990 pg. 466).

NON-PARAMETRIC DESIGN OF A 3-CLASS DIAGNOSIS MODEL

This Section is devoted to present the approach we use to design a classifier that is able to distinguish among non-neuropathic, asymptomatic neuropathic and symptomatic neuropathic subjects. To this end first the chosen classification algorithm is presented and then the experimental procedure is discussed.

An Introduction to Bayes Vector Quantization

In order to present the Bayes Vector Quantizer algorithm, as a first step we introduce the basic definitions about Labeled Vector Quantizers and to present the Bayes Vector Quantizer algorithm.

An Euclidean nearest neighbor Vector Quantizer (VQ) of dimension n and order Q is a function $\Omega : \mathbb{R}^n \to M$, $M = \{m_1, m_2, \ldots, m_Q\}$, $m_i \in \mathbb{R}^n$, $m_i \neq m_j$, which defines a partition of $\mathbb{R}^n$ into Q regions $\{V_1, V_2, \ldots, V_Q\}$, such that

$$V_i = \{x \in \mathbb{R}^n : \|x - m_i\|^2 < \|x - m_j\|^2 , j \neq i\},$$

M is called the *code*, and its elements are called *code vectors*. The region V_i is called the *Voronoi region* of the code vector m_i. Note that, the Voronoi region is completely defined by the code M. From the previous equation it turns out that the border of each Voronoi region is defined by the intersection of a finite set of hyperplanes.

A *Labeled* Vector Quantizer (LVQ) is a pair $< \Omega, \Gamma >$, where $\Omega : \mathbb{R}^n \to M$ is a vector quantizer, and $\Gamma : M \to C$ is a labeling function, assigning to each code vector a class label.

An LVQ defines a classification rule Ψ such that, $\Psi : \mathbb{R}^n \to C, x \to \Gamma(\Omega(x))$. .Note the nearest neighbor nature of this classification rule: each vector in $\mathbb{R}^n$ is assigned to the same class as its nearest code vector. Thus, decision regions are defined by the union of Voronoi regions of code vectors with the same label. Note also that decision borders are defined only by those hyperplanes separating code vectors having different labels.

The optimal situation is obtained when the LVQ produces the same classification rule as the multiclass Bayes (i.e. MAP) rule. To this end we can adapt a LVQ by means of the *Bayes Vector Quantizer(BVQ)* algorithm, which is a non-parametric learning algorithm devoted to find the best linear approximation of the true Bayes decision border. Here we briefly describe a simple version of the algorithm for the minimization of error probability, referring the interest reader to (Diamantini & Potena, 2009).

Let $\{(m_1, l_1), (m_2, l_2), \ldots, (m_Q, l_Q)\}$ be an LVQ, where $l_i \in C$ denotes the class of the code vector mi, and let TS=$\{(t1, u1), \ldots, (tT, uT)\}$ be the training set, where $t_i \in \mathbb{R}^n$ denotes the feature vector and $u_i \in C$ is the class the sample belongs to. The BVQ algorithm is an interactive punishing-rewarding adaptation schema. At each iteration, the algorithm considers a training sample randomly picked from *TS*. If the training sample turns out to fall ``on" the decision border, then the position of the two code vectors determining the border is updated, moving the code vector with the same label of the sample towards the sample itself and moving away that with a different label. Since the decision border is a null measure subspace of the feature space, we have zero probability to get samples falling exactly on it. Thus, an approximation of the decision border is made, considering those samples falling close to it (i.e., at a maximum distance of $\frac{\Delta}{2}$).

In the following the BVQ algorithm at the k-th iteration is given:

1. Randomly pick a training pair $(t^{(k)}, u^{(k)})$ from *TS*;
2. Find the code vectors m_i and m_j nearest to $t^{(k)}$;
3. $m_q^{(k+1)} = m_q^{(k)}$ for q ≠ i, j;
4. Compute $t_{i,j}^{(k)}$, the projection of $t^{(k)}$ on the hyperplane $S_{i,j}^{(k)}$ separating m_i and m_j regions;
5. If $t^{(k)}$ falls at a distance d≤Δ/2 from $S_{i,j}^{(k)}$, then

$$m_i^{(k+1)} = m_i^{(k)} - \gamma(k) \frac{\delta(u^{(k)} = l_j^{(k)}) - \delta(u^{(k)} = l_i^{(k)})}{\left\| m_i^{(k)} - m_j^{(k)} \right\|} \cdot (m_i^{(k)} - t_{i,j}^{(k)})$$

$$m_j^{(k+1)} = m_j^{(k)} + \gamma(k) \frac{\delta(u^{(k)} = l_j^{(k)}) - \delta(u^{(k)} = l_i^{(k)})}{\left\| m_i^{(k)} - m_j^{(k)} \right\|} \cdot (m_j^{(k)} - t_{i,j}^{(k)})$$

6. Else $m_q^{(k+1)} = m_q^{(k)}$ for q = i, j;

where $\delta(expr)$=1 if *expr* is true and 0 otherwise, and $\gamma(k)=\gamma(0)\cdot k^r$ defines the learning rate of the algorithm. More details on the algorithm can be found in (Diamantini & Potena, 2009).

Method of Work

The experimental protocol is the same as that described in Fioretti et al. (2010). The only difference is that the subject data set used for the present work has been increased: the same 37 subjects of the above cited paper have been considered and further 34 subjects, for a total of 71

patients, have been tested with the same protocol and under identical conditions. The protocol is here synthetically described. Seventy-one patients (30 females and 41 males) affected by type 2 diabetes mellitus have been tested: 23 diabetic non-neuropathic subjects, considered as control subjects (CNTR), 17 asymptomatic neuropathic subjects (AN), and 31 symptomatic ones (SN). The absence or presence of neuropathy was clinically assessed by determination of motor nerve, and sensory nerve, conduction velocities as described by Ziegler (2005). Neuropathic subjects were classified as symptomatic if they reported pain, numbness or paraesthesia in the lower limbs. All subjects gave their informed consent before the test. Exclusion criteria were:

1. Neuropathy other than of diabetic origin or neurological diseases;
2. Peripheral arterial disease;
3. Any medication potentially affecting peripheral nerve function.

The measurement protocol consisted in standing barefoot on a dynamometric platform (Kistler 9281 type) with ankle joint centres placed under the corresponding anterior-superior-iliac-spina. Multiple tests were performed both under eyes open (EO) and eyes closed (EC) conditions. Footprints were recorded so that feet were repositioned in the same way in the two trials. During EO condition subject had to look at a visual target placed 3m far at the height of subject's eyes. For each test, force-plate data were acquired for 60 seconds at a sampling frequency of 100 Hz. The anterior-posterior (AP) and medial-lateral (ML) COP coordinates were filtered with a cut-off frequency of 5 Hz by a 4-th order low-pass Butterworth filter. COP filtered data were processed according to classical and model-based approaches; in total 65 posturographic parameters were obtained for each test. Finally the dataset has been generated by averaging, for each experimental condition, all the tests performed on the same patient. Anthropometric parameters were recorded too, resulting in 12 further features.

For the LDA classification many parameters were submitted to a normalization procedure in order to take into account anthropometric or experimental factors such as height or base-of-support area; in the end, only 5 posturographic parameters satisfied all the conditions necessary for a proper LDA application and only the EC tests were considered as described in Fioretti et al.

Since non-parametric approaches do not require the fulfillment of the Normality assumption, in the experiments performed in this work, we consider all posturographic parameters excepting those clearly related each other, such as for instance polar and Cartesian representations of the same measure. Furthermore, anthropometric parameters were also considered as features, resulting in a 45 dimensions vector space.

For the BVQ classification we performed only the following normalization as data pre-processing:

$$x_i' = \frac{x_i - m_i}{M_i - m_i},$$

where x_i and x'_i, are respectively the ith feature of the original and the normalized datasets, m_i and M_i are respectively the minimum and maximum values of x_i. After this transformation, each feature is in the range [0; 1], giving equal importance to each feature during learning. The resulting dataset has 71 instances, 3 classes and 45 features.

We performed four experiments over two different sets of data: the whole dataset and a subset formed only by data used in Fioretti et al. Hereafter the subset will be denoted as A and the whole dataset will be called B. A is formed by 37 patients. Also, as said before, no further feature reduction was performed. On dataset A, 2-class and 3-class models have been built by BVQ. Experiments will be denoted by A2 and A3 respectively.

In the third experiment (B3), BVQ is trained over the dataset B for building a 3-class model. In B3 a feature reduction pre-processing is performed by NDA. Finally, we performed the same methodology proposed in Fioretti et al. on the dataset A for designing a 3-class classifier; such experiment is labeled A3$_{LDA}$. Since experiments are performed over a limited sample of patients, in order to evaluate the reliability of classification models in any experiments, the leave-one-out procedure was used to evaluate the error probability.

In A2, A3 and B3 experiments a simple initialization strategy has been adopted, by choosing the same number of code vectors for each class, and by selecting the first instances of each class as code vectors. We performed different experiments varying the number of code vectors, the value of Δ, the value of $\gamma(0)$, and the number of iterations. Let us note that, the higher the number of code vectors is, the more accurate piecewise linear approximation of the true border we get. On the other hand, more training samples are needed to properly train each code vector to avoid overfitting. In all the experiments it turns out that a good compromise has been reached with 9 code vectors (6 for 2-class experiments). The value Δ ranges from 0.1 to 1 with an incremental step of 0.1, and $\gamma(0)$ ranges from 0.1 to 0.5 with step of 0.1. Finally, the number of iterations ranges from 1,000 to 20,000.

Results

In Table 2 the confusion matrix for the A2 experiment is shown. The resulting misclassification error is 0.2703, which is twice the error reported in Fioretti et al. (2010), where only 5 subjects out of 37 were misclassified in the test set. Hence, when 2-class is considered, the linear model designed by LDA method has demonstrated better performances than the non-linear (i.e. piece-wise linear) classifier built by BVQ. Note however that no data pre-processing has been yet performed.

Situation turns in favor of BVQ when all classes are considered. The application of the LDA approach to the 3-class dataset has given rise to an error probability of 0.3784 (14 misclassified over 37). The related confusion matrix is shown in Table 3. Note that a significant contribution to the error is due to absence of correctly classified AN subjects. On the same dataset, BVQ has produced results that are shown in Table 4, where the error decreases to the value of 0.2973, having only 11 misclassified patients over 37. This results are obtained training the BVQ with $\Delta=0.4$, $\gamma(0)=0.1$, and only 2,000 iterations.

Note that if preventive normalization of posturographic parameters is not applied, $A3_{LDA}$ errors would increase considerably in an unacceptable manner from 0.3784 to 0.5676 (for the 2-class model from 0.1351 to 0.3784). This highlights the importance of a suitable feature reduction pre-processing, which has to be chosen on the basis of the adopted Statistical Pattern Recognition technique. As a matter of fact, best results are obtained when the NDA is exploited to reduce the feature space (see Table 5). In this experiment BVQ has run with $\Delta=0.2$, $\gamma(0)=0.1$, and 2,000 iterations. Only 8 patients over 71 were misclassified, returning an error probability of 0.1127. We like to note that, the 3-class model can be used as 2-class model as well, by aggregating AN and SN in the neuropathic class. The model reported in Table 5, when used to predict the two classes, gives an error that is smaller than the one obtained in 2-class LDA experiment. As a matter of fact, the error probability in the last experiment is 0.0845, that is due to the 2 AN and 3 SN patients classified as CNTR plus the single CNTR subject misclassified as belonging to SN.

Some remarks are due about the deployment of results reported in this Section. First, it is not necessary to build a classification model to predict the class of a symptomatic subject, which manifestly belongs to SN class. De facto, both $M_{SN,CNTR}$ and $M_{SN,AN}$ elements of the confusion matrix can be set to zero. Hence, the misclassification errors

Table 2. Confusion matrix of the A2 experiment: BVQ / Dataset A / 2-class

Real class membership	Predicted class membership		Total
	CNTR	Neuropathic	
CNTR	4	8	12
Neuropathic	2	23	25

Table 3. Confusion matrix of the $A3_{LDA}$ experiment: LDA / Dataset A / 3-class

Real class membership	Predicted class membership			Total
	CNTR	AN	SN	
CNTR	10	0	2	12
AN	2	0	6	8
SN	0	4	13	17

Table 4. Confusion matrix of the A3 experiment: BVQ / Dataset A / 3-class

Real class membership	Predicted class membership			Total
	CNTR	AN	SN	
CNTR	8	1	3	12
AN	2	5	1	8
SN	2	2	13	17

Table 5. Confusion matrix of the B3 experiment: BVQ / Dataset B / 3-class

Real class membership	Predicted class membership			Total
	CNTR	AN	SN	
CNTR	22	0	1	23
AN	2	13	2	17
SN	3	0	28	31

becomes 0.2703 (= 10/37) in $A3_{LDA}$, 0.1892 (= 7/37) in A3 and 0.0704 (= 5/71) in B3 respectively. The second comment regards the use of clinical tests (e.g. electromyography and nerve conduction studies) in order to improve the accuracy of the model. Note that both $M_{CNTR,SN}$ and $M_{AN,SN}$ represent subjects that clearly do not manifest neuropathic symptoms, but are classified as symptomatic; these patients result in recognizable errors, which can be corrected by means of clinical tests. Hence, the quality of a model can be also evaluated with respect to the overall testing costs, namely economic cost, time-to-diagnosis and not least induced pain. These costs are proportional to 8/37, 4/37 and 3/71 for $A3_{LDA}$, A3 and B3 experiments respectively. Finally, $M_{CNTR,AN}$ and $M_{AN,CNTR}$ are the non-detectable, and thus non-erasable, components of the error.

Concluding, results discussed in this Section highlight that the approach taken in B3 shows best performances from the point of view of both classification accuracy and deployment costs.

FUTURE RESEARCH DIRECTIONS

Various research directions can be investigated in order to improve the approach presented in this Chapter. First, we hope to be able to increase the number of patients in the study, thus improving the (already good) reliability of the approach and deploying the model as a diagnosis tool. Second, it is to be noted that the dataset used in this Chapter is imbalanced, that is the number of patients belonging to each class is not the same. Such is not an ideal situation for most of classification algorithms, which are usually defined to learn a classifier under the hypothesis of class equiprobability.

Furthermore, the dataset has a class distribution that is not representative of the true a-priori class probabilities: it is clear that in real world the number of non-neuropathic subjects is greater than the number of neuropathic patients. Hence, it

could be profitable to investigate the use of some mechanisms for properly taking into account such imbalance during learning. An efficient strategy proposed in the Literature is the cost-sensitive learning, which weighs differently the various misclassification errors, by assigning higher cost to the misclassification of smaller classes (Diamantini & Potena, 2009). In such algorithms, the classification problem moves from the minimization of the average error to the minimization of the average misclassification cost; when costs are symmetric cost-sensitive classification algorithms can be used in balanced problems. Indeed, BVQ is a cost-sensitive algorithm since it is guided by an objective function for the minimization of the average misclassification cost, and it has demonstrated good performances over real world datasets, even with a high degree of imbalance (Diamantini & Potena, 2009). Hence, we assume that results in this Chapter could be improved if BVQ is used in its cost-sensitive form; the experimental proof of this assumption will be the focus of future research.

Another research direction is the individuation of the borderline subjects, which are those patients for which the probability of misclassification is high. Performing a clinical test (e.g. electromyography) for each borderline subjects, we significantly reduce the overall misclassification error, with a small increase in the testing cost. From a geometric point of view, borderline subjects are points in the vector space that are closed to the decision border. Both LDA and BVQ allow recognizing borderline subjects. In particular, Diamantini and Potena (2008) reported that BVQ has shown a high accuracy in the individuation of the true (Bayes) decision border and, as a consequence, of borderlines.

Finally, further experimentations can be performed in order to study the robustness and the sensibility of both approaches proposed in this Chapter, with respect to the clinical protocol for data collection. For instance, it is interesting to evaluate: how results change if EO tests are considered too, how much model based on EO and EC tests are (dis-)similar, how the model depends on experimental conditions like, f.i., the size of the base of support and the foot placement. These analyses are in particular useful for discovering new and valid domain knowledge.

CONCLUSION

The results of the present study confirm that LDA applied to posturographic parameters might be a valid and reliable screening instrument for the early detection of peripheral neuropathy in diabetic patients but is not able to assess the severity of the disease, not allowing a valid method to distinguish between asymptomatic and symptomatic patients. Better performance has been revealed by the non-parametric approach in the 3-class model both in the case of datasets constituted by 37 and 71 subjects. In the case of 2-class model BVQ did not behave better than LDA probably for the significant difference in the cardinality of CNTR and of (AN+SN) classes.

In any case, notwithstanding the variability of posturographic parameters and the questions related to the ecologic validity of the posturographic tests to evaluate the complex dynamics of the postural control, it seems that the application of suitable classification techniques to posturographic signals can results in a valid and reliable technique to identify the presence of PN and to evaluate its severity.

REFERENCES

Baratto, L., Morasso, P. G., Re, C., & Spada, G. (2002). A new look at posturographic analysis in the clinical context: sway-density versus other parameterization techniques. *Motor Control*, *6*(3), 246–270.

Diamantini, C., & Potena, D. (2008). Borderline detection by Bayes vector quantizers. In *Proceedings of the 23rd Annual ACM Symposium on Applied Computing - Special Track on Data Mining,* Vol. 2, (pp. 904–908).

Diamantini, C., & Potena, D. (2009). Bayes vector quantizer for class-imbalance problem. *IEEE Transactions on Knowledge and Data Engineering, 21*(5), 638–651. doi:10.1109/TKDE.2008.187

Fioretti, S., Scocco, M., Ladislao, L., Ghetti, G., & Rabini, R. A. (2010). Identification of peripheral neuropathy in type-2 diabetic subjects by static posturography and linear discriminant analysis. *Gait & Posture, 32*(3), 317–320. doi:10.1016/j.gaitpost.2010.05.017

Fukunaga, K. (1990). *Introduction to statistical pattern recognition* (2nd ed.). San Diego, CA: Academic Press Professional, Inc.

Perkins, B. A., Olaleye, D., Zinman, B., & Bril, V. (2001). Simple screening tests for peripheral neuropathy in the diabetes clinic. *Diabetes Care, 24*(2), 250–256. doi:10.2337/diacare.24.2.250

Ziegler, D. (2005). Validation of a novel screening device (Neuroquick) for quantitative assessment of small nerve fiber dysfunction as an early feature of diabetic polyneuropathy. *Diabetes Care, 28*(5), 1169–1174. doi:10.2337/diacare.28.5.1169

KEY TERMS AND DEFINITIONS

Bayes Vector Quantizer: Is a supervised learning algorithm, which is based on an objective function for the minimization of the average misclassification cost. The BVQ trains a Labeled Vector Quantizer, which provides a piece-wise linear approximation of the Bayes decision border.

COP: Centre-of-Pressure is the point of application of the resultant force exchanged between feet and floor.

LDA: Linear Discriminant Analysis: is a method used in statistics, pattern recognition and machine learning to find a linear combination of features which characterize or separate two or more classes of objects or events. The resulting combination may be used as a linear classifier, or for dimensionality reduction.

Pattern Recognition: Is a discipline that studies methods and techniques for the discovery of regularities(i.e. patterns) in data.

Peripheral Neuropathy: Is a damage to nerves of peripheral nervous system, which may be caused by various diseases and in particular by diabetes. The most common form is symmetrical, peripheral, polyneuropathy, which mainly affects the feet and legs.

Posturography: Is a general term that covers all the techniques used to quantify postural control in upright stance in either static or dynamic conditions. In this paper we are dealing with static posturography and in particular to the techniques aimed at studying the effects of body oscillations on the ground reactions resultant force.

Chapter 3
Preprocessing MRS Information for Classification of Human Brain Tumours

C. J. Arizmendi
Universitat Politècnica de Catalunya, Spain & Universidad Autonoma de Bucaramanga, Colombia

A. Vellido
Universitat Politècnica de Catalunya, Spain

E. Romero
Universitat Politècnica de Catalunya, Spain

ABSTRACT

Brain tumours show a low prevalence as compared to other cancer pathologies. Their impact, both in individual and social terms, far outweighs such low prevalence. Their anatomical specificity also makes them difficult to explore and treat. The use of biopsies is limited to extreme cases due to the risks involved in the surgical procedure, and non-invasive measurements are the standard for diagnostic exploration. The usual measurement techniques come in the modalities of imaging and spectroscopy. In this chapter, the authors analyze magnetic resonance spectroscopy (MRS) data from an international database and illustrate the importance of data preprocessing prior to diagnostic classification.

DOI: 10.4018/978-1-4666-1803-9.ch003

INTRODUCTION

In neuro-oncology, diagnosis frequently relies on data acquired through non-invasive techniques of the imaging (e.g., Computed Tomography or Magnetic Resonance Imaging -MRI) and spectroscopy (MRS) modalities. In this chapter, we focus on the latter. MRS generates a wealth of quantitative data that can provide support for medical decision. Due to the complexity and variety of these data, clinicians should benefit from the use of computer-based medical decision support systems (MDSS).

The development and use of MDSS based on pattern recognition techniques holds the promise of substantially improving the quality of medical practice in diagnostic and prognostic tasks. The current chapter deals with the problem of diagnosis of a wide array of human brain tumour types from the biological signal obtained by MRS.

MRS is a signal in the frequency domain that peaks at specific frequencies or frequency bands, most of which are known to correspond to the resonances of specific metabolites present in the analyzed tissue. The signal profile is an indication of the quantities in which the components are present in the tissue. Therefore, those substances with substantial presence will have higher peaks associated than those present in lower concentrations.

One of the main characteristics of MRS data is their high dimensionality, as each measured frequency is considered as a data feature. It is well known that only a few of these frequencies (or short intervals of frequencies) are associated to identifiable metabolites present in the tumour tissue. On the other hand, it is also well known that some of those metabolites are informative as tumour type markers.

Additionally, there are several factors that make the MRS signal acquisition, processing and characterization non-trivial, such as signal degradation related to the sensitivity of the acquisition technique, thermal noise from the sample and noise from the electronic components, technical limitations when measuring the *in vitro* tissue, as well as time limitation during measurement. In general, *in vivo* MRS signals are characterized by a low signal-to-noise ratio (SNR), strong overlapping spectral components, and the presence of the residual water peak in ¹H-MRS, for which, even after presaturation, the residual water resonance dominates the proton free induction decay, causing baseline distortions in the frequency domain, particularly for resonances closer to the water peak.

To circumvent some of these limitations and provide an adequate representation of the raw signal, techniques in the field of signal processing can be used. In this chapter, we filter the signal and break it up in terms of decomposition coefficients using the Discrete Wavelet Transform (DWT) technique. In order to reduce the dimensionality of the system, a novel filter method called Moving Window and Variance Analysis (MWVA). Its results are compared with a traditional dimensionality reduction technique, namely Principal Components Analysis (PCA). Finally, classification is carried out using Artificial Neural Networks (ANN) with Bayesian regularization.

Classification problems in this context are treated as binary; that is, one tumour class against another. Multiple-class approaches are hindered by the limited number of MRS cases available. Furthermore, and as remarked in (Luts *et al.*, 2007), doctors frequently face situations of doubt between two different diagnosis, (i.e. types of tumour) in medical practice. Binary classification approaches are, therefore, more realistic than either multi-class or one-class-*vs*-the-rest approaches.

The following sections provide, first, some background on human brain tumours and the MRS data analyzed. This is followed by two main blocks. The first introduces the basics of the MWVA method and the results of a set of preliminary experiments in which ANNs were used as a classifier from a selection of frequencies. The second described the basics of DWT preprocessing and the subsequent classification with ANN from PCA and MWVA reductions of the preprocessed data.

BACKGROUND: HUMAN BRAIN TUMOURS

The tumours of the central nervous system (CNS) represent around the 2% of the total of cancers diagnosed around the world. Annually, about 175,000 people are diagnosed with tumours that affect the CNS (Stewart & Kleihues, 2003), out of which 29.000 are located in Europe. The incidence ratio of this pathology is of 7 persons per 100,000. Different studies have shown that the distribution of the tumours by age is bimodal, with a peak in infants and another in adults between 40 and 70 (Lantos, Vandenberg, & Kleihues, 2002). The most frequent types of tumours are those of neuroepithelial origin (60%); 28% are located in the meninges; 7,5% are located in the skull and spinal nerves, while lymphomas rate at 4%. The glioblastomas with neuroepithelial origin are the most frequent type of tumours. They are highly resistant to both radiation and chemotherapy, and are surgically incurable: only 3% of patients survive for more than three years.

The aetiology of brain tumours is still today a very open problem. Epidemiological studies have failed to discern with clarity if the causes of these pathologies are to be found in environmental and lifestyle factors (ICNIRP *et al.*, 2004), genetics, or a combination of some or all of them.

Brain Tumours: Diagnosis

Because the brain has no pain receptors, the tumours often grow unnoticed until by the effect of their own mass and the resulting high intracranial pressure begin generating visual disturbances, respiratory failures, epileptic events, or even episodes of coma. The manifestation of symptoms depends on how local the tumour is and on the cognitive functions it affects. The headache, for example, only appears as a symptom when the tumour infiltrates the meninges. When any of these symptoms is present, it is necessary to conduct a full radiological analysis. This may

include a Computerized Tomography (CT) scan and/or Magnetic Resonance Imaging (MRI) to accurately measure the size and location of the tumour. When a brain tumour appears on a CT or an MRI, additional *in vivo* tests, including MRS, are carried out to determine their exact type. The final diagnosis of a brain tumour, in terms of type and degree, can only be obtained by histopathological analysis of a brain biopsy (as a by-product of a surgical procedure, in which at least part of the tumour is removed). In some cases, there is no secure direct physical access to tumours that are found in deep areas of the brain. In these cases, a biopsy can only be carried out using minimally invasive techniques of three-dimensional orientation towards the tumour, from which cells are extracted by suction.

The development of Nuclear Magnetic Resonance (NMR) is an important milestone in the field of medical measurement techniques. While MRI allows exploring anatomic structure, MRS, a different variant of NMR that does not rely on imaging, enables the investigation of physiological processes through a characterization of the metabolism at molecular level.

MRS resorts to the use of strong magnetic fields for the generation of energy exchanges between the external magnetic field and the protons that are present in abundance in all living tissue. A radio-frequency machine picks up the energy exchanged, which is coded using sophisticated mathematical software. The result is a signal in the frequency domain that peaks at specific frequencies or frequency bands that are known to correspond to the resonances of specific chemical and biochemical components of the tissue. The wave profile is an indication of the quantities in which the components are present. Therefore, those substances that are present in big quantities in the tissue will have higher peaks associated than those present in lower concentrations, therefore MRS uses the principle that different chemical structures have different resonance patterns associated. Depending on the characteristics of the chemical structure of adjacent regions, and the interactions between these structures, MRS is able to detect the chemical composition of the tissue.

MRS has proven to be of great clinical significance, especially for the diagnosis and prognosis of malignant pathologies. MRS techniques can be used to:

- Provide a diagnostic assistance to expert radiologists.
- Help defining the type of tumour, its aggressiveness, as well as the relevance of the biochemical characterization of the pathology.
- Monitor changes in the tumour without the need for invasive surgery.
- Determine an early presence of the tumour and its possible recurrence.

Despite its potential, there is no clear consensus regarding what is the most appropriate technique for processing MRS data in order to carry out an optimal classification of the different pathologies.

INTERPRET: A MULTI-CENTER INTERNATIONAL DATABASE OF MRS BRAIN TUMOURS

All the analyses in this chapter rely on a database created under the framework of the European project INTERPRET, an international collaboration of centers from 4 different countries. More specifically, the data were collected by CDP (*Centre Diagnòstic Pedralbes*, Barcelona, España), IDI (*Institut de Diagnòstic per la Imatge*, Barcelona, España), SGHMS (St. George's Hospital Medical School, London, UK) and UMCN (University Nijmegen Medical Center, Nijmegen, Netherlands).

The original criteria for the selection of cases to be included in the database were: a) that the case had a single voxel short time of echo (TE), 1.5 T spectrum acquired from a nodular region of the tumour; b) that the voxel was located in the same region as where subsequent biopsy was obtained; c) that the short TE spectrum had not been discarded because of acquisition artifacts or other reasons; and d) that a histopathological diagnosis was agreed among a committee of neuropathologists. In those cases in which the spectra were obtained from normal volunteers with no pathology, or corresponded to abscesses or clinically proven metastases, biopsy was not required. For further details on data acquisition and processing, and on database characteristics, see, for instance, (Julià-Sapé *et al.*, 2006).

Class labeling was performed according to the World Health Organization (WHO) system for diagnosing brain tumours by histopathological analysis of a biopsy sample (Kleihues & Cavenee, 2000). The database consists of the types of tumours listed in Table 1.

Table 1. Contents of the INTERPRET database. The table includes a list of the tumour types and the number of cases in each of them for both acquisition TEs.

Tumour class	Number of cases	
	Short TE	Long TE
A2: Astrocytomas, grade II	22	20
A3: Astrocytomas, grade III.	7	6
Ab: Brain abscesses	8	8
Gl: Glioblastomas	86	78
Hb: Haemangioblastomas	5	3
Ly: Lymphomas	10	9
Me: Metastases	38	31
Mm: Meningiomas grade I	58	55
No: Normal cerebral tissue, white matter	22	15
Oa: Oligoastrocytomas grade II	6	6
Od: Oligodendrogliomas grade II	7	5
Pi: Pilocytic astrocytomas grade I.	3	3
Pn: Primitive neuroectodermal tumours and medulloblastomas	9	7
Ra: Rare tumours	19	18
Sc: Schwannomas	4	2

The database includes ^{1}H-MRS with removal of water obtained using PRESS and STEAM sequences. The long TE (266 patients) and short TE (304 patients) spectra were, in turn, acquired at 30-32ms and 135-136ms. The *time repetition* (TR) was set between 1500 and 2020 ms; the spectral bandwidth from 1000 Hz to 2500 Hz, and the total number of samples (frequencies) was set to 512.

FIRST BLOCK OF EXPERIMENTS: METHODOLOGY AND RESULTS USING MWVA WITH ANN CLASSIFICATION

Moving Window Variance Analysis

Moving Window (MW) is a technique in which a window of constant width (w) is selected from a signal $X[n]$. A mathematical function is applied to this data subset, obtaining a result (this can be used, for instance, to investigate the informativeness or relevance of a given signal region, or to perform either extraction or selection of features). Next, the window is displaced by one position, repeating the same operation. Figure 1 illustrates this idea. When $w = 1$, the MW is displaced along the signal, *travelling* from the first sample to the last. We thus obtain $m-w+1$ outlets (m is the number of attributes in the signal). The width of the window can vary from 1 to m, considering all possible intervals or adjacent sub-regions.

The MW has been used, in the field of computer networks, for error detection in the transmission of information, verification of parity, and cyclical redundancy. In the field of biomedical signal processing, MW has been used in the extraction of features from respiratory signals (Giraldo, *et al.*, 2006, Sá & Verbandt, 2002), for identification and detection in the direction of cardiorespiratory coupling (Rosenblum, *et al.*, 2002), and for the localization of epileptic activity in the electroencephalographic (EEG) signal

(Mohamed, Rubin, & Marwala, 2006), among other applications. The MW has also been used for the selection of variables from spectral signals, mostly focusing on the development of new methods for the selection of spectral regions to improve the predictive power (Du, *et al.*, 2004, Jiang, *et al.*, 2002, Shinzawa, *et al.*, 2006.)

The MWVA method consists of the combination of the MW technique in conjunction with the calculation of a standard ratio », defined as the quotient between the between-groups variance (BGV) and the within-groups variance (WGV) for a particular width w of the window, where:

$$\mathrm{WGV}(w,i) = \sum_{a=1}^{n1} \frac{\left\| c1_{a,w,i} - \mu c1_{w,i} \right\|^2}{n1\sqrt{w}} + \sum_{a=1}^{n2} \frac{\left\| c2_{a,w,i} - \mu c2_{w,i} \right\|^2}{n2\sqrt{w}} \qquad (1)$$

$$\mathrm{BGV}(w,i) = \frac{\left\| \mu c1_{w,i} - \mu c2_{w,i} \right\|^2}{\sqrt{w}} \qquad (2)$$

$$\lambda(w,i) = \frac{\mathrm{BGV}(w,i)}{\mathrm{WGV}(w,i)}. \qquad (3)$$

For every group, $c1_{a,w,i}$ and $c2_{a,w,i}$ are w-dimensional vectors that represent the window of width w of the element a that starts at position i. Here, the elements in the two groups (tumour types in this study) are represented in numerical matrices *X1* (of dimension $n1 \times n$) and *X2* (of dimension $n2 \times n$), where *n1* and *n2* are the number of elements in groups 1 and 2, respectively, and n is the input dimension. Therefore, $c1_{a,w,i}$ and $c2_{a,w,i}$ are the w-dimensional vectors in row a starting at column i of *X1* and *X2*, respectively. Vectors $\mu c1_{w,i}$ and $\mu c2_{w,i}$ are the mean w-dimensional vectors of $c1_{a,w,i}$ and $c2_{a,w,i}$ over a (the centroids of every group for a fixed width and starting point).

Figure 1. Schematic illustration of the moving window technique

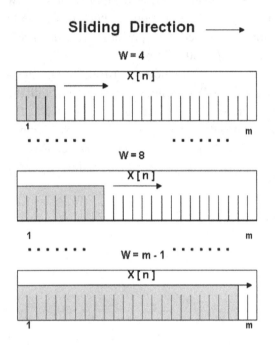

In order to determine the final width of the window, the values of $\lambda(w,i)$ are computed for increasing values of w (from 1 to n) and i (from 1 to $n-w+1$) and stored in a triangular matrix with zeros on its upper diagonal called Dissimilarity Index Matrix (DIM). Each value of λ is labeled with the coordinates k and l, where k indicates the position of the spectrum where the window starts and l indicates w used. Figure 2 illustrates this procedure.

Experiments with MWVA

A first study was carried out using a subset of patients from the database INTERPRET. We used the cases corresponding to classes *A3, Pn, Gl, Ly, Me, Mm, No, Od, Ab, A2* and *Oa* (see Table 2), acquired at short TE. As part of the pre-processing of the spectrum, prior to the computation of the MW, frequencies corresponding to the water reso-

nance (frequencies in positions 108 to 148, out of 512) were eliminated, and the uninformative area of each spectrum (frequencies in positions 346 to 512, out of 512) was replaced with the values generated by a normal random function, with mean and standard deviation equal to the average and standard deviation of the original noise. Figure 3 illustrates the figures of the mean and standard deviation of each of the types of tumours analyzed.

A visualization of the DIM was obtained for every experiment involving two types of tumours. Figure 4 is an illustrative example, and shows the DIM for *G2 vs Mm*. This figure shows three distinct zones: Zone 1 (Z1), which corresponds to artifacts associated with the beginnings of both the spectrum and the resonance frequency of water. Zone 2 (Z2) is the spectral band where most metabolic information resides and, therefore, should contribute the most to the discrimination between types of tumours. Zone 3 (Z3), finally, mostly contains noisy, irrelevant information. An analysis of λ values and a graphical representation of DIM provide us with interesting insights on the discrimination of tumour types. In brief:

- The highest values of the DIM in small bandwidths correspond to areas of the spectrum that, in previous studies, have been identified as most informative for the differentiation of the corresponding types of tumours. This reinforces the reliability of the proposed method.

- In contrast, in experiments aimed to discriminate between two classes where the percentage of correct classification was reported to stay between 60% and 70% (*Gl vs Me* and *A2 vs A3*), the values of λ in Z2 fall to levels very close to those obtained for Z1 and Z3, which are known to be completely uninformative (being Z2 the informative area). This shows the potential of the parameter λ as an indicator of the separation between types of tumour, compared with the experiments with high accuracy (e.g., *G2 vs Mm*).

Figure 2. Schematic illustration of the process of the computation of the DIM. You can observe the effect of increasing the dimensionality of the MW, which makes the values of the upper diagonal of DIM being zeros, and the lower diagonal correspond to values of lambda computations.

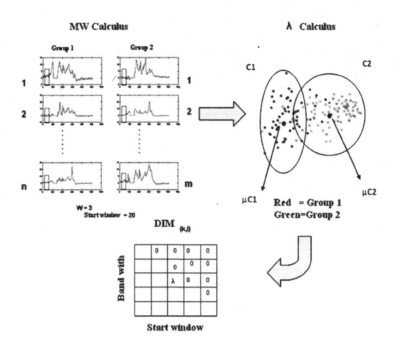

In all experiments, the largest values for λ were found for $w = 1$. Thus, window widths equal to 1 were used in subsequent experiments. The standard energies (E1, E2 and E3) were calculated for areas Z1, Z2 and Z3, in each experiment. The calculation of energy standardized by areas is given by:

$$E_i = \frac{\sum_{n=1}^{p} \| x_i[n] \|^2}{p} \qquad (4)$$

E_i corresponds to the calculation of the energy standard in zone i; $x_i[n]$ corresponds to the signal composed of discrete λ values with $w = 1$, of the zone i. Given that Z3 does not provide relevant information for classification, due to its direct correspondence with spectral zones modeled as random noise, it was decided to use the energy of this area to rescale the energy of zones Z_1 and Z_2 by E_3.

Feature Selection Based on Energy Criteria

As a preliminary step before the presentation of the patterns to a classifier, an initial feature selection was carried out, obtaining a ranking (in descending order) of the λ values of the starting window corresponding to zones Z_1 and Z_2. The variables were divided in groups corresponding to the set of variables whose energy gradually increased by 1% the total energy of the two zones E'_i / E_3, $i = \{1, \ldots\}$ (i.e., E'_3 corresponds to a 3% accumulated energy). When the energy of each group is gradually increased, the number of variables also increases, because the number of variables depends strongly of the energy level that everyone provides. Table 3 illustrates the computation of the ratio E'_i / E_3 (i = 1, ..., 10) for the 10 groups whose total energy is increased in steps of 1%.

Table 2. Calculation of the ratios E'/E_3 for the first 10 groups of discriminatory variables

Experiment	Groups									
	1%	2%	3%	4%	5%	6%	7%	8%	9%	10%
G1 vs G2	20.29	20.26	20.19	19.89	18.75	17.96	17.40	17.01	16.64	16.51
A2 vs G2	18.18	17.83	17.60	17.31	17.12	16.58	16.20	15.91	15.59	15.23
G1 vs Mm	12.89	12.67	12.5°	12.38	12.21	12.04	11.89	11.75	11.59	11.42
G2 vs Mm	21.16	21.01	20.80	20.58	20.34	20.11	19.91	19.47	19.06	18.76
Me vs Mm	20.67	20.29	19.90	19.61	19.34	18.87	18.53	18.20	17.93	17.60
Me vs No	31.16	30.20	29.70	29.41	29.08	28.78	28.41	27.88	27.41	26.91
Gl vs No	34.72	31.83	30.13	28.99	28.15	27.37	26.66	26.11	24.87	23.84
Gl vs Me	4.05	3.88	3.77	3.70	3.62	3.55	3.49	3.44	3.40	3.35
Od vs A2	5.50	4.65	4.40	4.27	4.13	3.99	3.90	3.81	3.74	3.65
Me vs Pn	11.65	11.47	11.31	11.14	10.99	10.86	10.55	10.17	9.86	9.52
Me vs Ly	6.03	5.90	5.79	5.68	5.56	5.47	5.40	5.31	5.22	5.14
A3 vs Pn	3.74	3.64	3.59	3.40	3.27	3.18	3.12	3.05	2.99	2.93
Gl vs A3	6.61	6.51	6.27	6.12	6.01	5.93	5.86	5.80	5.73	5.68
Gl vs Pn	9.45	9.36	9.14	8.92	8.73	8.52	8.33	8.15	8.00	7.85
Gl vs Ly	5.16	4.82	4.63	4.44	4.31	4.22	4.13	4.05	3.99	3.93
Mm vs Ab	15.41	13.60	12.25	11.66	11.22	10.92	10.68	10.51	10.37	10.2
A2 vs A3	2.92	2.84	2.76	2.70	2.66	2.62	2.58	2.55	2.51	2.47
Gl vs Ab	4.73	4.65	4.54	4.44	4.32	4.23	4.15	4.09	4.03	3.97
A2 vs Ly	7.70	7.52	7.39	7.22	6.88	6.60	6.38	6.20	6.02	5.87
A2 vs Oa	5.12	4.70	4.51	4.35	4.20	4.08	3.99	3.91	3.84	3.77

Classification Using ANN

Feed-forward neural networks with one hidden layer of neurons and one output layer were used for classification of the preprocessed data. A total of 200 networks were trained for the 20 experiments and 10 groups of discriminatory variables, from the group of variables that contained 1% of total energy to the one containing 10%. The input layer of every network was adjusted to the dimension of each set of variable group. Each network had 20 units in the hidden layer and one unit in the output layer. Logistic sigmoid and hyperbolic tangent sigmoid activation functions were used, in turn, in the hidden and output layers. Networks were trained with backpropagation and Bayesian regularization, using the Levenberg-Marquardt algorithm (MacKay, 1992; Foresee & Hagan, 1997). The initial weights were randomly generated with a normal distribution with mean 0 and unit standard deviation. One run of a 5-fold cross-validation was performed for each network, with a maximum of 150 epochs. The corresponding results are shown in Table 3.

Figure 5 shows that there is a relationship between λ and the percentage of classification reached for different experiments. Thus, the calculation of these ratios can be used as an indicator to find which frequencies or ranges of frequencies have the greatest ability to discriminate between types of tumor, as well as to investigate the degree of overlapping between types of tumour as a preliminary step before the presentation of the patterns to a classifier.

Figure 3. Mean ± standard deviation of the brain tumour spectra acquired by MRS for each type of tumour (whose name is shown in the title of each graph)

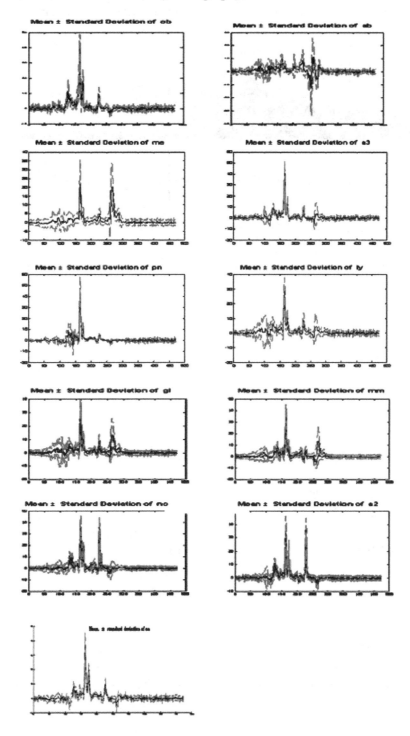

Figure 4. Graphic illustration DIM zones Z1, Z2, and Z3 of G2 vs Mm. The green stripes indicate the areas that generate the biggest differences between G2 and mm, corresponding to the highest values in the DIM. G2 is the union of the Me and Gl high-grade malignant types of tumour.

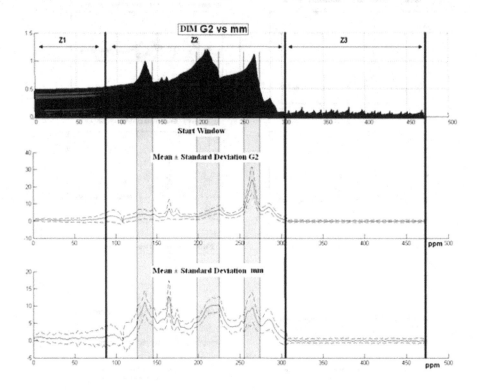

SECOND BLOCK OF EXPERIMENTS: METHODOLOGY AND RESULTS USING WAVELETS AND MWVA OR PCA, WITH ANN CLASSIFICATION

Determination of the Optimal Wavelet

In this block of experiments, we investigated an alternative MRS data pre-processing strategy, based on wavelet techniques. The selection of an adequate wavelet family for data processing is a crucial step in the application of wavelet analysis techniques.

In our experiments, the DWT was applied to the original SV-^{1}H-MRS data, taking the decomposition to the maximum allowable level. Different mother wavelets and, for each, different orders were used to implement the DWT: Biorthogonals (orders: 1.1, 1.3, 1.5, 2.2, 2.4, 2.6, 2.8, 3.1, 3.3, 3.5, 3.7, 3.9, 4.4, 5.5, 6, and 8), Coiflet (orders: 1 to 5), Daubechies (1 to 43), and Symlet (1 to 25). For every mother wavelet, the absolute values of the decomposition coefficients were sorted in descending order, and the signal of each spectrum was reconstructed by adding consecutive coefficients. The average mean square error (MSE) and signal-to-noise ratio (SNR) were calculated over the whole set of patients for each wavelet order r, together with the number of decomposition coefficients (NDC):

$$MSE = \frac{1}{n}\sum_{i=1}^{n}(x[i] - \hat{x}[i])^2 \qquad (5)$$

Table 3. Calculation of the ratios E'_i/E_3 for the first 10 groups of discriminatory variables

Experiments	E'_{10}/E_3	Classification percentage	
		Mean ± std. dev. of maximum values	Mean ± standard deviation of E'_{10}/E_3
A2 vs A3	2.478	82.000 ± 20.5	68.667± 18.5
Gl vs Me	3.356	75.695 ± 9.8	68.380 ± 9.0
Od vs A2	3.654	84.000 ± 16.7	68.000 ± 11.0
A2 vs Oa	3.771	84.667 ± 16.6	76.667 ± 9.4
Gl vs Ly	3.935	88.607 ± 5.5	82.043 ± 12.4
Gl vs Ab	3.970	95.294 ± 6.4	94.183 ± 5.9
Me vs Ly	5.144	82.500 ± 6.8	82.500 ± 16.8
Gl vs A3	5.681	94.000 ± 4.5	90.000 ± 8.4
A2 vs Ly	5.870	89.778 ± 10.0	81.778 ± 20.4
Gl vs Pn	7.853	97.647 ± 3.2	91.765 ± 8.9
Me vs Pn	9.529	93.143 ± 9.6	92.000 ± 8.2
Mm vs Ab	10.252	93.333 ± 8.6	91.000 ± 12.3
G1 vs Mm	11.425	100.000 ± 0.0	97.670 ± 3.2
A2 vs G2	15.275	94.510 ± 4.6	93.100 ± 3.7
G1 vs G2	16.354	94.286 ± 5.4	92.100 ± 3.0
Me vs Mm	17.685	98.000 ± 4.5	88.431 ± 9.2
G2 vs Mm	18.754	89.514 ± 4.9	88.333 ± 2.9
G1 vs No	23.884	100.000 ± 0.0	98.889 ± 2.5
Me vs No	26.962	98.000 ± 4.5	97.778 ± 5.0

$$SNR = 10log\left[\sum_{i=1}^{n} \frac{x[i]^2}{MSE * n}\right] \quad (6)$$

where $\hat{x}$ is the reconstructed signal. Finally, the $Q1$ index for the order r was computed with the mean of the aforementioned statistics, as follows:

$$Q1(r) = \frac{\overline{SNR_{Re}(r)}}{\overline{MSE_{Re}(r)} + \overline{NDC_{Re}(r)}} \quad (7)$$

The *Re* subindex corresponds to a rescaling of the data between the values 1 and 3. The maximum values of $Q1$ indicate the orders with the best reconstruction error using the minimum NDC. The two highest values of $Q1$ for each wavelet function are reported in Table 4.

The observed signal can be considered to consist of a real signal plus additive white noise. The denoising of the available MRS spectra was carried out according to three consecutive steps (Agoris *et al.*, 2004): *Threshold calculation* (using three methods: Universal threshold (*Sqtwolog*), Threshold applying the principle of Stein's Unbiased Risk (*Rigrsure*), and Threshold Minimax); *Threshold scaling* (again using three methods: *One*, *Sln* and *Mln*); and *Threshold implementation*. All the combinations of threshold estimation (*Sqtwolog*, *Rigrsure* and *Minimax*), threshold scaling (*Sln*, *One* and *Mln*), and *Hard* thresholding were implemented. The *Hard* function was used because it often yields smaller MSE than the *Soft* one and, furthermore, our results indicated that *Soft* thresholding could result in a decrease in the height of the resonance frequencies with a

Figure 5. Logarithmic adjustment (4th order) of λ values E'_{10}/E_3 vs. mean classification percentage of E'_{10}/E_3

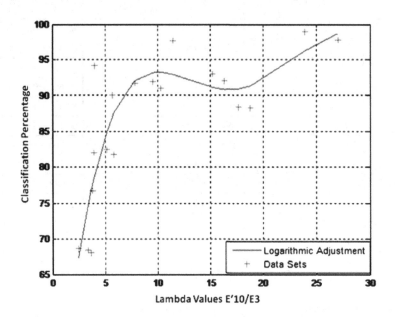

Table 4. Results of the different quality measures for the selection of the optimal mother wavelet

Wavelet	MSE	SNR	NDC	Q1
Symlet (2)	0.65	191.43	213	0.91
Symlet (3)	0.70	193.58	216	0.95
Coiflet (1)	0.66	192.75	216	0.50
Coiflet (2)	0.75	193.90	238	0.37
Daubichie (2)	0.62	191.58	213	0.93
Daubichie (3)	0.66	193.97	216	0.98
Biortogonal (1.3)	0.77	228.38	216	0.62
Biortogonal (3.3)	0.64	217.38	221	0.65

high degree of skewness, decreasing the importance of certain metabolites that are useful for classification (see details in Arizmendi *et al.*, 2010).

The results displayed in Figure 6 show that, for all wavelets, the lower MSE is achieved when applying the *Sln* weighting scheme, regardless of the threshold calculation. The MSE of the three types of thresholds when *Sln* scaling is applied

can be compared in Figure 6, which shows that the *Rigrsure-Sln-Hard* procedure yields the best results among all combinations.

In order to determine the final wavelet, the average values of several statistics were computed for the *Rigsure-Sln-Hard* combination. They include: SNR, Energy Preserved (EP), Percentage of Distortion (PD) and Compression Ratio (CR) defined as:

$$EP = \frac{\sum_{i=1}^{n} \hat{x}[i]^2}{\sum_{i=1}^{n} x[i]^2} *100\% \qquad (8)$$

$$PD = \sqrt{\frac{\sum_{i=1}^{n} (x[i] - \hat{x}[i])^2}{\sum_{i=1}^{n} x[i]^2}} *100\% \qquad (9)$$

$$CR = L_0 / L_c \qquad (10)$$

where *Lo* is the cardinality of the decomposition coefficients of the original signal, and *Lc* the cardinality of decomposition coefficients that are different from zero. This set of statistics has been used to choose the optimal wavelet in previous related works concerning ECG signal filtering (Olarte, & Sierra, 2007) and classification tasks (Rivas, Burgos, & García, 2009), among others. For a further objective criterion in choosing the optimal wavelet function, the *Q2* index was computed:

$$Q2(r) = \frac{\overline{SNR}_{Re}(r) + \overline{EP}_{Re}(r) + \overline{CR}_{Re}(r)}{\overline{MSE}_{Re}(r) + \overline{PD}_{Re}(r)} . \qquad (11)$$

Again, the *Re* subindex corresponds to a rescaling of the data between 1 and 3. The *Q2* values for the wavelet functions of Table 4 are shown in Table 5. The maximum value for this index was obtained for the Biortogonal (3.3) wavelet. Therefore, this wavelet was chosen for further experimentation.

Dimensionality Reduction with MWVA and PCA

After processing the MR spectra with wavelet Biortogonal (3.3) and filtering it with the combination *Rigsure-Sln-Hard*, we proceeded to reduce the dimensionality of the data using MWVA and PCA, taking as input variables the decomposition coefficients. The value of the optimal width *w* was found to be 1 (every window corresponds to a single variable).

The initial feature selection was carried out by obtaining a ranking (in descending order) of the values of λ. The variables were divided in groups corresponding to the set of variables whose energy gradually provided 1% of the total energy. Figure 7 provides the average of the λ ratio for the 20 tumour classification experiments investigated. The value of λ can be seen to decrease exponentially as new variables are added, starting its linear trend with the variable 26 (11% of the total energy). Therefore, variables added from this point are not likely to contribute significantly to the classification task.

For PCA, principal components were added one at a time until the differential cumulative variance between two consecutive components was less than 1%. An average of 10.15 and 13 variables were obtained for MWVA and PCA respectively.

Data Classification with ANN

Feed-forward ANNs were used in the classification experiments starting from the features selected and extracted through dimensionality reduction, as previously explained. Different network architectures between 5 and 40 units in the only hidden layer were employed. Given that all classifications are binary, one unit in the output layer does suffice. In order to avoid data overfitting, the networks were trained with Bayesian regularization (MacKay, 1992) as part of a back-propagation process. The adaptive weights and biases were updated according to the Levenberg-Marquardt algorithm (Foresee, & Hagan, 1997). One run of a 5-fold cross-validation was performed for each network, allowing a maximum of 500 epochs. To address the issue of class imbalance (the number of cases available from each tumour type is always small, but widely varying, as reported in Table 1), the original datasets were re-sampled, by over-

Figure 6. Figure 6a shows the MSE of the signal reconstructed by the implementation Sure. Figure 6b shows the MSE of the signal reconstructed by the implementation Minimax. Figure 6c shows the MSE of the signal reconstructed by the implementation Sqtwolog. Figure 6d shows the comparison of the MSE of the best top three thresholds when Sln is applied.

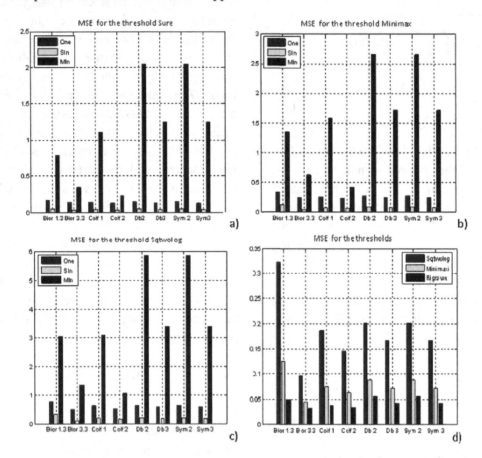

Table 5. Statistics for the final comparison of the performance of the best mother wavelets once the Rigrsure-Sln-Hard procedure has been selected

Wavelet	MSE	SNR	EP	PD	CR	Q2
Coiflet (1)	0.037	190.81	99.86	3.30	1.61	2.51
Coiflet (2)	0.033	192.86	99.86	3.08	1.43	2.78
Symlet (2)	0.056	188.23	99.78	3.78	1.68	1.18
Symlet (3)	0.042	191.94	99.83	3.28	1.63	2.10
Daubichie (2)	0.056	188.23	99.78	3.78	1.68	1.18
Daubichie (3)	0.042	191.94	99.83	3.29	1.63	2.10
Biortogonal (1.3)	0.050	182.73	99.92	4.47	1.68	1.25
Biortogonal (3.3)	0.032	193.62	99.81	3.02	1.55	3.20

sampling the minority class and under-sampling the majority class (Japkowicz, 2000).

Tables 6 and 7 show the detailed best results for all the analyzed problems. They include several quality indicators, including the balanced error rate (BER), the area under the ROC curve (AUC), and the accuracy for the balanced (B) and unbalanced (UB) groups.

Figures 8 and 9 provide a telling summary of the results for all problems. All indicators consistently show that dimensionality reduction using MWVA tends to achieve better and more homogeneous results than PCA throughout the experiments. This is an encouraging outcome, given that feature selection provides solutions that are easier to interpret clinically than those obtained with feature extraction (González-Navarro *et al.*, 2010). A Wilcoxon test was carried out to statistically compare the classification results corresponding to MWVA and PCA, looking for evidence of significant differences between the results obtained through both methods. Results of this test are reported in Table 8 and sustain the previous comments.

The few atypically poor results highlighted in these figures alert us of the special difficulty of some classification experiments. In some cases, such difficulty is well reported in the existing literature, as for astrocytomas of similar grade: a2 *vs.* a3 (see for instance, Ladroue, 2003), or high-grade malignant tumours: gl *vs.* me (see Romero *et al.*, 2009). In a few other cases (gl *vs.* ly, a3 *vs.* pn), such difficulty has not been reported.

The results obtained with balanced datasets are consistently better than those obtained with the original unbalanced datasets, although not in a statistically significant way, as evaluated through a Wilcoxon test. This holds both for feature selection with MWVA and extraction with PCA. These results can only justify to a certain extent the use of the class-balancing strategy.

Comparison with Other Studies Using the INTERPRET Database

Several binary classification problems including low grade gliomas (G1) *vs.* meningiomas (mm), glioblastomas (gl) *vs.* metastases (me), and me *vs.* mm were addressed in (García-Gómez *et al.* 2009). This study used a variation of the INTERPRET SET database also analyzed in the current chapter, which makes the comparison especially relevant. The authors reported a BER result of 0.91 for G1 *vs.* mm, with cross-validation, feature extraction with Independent Component Analysis (ICA) and a Least-Squares Support Vector Machine (LS-SVM) classifier (to be compared with a BER of 0.98 reported in Tables 6 and 7); a 100-BER result of 60% was reported for gl *vs.* me, with spectral Peak Integration (PI) and a Linear Discriminant Analysis (LDA) classifier (to be compared with a 100-BER of 77.24% reported in Table 7); finally, a 100-BER result of 95% was reported for me *vs.* mm, with PCA and a MLP classifier (to be compared with a 100-BER of 95.23% reported in Table 7). The difficult problem of discriminating between different grades of astrocytomas (a2 and a3) was addressed in (Ladroue, 2003). Here, PCA was used for dimensionality reduction and LDA, LS-SVM and K-Nearest Neighbor (K-NN) were used as classifiers. The author reports a mean test accuracy of just under 70% for 20 PCs and LS-SVM. This can be compared with our result of around 68% (although with a very high standard deviation of 17.9%), in Table 6. Another classically difficult problem: me *vs.* gl was also dealt with in (Ladroue, 2003). A maximum accuracy of only 55% was reported. This compares to our result of 71.23%, using MWVA for dimensionality reduction.

Figure 7. Mean ± standard deviation of, in descending order, as a function of the number of variables. The λ ratio and the number of variables corresponding to a total of energy of 11% are highlighted.

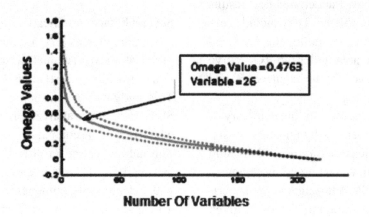

Table 6. Mean ± standard deviation of AUC and accuracy values for all balanced classification experiments

Experiments	MWVA AUC	PCA AUC	MWVA ACCURACY	PCA ACCURACY
G1 *vs* G2	0.97±0.04	0.91±0.07	93.19±5.04	88.74±2.52
G1 vs Mm	0.98±0.01	0.97±0.03	95.00±8.14	92.25±3.12
A2 vs A3	0.90±0.16	0.95±0.05	68.00±17.90	68.00±17.90
A2 vs G2	0.98±0.02	0.95±0.06	96.70±3.47	88.53±7.38
A2 vs Ly	1.00±0.00	0.95±0.04	92.00±10.90	84.00±21.90
A2 vs Oa	1.00±0.00	1.00±0.00	100.00±0.00	74.00±13.40
A3 vs Pn	1.00±0.00	0.70±0.00	93.33±14.90	53.33±29.80
G2 vs Mm	0.98±0.01	0.96±0.00	96.73±2.28	92.12±4.95
Gl vs A3	0.99±0.01	0.80±0.10	94.91±5.25	80.66±8.02
Gl vs Ab	1.00±0.00	0.80±0.12	97.50±3.42	84.66±7.72
Gl vs Ly	1.00±0.00	0.87±0.08	90.00±7.12	85.00±8.38
Gl vs Me	0.90±0.05	0.67±0.12	71.23±8.66	50.00±16.66
Gl vs No	1.00±0.00	1.00±0.00	100.00±0.00	93.33±12.00
Gl vs Pn	0.98±0.02	0.93±0.04	93.75±6.25	82.50±15.60
Me vs Ly	0.95±0.06	0.90±0.06	90.00±5.59	72.50±13.70
Me vs Mm	0.99±0.01	0.99±0.01	95.00±6.84	92.50±5.22
Me vs No	1.00±0.00	1.00±0.00	100.00±0.00	96.00±5.47
Me vs Pn	1.00±0.00	1.00±0.00	100.00±0.00	85.00±16.30
Mm vs Ab	1.00±0.00	1.00±0.00	100.00±0.00	78.18±15.21
Od vs A2	1.00±0.00	1.00±0.00	84.00±16.73	64.00±32.86

Table 7. Mean ± standard deviation of AUC and (100-BER) values for all unbalanced classification experiments

Experiments	MWVA.AUC	PCA.AUC	MWVA 100-BER	PCA 100-BER
G1 VS G2	0.97± 0.03	0.93± 0.06	90.22 ± 5.10	84.69± 10.76
G1 vs Mm	0.98 ± 0.02	0.96 ± 0.00	96.23 ± 3.67	92.12 ± 4.52
A2 vs A3	0.89 ± 0.11	1.00 ± 0.00	55.00 ± 10.55	66.67 ± 24.90
A2 vs G2	0.99 ± 0.00	0.90 ± 0.00	94.05 ± 1.18	91.58 ± 28.56
A2 vs Ly	1.00 ± 0.00	1.00 ± 0.00	86.67 ± 21.26	95.00 ± 21.38
A2 vs Oa	1.00 ± 0.00	0.95 ± 0.10	100.00 ± 15.42	70.84 ± 6.84
A3 vs Pn	1.00 ± 0.00	0.70 ± 0.00	85.00 ± 23.73	50.00 ± 9.77
G2 vs Mm	0.99 ± 0.00	0.98 ± 0.00	93.46 ± 22.36	93.06 ± 0.00
Gl vs A3	0.97 ± 0.00	0.93 ± 0.00	90.05 ± 0.00	83.01 ± 1.82
Gl vs Ab	0.99 ± 0.00	0.82 ± 0.14	93.62 ± 13.74	65.86 ± 21.54
Gl vs Ly	0.91 ± 0.00	0.88 ± 0.00	70.15 ± 18.18	75.24 ± 6.89
Gl vs Me	0.90 ± 0.00	0.70 ± 0.10	77.24 ± 7.18	56.96 ± 6.33
Gl vs No	1.00 ± 0.00	1.00 ± 0.00	100.00 ± 0.00	98.67 ± 20.62
Gl vs Pn	0.97 ± 0.00	0.97 ± 0.00	87.86 ± 5.46	76.62 ± 5.69
Me vs Ly	0.96 ± 0.00	0.92 ± 0.00	85.24 ± 0.00	76.19 ± 4.37
Me vs Mm	0.98 ± 0.00	0.98 ± 0.00	95.23 ± 3.36	93.89 ± 5.13
Me vs No	1.00 ± 0.00	1.00 ± 0.00	100.00 ± 12.24	95.24 ± 26.14
Me vs Pn	1.00 ± 0.00	0.98 ± 0.00	100.00 ± 0.00	87.39 ± 14.52
Mm vs Ab	1.00 ± 0.00	1.00 ± 0.00	99.00 ± 2.23	90.78 ± 7.47
Od vs A2	1.00 ± 0.00	0.85 ± 0.13	81.67 ± 20.75	60.84 ± 10.86

CONCLUSION

The diagnosis of neuro-oncology pathologies is a critical task for medical experts in clinical environments. Most decisions in this context bound to be made on the basis of a combination of doctors' experience and background knowledge, and information gathered through non-invasive measurement techniques.

Human brain tumours are a very diverse family of pathologies, and require an accurate diagnosis in order to select those tailored therapies that could maximize the chances of survival. The availability of tumour information in the form of signal and image makes the use of computer-based diagnostic assistance advisable. A sensitive stage in the computer-based analysis of tumour information is

that of data pre-processing. In this paper, we have outlined and evaluated diverse methods of MRS signal information pre-processing. The combination of DWT and dimensionality reduction has been shown to provide the best accuracy results over a wide array of classification experiments using Bayesian ANNs and concerning different types of tumours.

The comparison of the results obtained in our experiments with those previously reported in the recent scientific literature provides evidence of the adequacy of the proposed data pre-processing approach. To the best of the authors' knowledge, some of the classification experiments in which encouraging results have been obtained had never previously been investigated as a problem of binary classification. Such experiments should therefore

Figure 8. Box plot of the accuracy and 100-BER values corresponding to the unbalanced and balanced experiments. Each box represents the lower quartile (bottom line), median (line in the middle), and upper quartile (top line) values. The whiskers are lines extending from each end of the box to represent the extent of the rest of the data. Classification problems with atypical results are left outside the limits of the box plots.

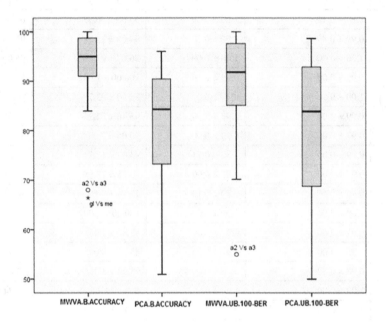

Figure 9. Box plots, represented as in Figure 8, of the AUC values corresponding to the unbalanced and balanced experiments

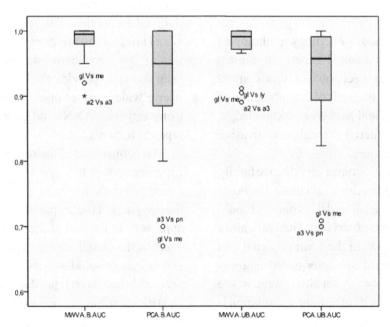

provide medical experts in neuro-oncology with some preliminary knowledge related to the discriminability of the concerned tumour pathologies on the basis of MRS information.

In this study, only MRS data acquired at short time of echo were analyzed. Future work should involve similar experiments with data acquired at long time of echo, or even with data obtained by combination of different acquisition times of echo.

ACKNOWLEDGMENT

This research was partially funded by Spanish MICINN R+D projects TIN2006-08114 and TIN2009-13895-C02-01. Authors gratefully acknowledge the former INTERPRET European project partners. Data providers: Dr. C. Majós (IDI), Dr. À. Moreno-Torres (CDP), Dr. F.A. Howe and Prof. J.Griffiths (SGUL), Prof. A. Heerschap (RU), Prof. L Stefanczyk and Dr J.Fortuniak (MUL) and Dr. J. Calvar (FLENI); data curators: Dr. M.Julià-Sapé, Dr. A.P. Candiota, Dr. I. Olier, Ms. T. Delgado, Ms. J. Martín and Mr. A. Pérez (all from GABRMN-UAB). GABRMN coordinator: Prof. C. Arús.

REFERENCES

Agoris, P. D., Meijer, S., Gulski, E., & Smit, J. J. (2004) Threshold selection for wavelet denoising of partial discharge data. In *Conference Record of the 2004 IEEE International Symposium on Electrical Insulation*, (pp. 62-65). IEEE.

Ahlbom, A., Green, A., Kheifets, L., Savitz, D., & Swerdlow, A. (2004). Epidemiology of health effects of radiofrequency exposure. *Environmental Health Perspectives*, *112*(17), 1741–1754. doi:10.1289/ehp.7306

Arizmendi, C., Hernández-Tamames, J., Romero, E., Vellido, A., & del Pozo, F. (2010). Diagnosis of brain tumours from magnetic resonance spectroscopy using wavelets and Neural Networks. In *Proceedings of the Engineering in Medicine and Biology Society (EMBC), Annual International Conference of the IEEE*, (pp. 6074-6077).

Du, Y. P., Liang, Y. Z., Jiang, J. H., Berry, R. J., & Ozaki, Y. (2004). Spectral regions selection to improve prediction ability of PLS models by changeable size moving window partial least squares and searching combination moving window partial least squares. *Analytica Chimica Acta*, *501*(2), 183–191. doi:10.1016/j.aca.2003.09.041

Foresee, F. D., & Hagan, M. T. (1997). Gauss-Newton approximation to Bayesian regularization. In *Proceedings of the International Joint Conference on Neural Networks, IJCNN 1997*, (pp. 1930-1935). Houston, Texas, USA.

García-Gómez, J. M., Luts, J., Julià-Sapé, M., Krooshof, P., Tortajada, S., & Robledo, J. V. (2009). Multiproject–multicenter evaluation of automatic brain tumor classification by magnetic resonance spectroscopy. *Magnetic Resonance Materials in Physics. Biologie Medicale*, *22*(1), 5–18.

Giraldo, B., Garde, A., Arizmendi, C., Jane, R., Benito, S., Díaz, I., & Ballesteros, D. (2006) Support vector machine classification applied on weaning trials patients. In *Proceedings of the Engineering in Medicine and Biology Society, EMBS'06, 28th Annual International Conference of the IEEE*, (pp. 5587-5590). IEEE.

González-Navarro, F. F., Belanche-Muñoz, L. A., Romero, E., Vellido, A., Julià-Sapé, M., & Arús, C. (2010). Feature and model selection with discriminatory visualization for diagnostic classification of brain tumors. *Neurocomputing*, *73*(4-6), 622–632. doi:10.1016/j.neucom.2009.07.018

Japkowicz, N. (2000). The class imbalance problem: Significance and strategies. In *Proceedings of the International Conference on Artificial Intelligence (ICAI 2000)*, Vol. 1, (pp. 111-117).

Jiang, J. H., Berry, R. J., Siesler, H. W., & Ozaki, Y. (2002). Wavelength interval selection in multicomponent spectral analysis by moving window partial least-squares regression with applications to mid-infrared and near-infrared spectroscopic data. *Analytical Chemistry, 74*(14), 3555–3565. doi:10.1021/ac011177u

Julià-Sapé, M., Acosta, D., Mier, M., Arús, C., & Watson, D. (2006). A multi-centre, web-accessible and quality control-checked database of in vivo MR spectra of brain tumour patients. *Magnetic Resonance Materials in Physics, Biology and Medicine. Magma (New York, N.Y.), 19*(1), 22–33. doi:10.1007/s10334-005-0023-x

Kleihues, P., & Cavenee, W.K. (2000). *Pathology and genetics of tumours of the nervous system.* World Health Organization Classification of Tumours. Lyon, France: IARCPress.

Ladroue, C., Howe, F. A., Griffiths, J. R., & Tate, A. R. (2003). Independent component analysis for automated decomposition of in vivo magnetic resonance spectra. *Magnetic Resonance in Medicine, 50*(4), 697–703. doi:10.1002/mrm.10595

Lantos, P. L., Vandenberg, S. R., & Kleihues, P. (1996). Tumours of the nervous system. In Graham, D. I., & Lantos, P. L. (Eds.), *Greenfield's neuropathology* (pp. 583–879). London, UK: Arnold.

Luts, J., Heerschap, A., Suykens, J. A. K., & Van Huffel, S. (2007). A combined MRI and MRSI based multiclass system for brain tumour recognition using LS-SVMs with class probabilities and feature selection. *Artificial Intelligence in Medicine, 40*(2), 87–102. doi:10.1016/j.artmed.2007.02.002

MacKay, D. J. C. (1992). The evidence framework applied to classification networks. *Neural Computation, 4*(5), 720–736. doi:10.1162/neco.1992.4.5.720

Mohamed, N., Rubin, D. M., & Marwala, T. (2006) Detection of epileptiform activity in human EEG signals using Bayesian neural networks. In *Proceedings of the IEEE 3rd International Conference on Computational Cybernetics, ICCC 2005*, (pp. 231-237). IEEE.

Olarte Rodríguez, O. J., & Sierra Bueno, D. A. (2010) Determinación de los parámetros asociados al filtro wavelet por umbralización aplicado a filtrado de interferencias electrocardiográficas (in Spanish). *Revista UIS Ingenierías, 6*(2).

Rivas, E., Burgos, J. C., & García-Prada, J. C. (2009). Condition assessment of power OLTC by vibration analysis using wavelet transform. *IEEE Transactions on Power Delivery, 24*(2), 687–694. doi:10.1109/TPWRD.2009.2014268

Romero, E., Vellido, A., Julià-Sapé, M., & Arús, C. (2009). Discriminating glioblastomas from metastases in a SV ¹H-MRS brain tumour database. In *Proceedings of the 26th Annual Meeting of the European Society for Magnetic Resonance in Medicine and Biology, ESMRMB 2009*, (p. 18). Antalya, Turkey.

Rosenblum, M. G., Cimponeriu, L., Bezerianos, A., Patzak, A., & Mrowka, R. (2002). Identification of coupling direction: Application to cardiorespiratory interaction. *Physical Review E: Statistical, Nonlinear, and Soft Matter Physics, 65*(4), 041909. doi:10.1103/PhysRevE.65.041909

Sá, R. C., & Verbandt, Y. (2002). Automated breath detection on long-duration signals using feedforward backpropagation artificial neural networks. *IEEE Transactions on Bio-Medical Engineering, 49*(10), 1130–1141. doi:10.1109/TBME.2002.803514

Shinzawa, H., Morita, S., Ozaki, Y., & Tsenkova, R. (2006). New method for spectral data classification: Two-way moving window principal component analysis. *Applied Spectroscopy, 60*(8), 884–891. doi:10.1366/000370206778062020

Stewart, B. W., & Kleihues, P. (2003). *World cancer report*. IARC Press.

KEY TERMS AND DEFINITIONS

Bayesian Artificial Neural Networks: A variant of classical feed-forward multi-layer perceptrons, defined within a Bayesian probability theory framework.

Brain Tumour: A tumour of the central nervous system. Tumours of this type have a rich and complex taxonomy.

Discrete Wavelet Transform: A wavelet-based technique for signal processing in discrete domains.

Medical Decision Support System: A computer-based system designed to provide at least semi-automated support in the form of operative knowledge for medical problems.

Moving Window Variance Analysis: A dimensionality reduction technique that consists of the combination of the MW technique in conjunction with the calculation of a standard ratio defined as the quotient between the between-groups variance (BGV) and the within-groups variance (WGV) for a particular width of the selected window.

Chapter 4
Semi–Supervised Clustering for the Identification of Different Cancer Types Using the Gene Expression Profiles

Manuel Martín-Merino
University Pontificia of Salamanca, Spain

ABSTRACT

DNA Microarrays allow for monitoring the expression level of thousands of genes simultaneously across a collection of related samples. Supervised learning algorithms such as k-NN or SVM (Support Vector Machines) have been applied to the classification of cancer samples with encouraging results. However, the classification algorithms are not able to discover new subtypes of diseases considering the gene expression profiles. In this chapter, the author reviews several supervised clustering algorithms suitable to discover new subtypes of cancer. Next, he introduces a semi-supervised clustering algorithm that learns a linear combination of dissimilarities from the a priory knowledge provided by human experts. A priori knowledge is formulated in the form of equivalence constraints. The minimization of the error function is based on a quadratic optimization algorithm. A L_2 norm regularizer is included that penalizes the complexity of the family of distances and avoids overfitting. The method proposed has been applied to several benchmark data sets and to human complex cancer problems using the gene expression profiles. The experimental results suggest that considering a linear combination of heterogeneous dissimilarities helps to improve both classification and clustering algorithms based on a single similarity.

DOI: 10.4018/978-1-4666-1803-9.ch004

INTRODUCTION

Classification techniques such as k-NN or Support Vector Machines (SVM) have been successfully applied to the identification of cancer samples using the gene expression profiles (Lanckriet, 2004; Martín-Merino, 2009b). This kind of supervised algorithms rely on a categorization of a subset of samples by human experts. Therefore, they are not able to discover new types of diseases which is usually more interesting for biologists. Besides, biological information provided by human experts is frequently very sparse and it is provided in the form of which pairs of objects are considered similar. This kind of information cannot be incorporated into classification techniques.

Clustering algorithms group similar objects without any supervision by human experts. They are able to discover new types of diseases but classical algorithms cannot incorporate a priori knowledge provided by human experts.

Clustering algorithms depend critically on the choice of a good dissimilarity (Xing, 2003). A large variety of dissimilarities have been proposed in the literature (Cox, 2001). However, in real applications no dissimilarity outperforms the others because each dissimilarity reflects often different features of the data (Martín-Merino, 2009a). Instead of using a single dissimilarity it has been recommended in (Lanckriet, 2004; Martín-Merino, 2009b) to consider a linear combination of heterogeneous dissimilarities and data sources.

Therefore, new clustering algorithms should be developed that are able to adapt the metric to the problem at hand considering the a priori information provided by human experts in the form of similarity/dissimilarity constraints.

Several authors have proposed techniques to learn a linear combination of kernels (similarities) from the data (Lanckriet, 2004; Martín-Merino, 2009b; Soon Ong, 2005; Xiong, 2006). These methods are designed for classification tasks and assume that the class labels are available for the training set. However, for certain applications such as Bioinformatics, domain experts provide only incomplete knowledge in the form of which pairs of samples or genes are related (Huang, 2006). This a priory information can be incorporated via semi-supervised metric learning algorithms using equivalence constraints (Bar-Hillel, 2005). Thus, (Xing, 2003) proposed a distance metric learning algorithm that incorporates such similarity/dissimilarity information using a convex programming approach. The experimental results show a significant improvement in clustering results. However, the algorithm is based on an iterative procedure that is computationally intensive particularly, for high dimensional applications. To avoid this problem, (Bar-Hillel, 2005; Kwok, 2003; Wu, 2005) presented more efficient algorithms to learn a Mahalanobis metric. However, these algorithms are not able to incorporate heterogeneous dissimilarities and rely on the use of the Mahalanobis distance that may not be appropriate for certain kind of applications (Martín-Merino, 2009a; Martín-Merino 2009b).

The approach introduced in this chapter, considers that the integration of dissimilarities that reflect different features of the data should help to improve the performance of clustering and classification algorithms. To this aim, a linear combination of heterogeneous dissimilarities is learnt considering the relation between kernels and distances (Pekalska, 2001). A learning algorithm is proposed to estimate the optimal weights considering the similarity/dissimilarity constraints available. The method proposed is based on a convex quadratic optimization algorithm and incorporates a smoothing term that penalizes de complexity of the family of distances avoiding overfitting.

The metric learning algorithm proposed has been applied to a wide range of practical problems. The empirical results suggest that the method proposed helps to improve pattern recognition algorithms based on a single dissimilarity and a widely used metric learning algorithm proposed in the literature.

BACKGROUND

Supervised learning algorithms such as k-NN or SVM (Support Vector Machines) (Vapnik, 1998) have been applied to the classification of cancer samples with encouraging results (Martín-Merino, 2009b). However, classification algorithms are not able to discover new subtypes of diseases considering the gene expression profiles. This goal is often more interesting for human experts.

Clustering algorithms, allow us to discover new types of cancer that have not been previously identified by human experts. Given a finite set of samples $X = \{\vec{x}_1, \ldots, \vec{x}_n\}$ clustering techniques look for a partition $S = \{S_1, S_2, \ldots, S_g\}$ such that similar objects according to a given dissimilarity are assigned to the same group while dissimilar ones are assigned to different groups. Thus, in order to cluster a set of patterns, we have to choose a dissimilarity that reflects the proximities among the objects. Next we have to define an error function that evaluates the quality of the partition obtained. Finally, an optimization algorithm should be considered depending on the problem at hand.

A large variety of algorithms have been proposed in the last years that exhibit different properties (Shawe-Taylor, 2004). Perhaps, the most popular is k-means clustering algorithm because it is easy to understand, efficient computationally and gives good results for a wide range of real problems.

k-means clustering looks for a partition of the data into g clusters $S = \{S_1, S_2, \ldots, S_g\}$ such that the within-group sum of squares is minimized.

$$\mathbf{J} = \frac{1}{n} \sum_{j=1}^{g} \sum_{\vec{x}_i \in S_j} |\vec{x}_i - \vec{m}_j|^2 \tag{1}$$

where $\vec{m}_j = \frac{1}{N_j} \sum_{\vec{x}_i \in S_j}^{N_j} \vec{x}_i$ is the usual mean of the cluster j, N_j denotes the number of patterns assigned to the cluster j and n is the number of patterns.

The optimization of this error function is usually carried out by an iterative algorithm in two steps:

1. Assign each object $\vec{x}_i$ to the nearest mean in the Euclidean sense. That is,

$$k = \arg \min_j \| \vec{x}_i - \vec{m}_j \| \tag{2}$$

2. Computation of new means based on the pattern assignments.

$$\vec{m}_j = \frac{1}{N_j} \sum_{\vec{x}_i \in S_j}^{N_j} \vec{x}_i \tag{3}$$

The previous algorithm suffers from several drawbacks for the applications we are dealing with. First, in genomics applications a priori knowledge is frequently available in the form of which pairs of genes or samples are related. Considering this knowledge, may help to improve significantly the clustering results. Therefore, k-means must be modify to take into account this kind of supervised information. Besides, clustering results depend strongly on the dissimilarity considered to evaluate the sample proximities. Several dissimilarities are usually available that may come from different object representations or from different data sources. Each dissimilarity provides frequently complementary information about the problem and therefore, choosing a single dissimilarity may become meaningless. Recently, it has been suggested in the literature (Lanckriet, 2004; Martín-Merino, 2009b) that the integration of several dissimilarities and data sources helps to reflect more accurately which is similar for the problem at hand. Learning algorithms should be developed that are able to obtain an optimal combination of measures from the a priori knowledge provided by human experts.

Several authors have proposed semi-supervised clustering algorithms that adapt the metric to the data (Xing, 2003; Bar-Hillel, 2005; Kwok,

2003). Next, we introduce the algorithm proposed by Xing in order to learn a Mahalanobis parametrized metric from a set of similarity/dissimilarity constraints.

Let $\{\vec{x}_i\}_{i=1}^n \in R^d$ be the input patterns. We are given side-information in the form of pairs that are considered similar or dissimilar for the application at hand. Let S and D be the subset of pairs of patterns known to be similar/dissimilar defined as:

$$S = \{(\vec{x}_i, \vec{x}_j) : \vec{x}_i \text{ is similar to } \vec{x}_j\} \qquad (4)$$

$$D = \{(\vec{x}_i, \vec{x}_j) : \vec{x}_i \text{ is dissimilar to } \vec{x}_j\} \qquad (5)$$

Consider the Mahalanobis distance parametrized by the matrix $\mathbf{A}$:

$$d(\vec{x}, \vec{y}) = d_{\mathbf{A}}(\vec{x}, \vec{y}) = \| \vec{x} - \vec{y} \|_{\mathbf{A}} = \sqrt{(\vec{x} - \vec{y})^T \mathbf{A}(\vec{x} - \vec{y})} \qquad (6)$$

To ensure this metric to be non-negative and that it satisfies the triangle inequality we should constraint the matrix $\mathbf{A}$ to be positive semi-definite, $\mathbf{A} \succeq 0$. If the matrix $\mathbf{A}$ is diagonal, learning the metric is equivalent to rescale the data giving different weight to each axe. In particular, setting $\mathbf{A} = I$ corresponds to the Euclidean distance.

A good metric for clustering applications should become small for pairs of patterns considered similar by human experts, $(\vec{x}_i, \vec{x}_j) \in S$. Therefore, the metric learnt should minimize $\sum_{(\vec{x}_i, \vec{x}_j) \in S} \| \vec{x}_i - \vec{x}_j \|_{\mathbf{A}}^2$.

The optimization problem can be written as follows:

$$\min_{\mathbf{A}} \sum_{(\vec{x}_i, \vec{x}_j) \in S} \| \vec{x}_i - \vec{x}_j \|_{\mathbf{A}}^2 \qquad (7)$$

$$s.t. \sum_{(\vec{x}_i, \vec{x}_j) \in D} \| \vec{x}_i - \vec{x}_j \|_{A} \geq 1, \qquad (8)$$

$$\mathbf{A} \succeq 0 \qquad (9)$$

The first constraint in the optimization problem avoids the trivial solution corresponding to $\mathbf{A} = 0$. The choice of the constant 1 is not relevant because changing it to another positive constant c is equivalent to multiply the matrix $\mathbf{A}$ by c^2. Both, the objective function and the constraints are convex, which allow us to develop optimization algorithms that converge to a global minimum.

In order to solve the optimization problem we are going to consider two cases. If the matrix $\mathbf{A}$ is diagonal, the original problem is equivalent to minimize the following error function:

$$g(\mathbf{A}) = \sum_{(\vec{x}_i, \vec{x}_j) \in S} \| \vec{x}_i - \vec{x}_j \|_{\mathbf{A}}^2 - \log\left(\sum_{(\vec{x}_i, \vec{x}_j) \in D} \| \vec{x}_i - \vec{x}_j \|_{\mathbf{A}}\right) \qquad (10)$$

$$s.\, t. \quad A \geq 0 \qquad (11)$$

that can be solved efficiently by a Newton-Raphson algorithm.

When we have to learn a full matrix $\mathbf{A}$ the constraint $\mathbf{A} \succeq 0$ is more trickier to enforce and the Newton's method become computationally intensive. To avoid this, the following optimization problem is solved:

$$\max_{\mathbf{A}} g(\mathbf{A}) = \sum_{(\vec{x}_i, \vec{x}_j) \in D} \| \vec{x}_i - \vec{x}_j \|_{\mathbf{A}} \qquad (12)$$

$$s.t. \quad f(A) = \sum_{(\vec{x}_i, \vec{x}_j) \in S} \left\| \vec{x}_i - \vec{x}_j \right\|_A^2 \leq 1 \qquad (13)$$

$$\mathbf{A} \succeq 0 \qquad (14)$$

This problem can be solved by gradient ascent of g, $\mathbf{A} = \mathbf{A} + \alpha \nabla_A g(\mathbf{A})$ and, projecting repeatedly the matrix $\mathbf{A}$ on to the sets $C_1 = \{\mathbf{A} : \sum_{(\vec{x}_i, \vec{x}_j) \in S} \| \vec{x}_i - \vec{x}_j \|^2 \leq 1\}$ and $C_2 = \{\mathbf{A} : \mathbf{A} \succeq 0\}$ to enforce the two constraints. The projection step can be solved efficiently via a quadratic programming and a singular value decomposition approach respectively (Bar-Hillel, 2005).

The previous algorithm suffers from several drawbacks. First, it is very intensive computationally particularly for high dimensional problems. Next, it relies only on a Mahalanobis metric, which may not be appropriate to model the sample proximities in many problems. Finally, it doesn't allow to integrate several data sources.

To avoid the first problem it has been proposed in (Bar-Hillel, 2005) the Relevant Component Analysis algorithm (RCA). This technique, applies a global linear transformation to the data assigning large weights to "relevant dimensions" and small weights to the "irrelevant ones". The relevant dimensions are identified considering "chunklets", that is, small subsets of points that are known to belong to the same group although the class label is usually unknown. The algorithm is shown next.

1. Let $X = \{\vec{x}\}_{i=1}^{N}$ the dataset and $C_j = \{x_{ji}\}_{i=1}^{n_j}$, $j = 1,\dots,n$ the chunklets of size n_j

2. Compute the within chunklet covariance matrix

$$\hat{C} = \frac{1}{N} \sum_{j=1}^{n} \sum_{i=1}^{n_j} (x_{ji} - m_j)(x_{ji} - m_j)^T \quad (15)$$

where m_j denotes the mean of the $j'th$ chunklet.

3. Reduce the dimensionality of the data using PCA or Fisher Linear Discriminant Analysis over $\hat{C}$

Compute the dissimilarities using the Mahalanobis distance induced by $\hat{C}$

$$d(\vec{x}_1, \vec{x}_2) = (\vec{x}_1 - \vec{x}_2)^T \hat{C}^{-1} (\vec{x}_1 - \vec{x}_2) \quad (16)$$

The first step in the algorithm is the identification of chunklets and the computation of the

within chunklet covariance matrix. If $\vec{x}_1$ is related to $\vec{x}_2$ by a similarity constraint and $\vec{x}_2$ is also related to $\vec{x}_3$ then $\{\vec{x}_1, \vec{x}_2, \vec{x}_3\}$ form a chunklet. RCA considers only positive constraints because they are more informative than negative constraints and the last ones are much harder to use computationally. The RCA algorithm requires only to compute the pseudoinverse of the covariance matrix $\hat{C}$. Considering negative constraints leads to non-linear optimization problems such as the one solved by (Xing, 2003) that are intensive computationally and more unstable.

The Mahalanobis distance learnt by the RCA algorithm is equivalent to transform linearly the data using the matrix $W = \hat{C}^{-\frac{1}{2}}$. The coordinates in the new axes are given by: $X_{new} = WX$. The whitening transformation W gives smaller weight to directions of large variability, because this variability is mainly due to changes within chunklets and are irrelevant for clustering purposes. This transformation will reduce the variability withing clusters and will increase the separation among different clusters. However, when the irrelevant noise is distributed among many dimensions with small amplitude, whitening may amplify these noisy directions with undesirable effects. Therefore, when we are dealing with high dimensional problems, X is previously projected to a subspace of smaller dimension. To this aim, dimensions with low total variability with respect to the within chunklet variability are removed. This can be accomplished by a variant of Fisher Linear Discriminant Analysis where the withing class covariance matrix is substituted by the withing chunklet covariance matrix employed by RCA. See (Bar-Hillel, 2005) for more details.

RCA have two interesting properties that are worth to mention:

- The algorithm has a strong theoretical foundation. In particular, the linear transformation carried out by RCA, $\mathbf{Y} = \mathbf{WX}$

seeks to maximize the mutual information between the input $\mathbf{X}$ and the new representation $\mathbf{Y}$ under suitable constraints. Therefore, RCA transformation preserves as much as possible clustering information. Besides, the optimization problem can be reformulated in terms of the within chunklet squared distances. Thus, RCA looks for a Mahalanobis metric such that it minimizes the sum of all within chunklet squared distances with a constraint to avoid the trivial solution. This interpretation, allow us to understand the connection between the method proposed by (Xing, 2003) and RCA.

- RCA is based on a lineal algebra operation that can be carried out efficiently.

Finally, we comment the main differences between the method proposed by (Xing, 2003) and RCA. Both methods minimize the sum of squared distances between objects related by positive constraints. However, the constraints proposed by (Xing, 2003) are based on the squared distances of dissimilar objects. The constraints in RCA formulation avoid the volume of the Mahalanobis distance to shrink indefinitely. As a result, the method proposed by *Xing* addresses a much harder non-linear optimization problem but it allow us to incorporate negative constraints.

Other approaches that have been proposed to learn the metric from the data are based on kernel alignment formalism (Kwok, 2003; Wu, 2005). Here, we focus on the method proposed by the first author. First an ideal kernel matrix is defined considering positive and negative constraints.

$$K_{ij}^* = \begin{cases} 1 & (\vec{x}_i, \vec{x}_j) \in S \\ 0 & (\vec{x}_i, \vec{x}_j) \in D \end{cases} \qquad (17)$$

Next, an idealized kernel matrix can be defined such that the original kernel becomes more similar to the ideal kernel:

$$\hat{K} = K + \frac{\gamma}{2} K^*, \qquad (18)$$

It is shown in the original paper that this definition increases the alignment between the idealized kernel and the ideal kernel (Kwok, 2003). Considering the relation between the Euclidean distance and kernels $\hat{d}_{ij} = \hat{K}_{ii} + \hat{K}_{jj} - 2\hat{K}_{ij}$ (Vapnik, 1998), the idealized distance that we should learn is defined as follows:

$$d_{ij}^{*2} = \begin{cases} d_{ij}^2 & (\vec{x}_i, \vec{x}_j) \in S \\ d_{ij}^2 + \gamma & (\vec{x}_i, \vec{x}_j) \in D \end{cases} \qquad (19)$$

Let $s_{ij} = \vec{x}_i^T \vec{x}_j$ the scalar product. If we incorporate input feature weights the inner product can be written as:

$$\hat{s}_{ij} = \vec{x}_i^T \mathbf{A} \mathbf{A}^T \vec{x}_j \qquad (20)$$

and the corresponding distance metric becomes:

$$\hat{d}_{ij}^2 = (\vec{x}_i - \vec{x}_j)^T \mathbf{A} \mathbf{A}^T (\vec{x}_i - \vec{x}_j) \qquad (21)$$

where notice that the metric to be learnt $\mathbf{A} \mathbf{A}^T$ is always positive semi-definite.

The goal is now to look for a matrix $\mathbf{A}$ such that the corresponding distance metric (21) verifies:

$$\hat{d}_{ij}^2 \begin{cases} \leq d_{ij}^2 & (\vec{x}_i, \vec{x}_j) \in S \\ \geq d_{ij}^2 + g & (\vec{x}_i, \vec{x}_j) \in D \end{cases} \qquad (22)$$

Considering the new metric, distances among similar patterns should become smaller while distances between dissimilar ones should get larger.

The matrix $\mathbf{A}$ can be learnt through the following optimization problem.

$$\min_{\mathbf{A},\gamma,\xi_{ij}} \frac{1}{2} \parallel \mathbf{A}\mathbf{A}^T \parallel^2 + \frac{C_S}{N_S} \sum_{(x_i,x_j) \in S} \xi_{ij} + \frac{C_D}{N_D} \sum_{(x_i,x_j) \in D} \xi_{ij}$$

(23)

$$s.\,t.\ d_{ij}^2 \geq \hat{d}_{ij}^2 - \xi_{ij} \qquad \forall\, (\vec{x}_i, \vec{x}_j) \in S \qquad (24)$$

$$\hat{d}_{ij}^2 - d_{ij}^2 \geq \gamma - \xi_{ij} \qquad \forall\, (\vec{x}_i, \vec{x}_j) \in D \qquad (25)$$

$$\xi_{ij} \geq 0 \quad \gamma \geq 0 \qquad\qquad (26)$$

The first term in (23) determines the complexity of the linear transformation, while the second and third correspond to the training error of the idealized metric approximation. ξ_{ij} are the slack variables that allows for errors in the constraints, C_S and C_D are regularization parameters that achieve a compromise between training error the complexity of the linear transformation. Finally, γ is a non negative parameter similar to the one employed in ν -SVM (Vapnik, 1998).

The previous problem can be solved in the dual using a standard quadratic programming approach. Therefore, the computational complexity depends on the number of constraints rather than on the dimensionality of the original space as it happens in the method proposed by (Xing, 2003). Besides, the error function doesn't have local minima.

Finally, some authors have proposed semi-supervised clustering algorithms that learn a Mahalanobis metric from the data and also modify the error function to incorporate constraint violations (Bilenko, 2004). Besides, different metrics are considered for each cluster. However, although clustering performance is slightly improved, this results in complex optimization problems that are too expensive for real applications.

MAIN FOCUS OF THE CHAPTER

In the background section, we introduced several semi-supervised clustering algorithms that are able incorporate a priori knowledge provided by human experts. Most of the algorithms, learn a Mahalanobis metric from a set of equivalence constraints given in the form of which pairs of objects are considered similar or dissimilar. However, the algorithms presented rely on the use of a single dissimilarity matrix such as the Mahalanobis metric. But, Mahalanobis based distances may not be appropriate for instance, to model the proximities between genes in Bioinformatics applications (Martín-Merino, 2009b). Besides, there are other dissimilarities that may come from different representations of the objects or from different data sources that provide complementary information to the classical Mahalanobis distance. Therefore, new clustering algorithms are needed that are able to incorporate different dissimilarities and data sources.

The problem of combining heterogeneous dissimilarities has been widely studied in the context of classification using kernel methods (see for instance (Lanckriet, 2004; Martín-Merino, 2009b). In clustering applications, the supervision is very sparse and it is usually provided in the form of equivalence constraints. Thus, learning algorithms that integrate heterogeneous dissimilarities are more difficult to develop and have been hardly studied. In this section, we introduce an algorithm to learn a combination of heterogeneous dissimilarities from a set of equivalence constraints.

Solutions and Recommendations

Let $\{d_{ij}^l\}_{l=1}^M$ be the set of heterogeneous dissimilarities considered. Each dissimilarity can be embedded in feature space via the empirical kernel map (Pekalska, 2001) introduced in appendix A. Let K_{ij}^l be the kernel matrix that represents the dissimilarity matrix $(d_{ij}^l)_{i,j=1}^n$. The kernel function can be written as an inner product in feature space (Vapnik, 1998) $k(\vec{x}_i, \vec{x}_j) = <\phi(\vec{x}_i), \phi(\vec{x}_j)>$ and therefore, it can be considered a similarity measure (Wu, 2005).

The ideal similarity (kernel) should be defined such that it becomes large for similar patterns and small for dissimilar ones. Mathematically, the ideal kernel is defined as follows:

$$k_{ij}^* = \begin{cases} \max_l \{k_{ij}^l\} & \text{If } (\vec{x}_i, \vec{x}_j) \in S \\ \min_l \{k_{ij}^l\} & \text{If } (\vec{x}_i, \vec{x}_j) \in D \end{cases} \tag{27}$$

The idealized kernel introduced in this section is related to the one proposed by (Cristianini, 2002) for classification purposes: $k(x_i, x_j) = 1$ if $y_i \neq y_j$ and zero otherwise. However, there are two differences that are worth to mention. First, the ideal kernel proposed by (Cristianini, 2002) doesn't take into account the structure and distribution of the data, missing relevant information particularly for clustering applications. The idealized kernel defined here, collect information from a set of similarity measures and hence considers the spatial distribution of the data. Second, the kernel proposed by (Cristianini, 2002) can be considered an extreme case of the idealized kernel defined earlier and thus, more prone to overfitting.

Considering the relation between distances and kernels (Vapnik, 1998), the idealized distance between $\vec{x}_i$ and $\vec{x}_j$ can be written in terms of kernel evaluations as:

$$d^{2*}(\vec{x}_i, \vec{x}_j) = \| \phi(\vec{x}_i) - \phi(\vec{x}_j) \|^2 \tag{28}$$

$$= k^*(\vec{x}_i, \vec{x}_i) + k^*(\vec{x}_j, \vec{x}_j) - 2k^*(\vec{x}_i, \vec{x}_j) \tag{29}$$

The idealized dissimilarity improves the separability among different groups in the data set. However, this dissimilarity may increase the overfitting. Hence, robust learning algorithms

should be developed that achieve a balance between the complexity of the family of distances and the separability among different clusters.

In this section, we present a learning algorithm to estimate the optimal weights of a linear combination of kernels from a set of similarity/dissimilarity constraints.

Let $\{k_{ij}^l\}_{l=1}^M$ be the set of kernels obtained from a set of heterogeneous dissimilarities via the empirical kernel map introduced in (Pekalska, 2001). If non-linear kernels with different parameter values are considered, we get a wider family of measures that includes non-linear transformations of the original dissimilarities. The kernel sought is defined as:

$$k_{ij} = \sum_{l=1}^M \beta_l k_{ij}^l, \tag{30}$$

where the β_l coefficients are constrained to be ≥ 0. This non negative constraint on the weights helps to interpret the results and guarantees that provided all the individual kernels are positive semi-definite the combination of kernels is convex and positive semi-definite (Soon Ong, 2005).

The optimization problem in the primal may be formulated as follows:

$$\min_{\vec{\beta}, \xi} \frac{1}{2} \| \vec{\beta} \|^2 + \frac{C_S}{N_S} \sum_{(x_i, x_j) \in S} \xi_{ij} + \frac{C_D}{N_D} \sum_{(x_i, x_j) \in D} \xi_{ij} \tag{31}$$

$$s.t. \quad \vec{b}^T \vec{K}_{ij} \geq K_{ij}^* - \xi_{ij} \quad \forall (\vec{x}_i, \vec{x}_j) \in S \tag{32}$$

$$\vec{\beta}^T \vec{K}_{ij} \leq K_{ij}^* + \xi_{ij} \quad \forall (\vec{x}_i, \vec{x}_j) \in D \tag{33}$$

$$\beta_l \geq 0 \quad \xi_{ij} \geq 0 \quad \forall l = 1, ..., M \tag{34}$$

where the first term in Equation (31) is a regularization term that penalizes the complexity of the family of distances, C_S and C_D are regularization parameters that give more relevance to the similarity or dissimilarity constraints. N_S, N_D are the number of pairs in S and D, $\vec{K}_{ij} = [K_{ij}^1, \ldots, K_{ij}^M]^T$, K_{ij}^* is the idealized kernel matrix introduced earlier and, ξ_{ij} are the slack variables that allows for errors in the constraints.

To solve this constrained optimization problem the method of Lagrange Multipliers is used. The dual problem becomes:

$$\max_{\alpha_{ij},\gamma} -\frac{1}{2} \sum_{\substack{(x_i,x_j)\in S \\ (x_k,x_l)\in S}} \alpha_{ij}\alpha_{kl}\mathbf{K}_{ij}^T\mathbf{K}_{kl} - \frac{1}{2} \sum_{\substack{(x_i,x_j)\in D \\ (x_k,x_l)\in D}} \alpha_{ij}\alpha_{kl}\mathbf{K}_{ij}^T\mathbf{K}_{kl} \tag{35}$$

$$+ \sum_{\substack{(x_i,x_j)\in S, \\ (x_k,x_l)\in D}} \alpha_{ij}\alpha_{kl}\mathbf{K}_{ij}^T\mathbf{K}_{kl} - \sum_{(x_i,x_j)\in S} \alpha_{ij}\gamma^T\mathbf{K}_{ij} - \frac{1}{2}\gamma^T\gamma \tag{36}$$

$$+ \sum_{(x_i,x_j)\in D} \alpha_{ij}\gamma^T\mathbf{K}_{ij} + \sum_{(x_i,x_j)\in S} \alpha_{ij}K_{ij}^* - \sum_{(x_i,x_j)\in D} \alpha_{ij}K_{ij}^*, \tag{37}$$

subject to:

$$0 \leq \alpha_{ij} \leq \begin{cases} \dfrac{C_S}{N_S} & \text{for } (\vec{x}_i,\vec{x}_j) \in S \\[2mm] \dfrac{C_D}{N_D} & \text{for } (\vec{x}_i,\vec{x}_j) \in D \end{cases} \tag{39}$$

$$\gamma_l \geq 0 \quad \forall l = 1,\ldots,M, \tag{40}$$

where α_{ij} and γ_l are the lagrange multipliers. This is a standard quadratic optimization problem similar to the one solved by the SVM. The computational burden does not depend on the dimensionality of the space and it avoids the problem of local minima.

Once the α_{ij} and γ_l are computed, the weights β_l can be obtained considering $\partial L / \partial \vec{\beta} = 0$:

$$\vec{\beta} = \sum_{(x_i,x_j)\in S} \alpha_{ij}\mathbf{K}_{ij} - \sum_{(x_i,x_j)\in D} \alpha_{ij}\mathbf{K}_{ij} + \vec{\gamma}. \tag{41}$$

The weights β_l can be substituted in Equation (30) to get the optimal combination of heterogeneous kernels. Next, a clustering or classification algorithm based on kernels may be applied.

The metric learning algorithm proposed allows to incorporate into kernel clustering algorithms a priory knowledge given in the form of equivalence constraints. However, it can also be applied to integrate a linear combination of heterogeneous dissimilarities and data sources into kernel based classifiers.

Several techniques related to the one proposed here, have been studied in section 2. In (Xing, 2003) it has been proposed an algorithm to learn a full or diagonal Mahalanobis metric from similarity information. The optimization algorithm is based on an iterative procedure that is more costly particularly for high dimensional problems. (Bar-Hillel, 2005) and (Kwok, 2003; Wu, 2005) have proposed more efficient algorithms to learn a Mahalanobis metric from equivalence constraints. The first one (Relevant Component Analysis), can only take into account similarity constraints and when there is no labels, the chunklets created from equivalence constraints are not well defined. All of them, rely solely on a Mahalanobis metric that may fail to reflect appropriately the sample proximities for certain kind of applications (Martín-Merino, 2009a; Martín-Merino, 2009b). Hence, they are not able to integrate heterogeneous measures that convey complementary information. Finally, (Zhao, 2009) has proposed a modification of the maximum margin clustering that is able to learn a linear combination of kernels. However, this algorithm is unsupervised and can not incorporate a priory information in a semi-supervised way. Besides, it can not be extended to other clustering and classification algorithms based on dissimilarities or kernels as the method proposed here.

Experimental Results

The algorithm proposed has been evaluated considering a wide range of applications. First, several clustering problems have been addressed. Table 1 shows the features of the different data sets. We have chosen problems with a broad range of signal to noise ratio (Var/Samp.), varying number of samples and classes. The first three problems correspond to benchmark data sets obtained from the UCI database http://archive.ics.uci.edu/ml/datasets/. The last ones aim to the identification of complex human cancer samples using the gene expression profiles. They are available from http://bioinformatics2.pitt.edu.

Finally, we apply the metric learning algorithm proposed to the prediction of protein subcellular location (Lanckriet, 2004) considering a set of heterogeneous data sources. We use as a gold standard the annotation provided by the MIPS comprehensive yeast genome database (CYGD). CYGD assigns subcellular locations to 2138 yeast proteins. The primary input for the learning algorithm is a collection of seven kernel matrices obtained from different data sources. For a detailed description of the sources and kernels employed see (Lanckriet, 2004b).

All the data sets have been standardised subtracting the median and dividing by the interquantile range.

For high dimensional problems such as gene expression data sets, dimension reduction helps to improve significantly the clustering results (Jeffery, 2006). Therefore, for the algorithms based on a single dissimilarity we have considered different number of genes $280, 146, 101, 56$ and 34 obtained by feature selection (Martín-Merino, 2009b). We have chosen the subset of genes that gives rise to the smallest error. Genes have been ranked according to the interquantile range. As we are addressing clustering problems, feature selection methods that take into account the class

Table 1. Features of the different data sets considered

	Samples	Variables	Var./Samp.	Classes
Wine (UCI)	177	13	0.17	3
Ionosphere (UCI)	351	35	0.01	2
Breast Cancer (UCI)	569	32	0.056	2
Lymphoma	96	4026	41.9	2
Colon Cancer	62	2000	32	2

labels are discarded. Regarding the algorithm proposed to integrate several dissimilarities, we have considered all the dissimilarities obtained for the whole set of dimensions.

The similarity/dissimilarity constraints are obtained as in (Xing, 2003). S is generated by picking a random subset of all pairs of points sharing the same class label. The size is chosen such that the number of connected components is roughly 20% of the size of the original data set. D is chosen in a similar way although the size in this case is less relevant. Twenty independent random samples for S and D are considered and the average error is reported.

Regarding the value of the parameters, the number of clusters is set up to the number of classes, C_S and C_D are regularization parameters and the optimal value is determined by cross-validation over the subset of labeled patterns. Finally, kernel k-means is restarted randomly 20 times and the errors provided are averages over 20 independent trials.

Clustering results have been evaluated considering two objective measures. The first one is the accuracy. It determines the probability that the clustering agrees with the "true" clustering in the sense that the pair of patterns belong to the same or different clusters. It has been defined as in (Xing, 2003):

$$accuracy = \sum_{i>j} \frac{1\{1\{c_i = c_j\} = 1\{\hat{c}_i = \hat{c}_j\}\}}{0.5m(m-1)}, \quad (42)$$

where c_i is the true cluster label for pattern x_i, $\hat{c}_i$ is the corresponding label returned by the clustering algorithm and m is the number of patterns. One problem of the accuracy is that the expected value for two random partitions is not zero. Therefore, we have computed also the adjusted randindex defined in (Hubert, 1985) that avoids this problem. This index is also normalized between zero and one and larger values suggest better clustering.

Tables 2 and 3 show the accuracy and the adjusted randindex for the clustering algorithms evaluated. We have compared with a standard metric learning strategy proposed by (Xing, 2003), k-means clustering based on the Euclidean distance and k-means considering the best dissimilarity out of ten different measures. Both tables indicates which is the best distance for each case.

From the analysis of Tables 2 and 3, the following conclusions can be drawn:

- The combination of dissimilarities improves significantly a standard metric learning algorithm for all the data sets considered. Our method is robust to overfitting and outperforms the algorithm proposed by (Xing, 2003) in high dimensional data sets such as Colon cancer and Lymphoma. These data sets exhibit a high level of noise. We can explain this because the algorithm based on a combination of dissimilarities allows to integrate distances computed for several dimensions discarding the noise and reducing the errors.

- The combination of dissimilarities improves usually kernel k-means based solely on the best dissimilarity. This suggests that the integration of several dissimilarities allows to extract complementary information that may help to improve the performance. Besides, the algorithm proposed always achieves at least the same performance that k-means based on the best dissimilarity. Only for lymphoma and polynomial kernel we get worst results, probably

Table 2. Accuracy for k-means clustering considering different dissimilarities. The results are averaged over twenty independent random subsets S and D

Technique	Kernel	Wine	Ionosphere	Breast	Colon	Lymphoma
k-means (Euclidean)	linear	0.92	0.72	0.88	0.87	0.90
	pol. 3	0.87	0.73	0.88	0.88	0.90
k-means (Best diss.)	linear	0.94	0.88	0.90	0.88	0.94
	pol. 3	0.94	0.88	0.90	0.88	0.93
		χ^2	Maha.	Manha.	Corr./euclid.	χ^2
Comb. dissimilarities	linear	0.94	0.90	0.92	0.89	0.95
	pol. 3	0.96	0.89	0.92	0.90	0.92
Metric learning (Xing)	linear	0.87	0.74	0.85	0.87	0.90
	pol. 3	0.51	0.74	0.86	0.88	0.90

Table 3. Adjusted RandIndex for k-means clustering considering different dissimilarities. The results are averaged over twenty independent random subsets S and D

Technique	Kernel	Wine	Ionosphere	Breast	Colon	Lymphoma
k-means (Euclidean)	linear	0.79	0.20	0.59	0.59	0.65
	pol. 3	0.67	0.21	0.60	0.59	0.65
k-means (Best diss.)	linear	0.82	0.58	0.66	0.59	0.77
	pol. 3	0.81	0.58	0.66	0.59	0.76
		χ^2	Maha.	Manha.	Corr./euclid.	χ^2
Comb. dissimilarities	linear	0.82	0.63	0.69	0.60	0.79
	pol. 3	0.85	0.60	0.69	0.63	0.73
Metric learning (Xing)	linear	0.68	0.23	0.50	0.54	0.66
	pol. 3	0.50	0.23	0.52	0.58	0.65

because the value assigned to the regularization parameters overfit the data. We remark that the algorithm proposed, helps to overcome the problem of choosing the best dissimilarity, the kernel and the optimal dimension. This a quite complex and time consuming task for certain applications such as Bioinformatics.

Finally, the combination of dissimilarities improves always the standard k-means clustering based on the Euclidean measure.

- Tables 2 and 3 show that the best distance depends on the data set considered. Moreover, we report that the performance of k-means depends strongly on the particular measure employed to evaluate the sample proximities.

Figures 1(a) and (b) show a boxplot diagram for the accuracy and adjusted randindex coefficients. Twenty independent random samples for S and D are considered. Odds numbers correspond to the combination of dissimilarities and the even ones to the metric learning algorithm proposed by (Xing, 2003). We can see that the differences between the method proposed here and the one proposed by (Xing, 2003) are statistically significant at 95% confidence level for all the data sets considered.

Regarding the identification of membrane protein classes, a linear combination of seven heterogeneous kernels (data sources) is learnt considering only similarity constraints. The size of S is chosen such that the number of connected components is roughly 10% of the number of patterns. Once the kernel is learnt, a k-NN algorithm is run and the accuracy is estimated by ten-fold cross-validation. We have compared with k-NN based solely on a single data source and with the Lanckriet formalism (Lanckriet, 2004b). Notice that the method proposed by Lanckriet is not able to work from similarity constraints only and needs the class labels. Besides, it is only applicable for SVM classifiers.

Table 4 shows that our algorithm improves k-NN based on a single kernel (source) by at least

Figure 1(a). Boxplots that compare the combination of dissimilarities with the metric learning algo-rithm proposed by Xing according to accuracy. All the boxplots consider linear kernels. (b). Boxplots that compare the combination of dissimilarities with the metric learning algorithm proposed by Xing according to Adjusted RandIndex. All the boxplots consider linear kernels.

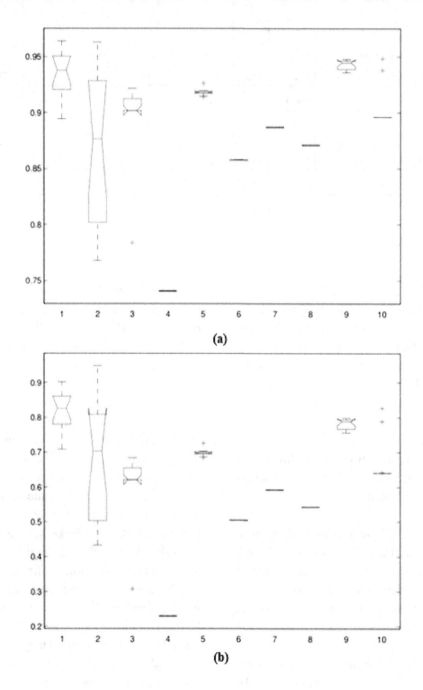

(a)

(b)

Table 4. Accuracy of k-NN considering the best data sources and learning the optimal weights of a combination of heterogeneous data sources. Only five sources with non-null β_l are shown

Source	Gen. Expre.	BLAST	Pfam	Hydropho.	Difussion	Combination	Lanckriet
Accuracy	73.30%	79.98%	82.48%	77.01%	80.16%	86.68%	88.66%
β_l	0.24	0.15	0.29	0.62	4.45	-	-

4%. The β_l coefficients are larger for the diffusion and Hydrophobicity FFT kernels which is consistent with the analysis of (Lanckriet, 2004b) that suggests that diffusion kernels perform the best. Kernels removed correspond to redundant kernels and not to the less informative as suggested by (Hulsman, 2009). Our method performs similarly to the algorithm proposed by Lanckriet although we use only 10% of similarity constraints. Finally, we have incorporated a random kernel (source) to check the robustness against noise. The accuracy is similar (86.75%) which suggests that the combination algorithm tolerates high level of noise.

FUTURE RESEARCH DIRECTIONS

In this chapter, we have introduced several clustering algorithms that are able to adapt the metric to the data considering the a priori knowledge provided by human experts. However, modern applications such as genomics or proteomics pose several challenges that require the development of new machine learning techniques. Next, we outline several issues that should be addressed in the future.

First, more complex combinations of dissimilarities should be studied in order to model complex relationships in bioinformatics applications. To this aim, (Woznica, 2007) have proposed a method to learn non-linear combinations of dissimilarities. (Gehler, 2008) have developed a framework that may allow to consider infinite families of dissimilarities and powerfull transformations of them. Currently, this method is only applicable to classification techniques based on kernel methods, but it may be adapted for clustering applications.

Although we have assumed that the a priori knowledge provided by human experts has no probability of error, this is not true in general. For instance, the classification of certain cancer types is likely to be wrong, due to the lack of information, errors in the technology considered etc. Therefore, clustering algorithms should incorporate the a priori knowledge considering a certain probability of error. Several authors have addressed this problem (Stempfel, 2009) but in the context of classification rather than for clustering.

In biological applications, human experts provide often a priori knowledge using different types of constraints. Therefore, new semi-supervised clustering algorithms should be developed that are able to integrate different types of constraints.

Finally, modern applications such as genomics and proteomics require the development of hybrid techniques that exploit the advantages of clustering and classification algorithms. For this kind of applications, some classes may be known, others may be unknown or may correspond to a highly heterogeneous set of objects. Supervision may be formulated in the form of labels, different types of constraints etc. Therefore, a new class of machine learning techniques are needed that take advantage of all this supervised information.

CONCLUSION

In this chapter, we have introduced several semi-supervised clustering algorithms that are able to adapt the metric to the data considering the a priori knowledge provided by human experts. Next, a semi-supervised algorithm is proposed that is able to learn a combination of dissimilarities from a set of equivalence constraints. The error function includes a penalty term that controls the complexity of the family of distances considered and the optimization is based on a robust quadratic programming approach that does not suffer from the problem of local minima.

The experimental results suggest that the combination of dissimilarities improves almost always the performance of clustering and classification algorithms based solely on a single dissimilarity. Besides, the algorithm proposed improves significantly a standard metric learning algorithm for all the data sets considered in this chapter and is robust to overfitting.

REFERENCES

Bar-Hillel, A., Hertz, T., Shental, N., & Weinshall, D. (2005). Learning a Mahalanobis metric from equivalence constraints. *Journal of Machine Learning Research*, 6, 937–965.

Bilenko, M., Basu, S., & Mooney, R. J. (2004). Integrating constraints and metric learning in semi-supervised clustering. *Proceedings of the 21 International Conference on Machine Learning* (pp. 81-88). Banff, Canada.

Cox, T. F., & Cox, M. A. A. (2001). *Multidimensional scaling* (2nd ed.). USA: Chapman & Hall/CRC.

Cristianini, N., Kandola, J., Elisseeff, J., & Shawe-Taylor, A. (2002). On the kernel target alignment. *Journal of Machine Learning Research*, 1, 1–31.

Gehler, P. V., & Nowozin, S. (2008). Infinite kernel learning. *Proceedings of the NIPS 2008 Workshop on Kernel Learning: Automatic Selection of Optimal Kernels.*

Huang, D., & Pan, W. (2006). Incorporating biological knowledge into distance-based clustering analysis of microarray gene expression data. *Bioinformatics (Oxford, England)*, 22(10), 1259–1268. doi:10.1093/bioinformatics/btl065

Hubert, L., & Arabie, P. (1985). Comparing partitions. *Journal of Classification*, 2(1), 193–218. doi:10.1007/BF01908075

Hulsman, M., Reinders, M. J. T., & de Ridder, D. (2009). Evolutionary optimization of kernel weights improves protein complex comembership prediction. *IEEE/ACM Transactions on Computational Biology and Bioinformatics*, 6(3), 427–437. doi:10.1109/TCBB.2008.137

Jeffery, I. B., Higgins, D. G., & Culhane, A. C. (2006). Comparison and evaluation methods for generating differentially expressed gene list from microarray data. *BMC Bioinformatics*, 7(359), 1–16.

Kwok, J. T., & Tsang, I. W. (2003). Learning with idealized kernels. *Proceedings of the Twentieth International Conference on Machine Learning*, (pp. 400-407). Washington, DC.

Lanckriet, G., Cristianini, N., Barlett, P., El Ghaoui, L., & Jordan, M. (2004). Learning the kernel matrix with semidefinite programming. *Journal of Machine Learning Research*, 3, 27–72.

Lanckriet, G. R. G., De Bie, T., Cristianini, N., Jordan, M. I., & Stafford Noble, W. (2004b). A statistical framework for genomic data fusion. *Bioinformatics (Oxford, England)*, 20(16), 2626–2635. doi:10.1093/bioinformatics/bth294

Martín-Merino, M., & Blanco, A. (2009a). A local semi-supervised Sammon algorithm for textual data visualization. *Journal of Intelligent Information Systems, 33*(1), 23–40. doi:10.1007/s10844-008-0056-5

Martín-Merino, M., Blanco, A., & De Las Rivas, J. (2009b). Combining dissimilarities in a hyper reproducing kernel Hilbert space for complex human cancer prediction. *Journal of Biomedicine & Biotechnology, 2009*, 1–9. doi:10.1155/2009/906865

Pekalska, E., Paclick, P., & Duin, R. (2004). A generalized kernel approach to dissimilarity-based classification. *Journal of Machine Learning Research, 2*, 175-211, 2001.

Shawe-Taylor, J., & Cristianini, N. (2004). *Kernel methods for pattern analysis.* Cambridge University Press. doi:10.1017/CBO9780511809682

Soon Ong, C., Smola, A., & Williamson, R. (2005). Learning the kernel with hyperkernels. *Journal of Machine Learning Research, 6*, 1043–1071.

Stempfel, G., & Ralaivola, L. (2009). Learning SVMs from sloppily labeled data. *International Conference on Artificial Neural Networks*, Vol. 1, (pp. 884-893).

Vapnik, V. (1998). *Statistical learning theory.* New York, NY: John Wiley & Sons.

Woznica, A., Kalousis, A., & Hilario, M. (2007). Learning to combine distances for complex representations. In *Proceedings of the 24th International Conference on Machine Learning*, (pp. 1031-1038). Corvallis, USA.

Wu, G., Chang, E. Y., & Panda, N. (2005). *Formulating distance functions via the kernel trick* (pp. 703–709). Chicago: ACM SIGKDD.

Xing, E., Ng, A., Jordan, M., & Russell, S. (2003). Distance metric learning, with application to clustering with side-information. *Advances in Neural Information Processing Systems, 15*, 505–512.

Xiong, H., & Chen, X.-W. (2006). Kernel-based distance metric learning for microarray data classification. *BMC Bioinformatics, 7*(299), 1–11.

Zhao, B., Kwok, J. T., & Zhang, C. (2009). Multiple kernel clustering. *Proceedings of the Ninth SIAM International Conference on Data Mining*, (pp. 638-649). Nevada.

KEY TERMS AND DEFINITIONS

Clustering: Algorithms that identify groups of similar objects without external supervision.

Mercer Kernel: Positive definite function that transforms non-linearly the data to feature space and that can be written in terms of a scalar product.

Metric: A function that evaluates the proximities among the objects and that obeys three mathematical properties, non-negative, symetry and triangle inequality.

Metric Learning: The process of adapting the metric to the particular data considered.

Microarrays: Synthetic chip that allows to monitor the expression levels of thousands of genes simultaneously.

Prototype: The best representative for a group of objects.

Semi-Supervised Learning: Particular case of learning in which the algorithm takes into account non-labeled data in order to improve the parameter estimation.

Support Vector Machines: Non-linear classifiers with high generalization ability and that rely on a robust quadratic optimization algorithm.

APPENDIX A

This appendix introduces shortly the Empirical Kernel Map that allow us to work with non-Euclidean dissimilarities considering kernel methods (Pekalska, 2001).

Let $d: X \times X \to R$ be a dissimilarity and $R = \{\vec{x}_1, \ldots, \vec{x}_n\}$ a subset of representatives drawn from the training set. Define the mapping $\phi: F \to R^n$ as:

$$\phi(z) = D(z, R) = [d(z, \vec{x}_1), d(z, \vec{x}_2), \ldots, d(z, \vec{x}_n)]$$
(42)

This mapping defines a dissimilarity space where feature i is given by $d(., \vec{x}_i)$. The set of representatives R determines the dimensionality of the feature space.

The kernel of dissimilarities can be defined as the dot product of two dissimilarity vectors in feature space.

$$k(\vec{x}, \vec{x}') = < \phi(\vec{x}), \phi(\vec{x}') > = \sum_{i=1}^{n} d(\vec{x}, p_i) d(\vec{x}', p_i) \quad \forall \vec{x}, \vec{x}' \in X.$$
(43)

The resulting kernel matrix is positive definite which is interesting in order to obtain convex optimization problems. Any algorithm based on kernels can be extended to work with a given dissimilarity matrix considering the kernel of dissimilarities defined by equation (43).

Chapter 5
Real–Time Robust Heart Rate Estimation Based on Bayesian Framework and Grid Filters

Radoslav Bortel
Czech Technical University in Prague, Czech Republic

Pavel Sovka
Czech Technical University in Prague, Czech Republic

ABSTRACT

In this chapter, the authors discuss derivation, implementation, and testing of a robust real-time algorithm for the estimation of heart rate (HR) from electrocardiograms recorded on subjects performing vigorous physical activity. They formulate the problem of HR estimation as a problem of inference in a Bayesian network, which utilizes prior information about the probability distribution of HR changes. From this formulation they derive an inference procedure, which can be implemented as a grid filter. The resulting algorithm can then follow even a rapidly changing HR, whilst withstanding a series of missed or false QRS detections. Also, the HR estimate is complete with confidence intervals to allow the identification of the moments, where the precision of HR estimation is lowered. Additionally, the computational complexity of this algorithm is acceptable for battery powered portable devices.

INTRODUCTION

In many hazardous occupations (e.g. soldiers, fire-fighters) the chance of a failure increases with the stress levels under which an individual performs. High stress levels can diminish person's ability to carry out even simple tasks, which can endanger the individual or the group this individual is a part of. It is therefore desired to assess and follow the stress levels of individuals performing under harsh conditions, and to withdraw them if they become unfit for their job.

DOI: 10.4018/978-1-4666-1803-9.ch005

One way to estimate stress levels is by measuring the heart rate (HR). Once a person is highly aroused, the sympathetic branch of his/her autonomous neural system becomes active, which influences the heart, and increases HR to high levels (Andreassi, 2000).

There are several physiological measures, from which HR can be estimated. In this chapter we will describe a method based on electrocardiograms (ECG), in which we detect QRS complexes, compute the distance between two successive QRS complexes, i.e. so called R-R interval, and then estimate the HR as the inverse of this R-R interval.

The main problem of this approach is that the detection of QRS complexes can be quite unreliable if the measured subject is intensely moving. Under such circumstances the ECG record can be often heavily corrupted by various artifacts caused by electrode movement, activity of skeletal muscles or external electromagnetic interference. Additionally, HR changes can be rapid and wide, ranging from resting to the maximum HR. Under these conditions even the best of QRS complex detectors are not guaranteed to correctly identify all the heartbeats. Faulty detections can occur, and QRS complexes can be missed in time intervals stretching over several tens of seconds. It is therefore necessary to further process QRS complex detections, and device a robust estimator that can reconstruct HR in a stable and reliable way.

In this chapter we will present an approach to a real-time HR estimation based on a Bayesian framework. This problem will be formulated as a Bayesian network, which utilizes prior information about the probability distribution of HR changes. From this formulation we will derive an inference procedure that can be implemented as a grid filter. The resulting algorithm can then follow even a rapidly changing HR, whilst withstanding a series of missed or false QRS detections. Also, we will suggest a procedure for the computation of confidence intervals to allow the identification of moments, where the precision of HR estimation is lowered. Additionally, the algorithm is designed

so that its computational complexity is acceptable for battery powered portable devices.

We will also present results of real-life tests using ECG data obtained from subjects performing bouts of vigorous physical exercises. We will show that despite all the difficulties and ECG signal corruption, the algorithm is capable to estimate the HR with fair reliability.

BACKGROUND

The signal processing chain for the HR estimation is shown in Figure 1. First, the electric potentials created by the heart are measured, amplified and digitized. After, an algorithm commonly termed as a QRS complex detector, or simply QRS detector, searches the ECG signal, and identifies all the recognizable QRS complexes. Last, the positions of the QRS complexes are used to estimate the HR of the measured subject.

Even though in this chapter we will concentrate chiefly on the last stage - the HR estimation - it is important to understand characteristics of data we are going to process. Therefore, in this section we will provide a brief overview of all the abovementioned signal processing stages. Namely, we will comment on heart activity, ECG signal measurement, QRS complex detection, current state of the art of a robust HR estimation, and also on the Bayesian framework that we are going to use in the design our HR estimator.

Heart Activity

Being controlled by both sympathetic and parasympathetic branches of the nervous system, the heart activity adjusts to meet the blood supply needs of a human body, and is affected by emotional stimuli. For the purpose of the HR estimation it is important to note that HR changes can be quite variable. Mostly, the HR is fairly stable or changing slowly (e.g. during rest, or sustained physical activity). However, sometimes a strong

Figure 1. The signal processing chain used for the heart rate estimation

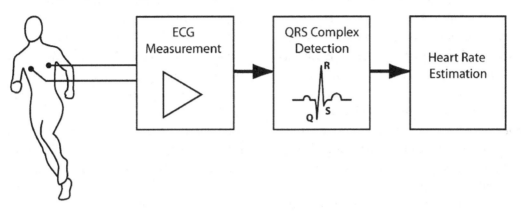

stressful stimulus, or a sudden onset of physical activity (or a combination of both), can cause a rapid change of HR. These rapid changes, however, are somewhat less frequent than the stable heart operation; therefore, the HR estimate can be expected to contain intervals of stable or slowly changing HR, punctuated by irregular occurrence of rapid HR changes. However, the rapid HR changes are important indicators of changes in the state of the monitored subjects; therefore, our HR estimation algorithm will be developed so that it can track rapid HR changes well.

For a more detailed discussion of HR and heart physiology see (Andreassi, 2000; Cacioppo at al., 2007).

ECG Measurement

An ECG signal is normally measured by at least two electrodes, which are placed directly on the subject's skin. The signal is amplified, and subsequently digitized for further digital signal processing. The chief problem of this process is that the measured potential is not created merely by the heart activity, but there are other interfering contributions, commonly referred to as *artifacts*.

First, the electrode skin contact can create potentials that are many times greater than the amplitude of ECG. This is especially true if the subject is moving so vigorously that s/he causes

the movement of the electrodes. Mechanical movement of the electrodes can create instability of their electrochemical potentials, which can shift the baseline of ECG by amount many times exceeding the amplitude of QRS complexes. This phenomenon is commonly called *baseline wander*, and if it gets excessive, it can cause saturation of the measurement amplifiers and consequent corruption of the ECG signal (examples of ECG corrupted by saturation caused by baseline wander are presented towards the end of this chapter).

Another, source of artifacts is the omnipresent power noise interference, which gets more prominent as the quality (i.e. conductance) of the electrode-skin contact decreases.

Yet another source of artifacts is the electrical activity of skeletal muscles underneath the electrodes. These artifacts can usually be mitigated by a suitable placement of the electrodes.

QRS Detection

A QRS detector is an algorithm, which analyzes an ECG signal, and tries to identify the positions of all QRS complexes. Additionally, a QRS detector may also supplement the position of each QRS complex with an indication of certainty, with which this QRS complex was detected.

The algorithm presented in this chapter is supposed to operate on results of a general QRS detector; therefore, the problem of the QRS detection itself is not within our scope. However, to guide a reader who would be interested in this topic, we provide a brief comment on various types of QRS detectors (note that this section is not meant to provide a review of the current state of the art of the QRS detection algorithms; we only point out a few representative works that can provide an interested reader a basic overview of the topic). For more detailed review we recommend consulting (Kohler, 2002).

The research of QRS detection has grown wide, and provided a great variety of various principles, among which it is possible to recognize the following approaches. First, it is so called filtering approach, in which the ECG is filtered to some band of interest, and then QRS complexes are detected as a rise of power in this filtered signal (e.g. Fiersen, 1990; Pan, 1985). Next, so called correlation approach computes a correlation of ECG with a template QRS complex, detecting QRS occurrences as spikes in the correlation function (e.g. Ruha, 1997). More complex methods can detect QRS complexes using neural networks (e.g. Barro, 1998; Dokur, 1997), filter banks (e.g. Alfonso, 1995; Alfonso, 1999), adaptive filters (e.g. Hamilton, 1988), hidden Markov models (e.g. Coast, 1990) and several other techniques.

Note that in the following text, we will refer to the act of QRS detection as a measurement.

Robust HR Estimation

So far only limited work has been done in the field of robust HR estimation from corrupted detection of QRS complexes. Most commonly, the HR was estimated directly by mere inversion of R-R intervals, and the only correction was the exclusion of physiologically unfeasible data (e.g. Pan, 1985).

A simple attempt for a more robust approach that can cope with noisy data was presented by Cheng (2006). In this work the HR was estimated based on the R-R interval most commonly occur-

ring in a given time window. Specifically, after the detection of QRS complexes, the R-R intervals were computed, and physiologically implausible values were excluded. The rest of the R-R intervals were used to construct a histogram (using 34 bins spanning from 40 to 209bpm). The maximum of this histogram was identified, and its position was used to derive the most probable value of the R-R interval and the corresponding HR for the given segment. This algorithm was shown to provide a certain level of robustness; however, there are some shortcomings: This algorithm derives the HR as a characteristic of a data segment, which, for reliable operation, needs to contain a certain number of heart beats. Therefore, this algorithm will provide the HR estimate only *after* collecting all these heart beats, thus introducing an unpleasant time delay. Moreover, the averaging nature of this algorithm will diminish its ability to track rapid HR changes. Also, no confidence limits of the HR estimate are provided.

Yet another simple attempt for robust HR estimation was suggested by Piotrowski (2010). In this paper it was suggested to compute the autocorrelation function of a filtered and segmented ECG, and estimate the HR from the maximum of this autocorrelation function. We admit that such approach could provide certain robustness against artifacts if the segment from which the autocorrelation function is estimated is sufficiently long, and the HR in this segment is stable. However, to account for changing HR the ECG segment would have to be shortened, in which case the autocorrelation function would no longer be robust against artifacts. Therefore, this approach does not allow estimation of changing HR from ECG signal corrupted by artifacts.

A more complex approach to HR estimation was suggested by Stegle (2008). This work presented an algorithm, which was constructed for a long-term HR estimation, and was designed to be resistant against outliers and noise bursts. This algorithm involves two steps: unsupervised clustering followed by a Bayesian regression. The

Gaussian process (GP) regression model uses the results of the clustering as prior information, and also incorporates additional expert knowledge about the physiology of the heart. The prior knowledge specifies smoothness assumptions about typical properties of the HR. Two periodicities are taken into account: the circadian rhythm and 2-3 minute periodicities. It is not assumed that the HR would manifest any rapid changes (i.e. substantial changes within a few heart beats). Additionally, this algorithm does not use the measurements of the individual R-R intervals directly, but merely uses data pre-processed by wearable heart monitors. Specifically, this algorithm operates on the trimmed mean HR estimate based on the 16 most recent R-R intervals and additional auxiliary data such as two longest and shortest R-R intervals. Therefore, even though this algorithm manifests some robust performance, it is mostly suitable for off-line processing and for prediction of the latent HR from the long-term (several days) recordings.

Overall, none of the above-mentioned algorithms seems to be suitable to track HR under the conditions of our interest. Therefore, we have decided to devise a new algorithm that would be able to promptly track rapid HR changes, while retaining its robustness even if the function of a QRS detector is impaired by a strong corruption of the analyzed ECG signal.

Bayesian Networks

Bayesian networks are structures that allow to graphically describe dependences (and independences) of a higher number of random variables. Loosely speaking a Bayesian network describes the joint distribution of a set of random variables as a directed acyclic graph (DAG), where conditional dependences between the individual random variables are represented as directed edges.

A formal definition of a Bayesian network follows:

Let $\mathbf{V} = \{v_1, \ldots, v_N\}$ be a set of random variables v_n with the joint probability distribution $p(v_1, \ldots, v_N)$, and $G = (V, E)$ be a DAG, with nodes $\mathbf{V}$ and edges $\mathbf{E}$. Further, let $(\mathbf{G}, p)$ be a pair such that each $v \in \mathbf{V}$ is conditionally independent of the set of all its nondescendants given the set of all its parents

$$P(v \mid \mathbf{ND}_v, \mathbf{PA}_v) = P(v \mid \mathbf{PA}_v), \qquad (1.1)$$

where $P(. \mid .)$ denotes the conditional probability operator, $\mathbf{ND}_v$ denotes the set of all nondescendants of v in $\mathbf{G}$, and $\mathbf{PA}_v$ denotes the set of all parents of v in $\mathbf{G}$. Then, we say that $(\mathbf{G}, p)$ satisfies so called Marcov condition, and $(\mathbf{G}, p)$ is a *Bayesian network*.

An important concept in the theory of Bayesian networks is so called d-separation that allows us to identify independencies among the individual random variables based on the examination of the graph $\mathbf{G}$.

This is a formal definition of d-separation:

Let $\mathbf{G}$ be a DAG with nodes $\mathbf{V}$ and edges $\mathbf{E}$, $\mathbf{A}$ be a subset of $\mathbf{V}$, $x, y \in \mathbf{V} - \mathbf{A}$ be two distinct nodes, and q be a chain (i.e. a path with edges in an arbitrary direction) between x and y. Then, q is d-separated by $\mathbf{A}$ if one of the following holds:

1. There is a node $z \in \mathbf{A}$ on the chain q, and this node connects one incoming and one outgoing edge of q.
2. There is a node $z \in \mathbf{A}$ on the chain q, and this node connects two outgoing edges of q.
3. There is a node z on the chain q, such that z and all of its descendents are not in $\mathbf{A}$, and this node connects two incoming edges of q.

If every chain between x and y is d-separated by $\mathbf{A}$, we say that x and y are d-separated by $\mathbf{A}$.

If $\mathbf{A}$, $\mathbf{B}$ and $\mathbf{C}$ are mutually disjoint subsets of $\mathbf{V}$, and each element of $\mathbf{A}$ is d-separated from each element of $\mathbf{B}$ by $\mathbf{C}$, then we say that $\mathbf{A}$ and $\mathbf{B}$ are d-separated by $\mathbf{C}$.

If $(\mathbf{G}, p)$ is a Bayesian network, $\mathbf{A}$, $\mathbf{B}$ and $\mathbf{C}$ are mutually disjoint subsets of $\mathbf{V}$, and $\mathbf{A}$ and $\mathbf{B}$ are d-separated by $\mathbf{C}$, then $\mathbf{A}$ and $\mathbf{B}$ are independent given $\mathbf{C}$

$$P(\mathbf{A} \mid \mathbf{B}, \mathbf{C}) = P(\mathbf{A} \mid \mathbf{C}). \qquad (1.2)$$

For proof see (Verma & Pearl, 1990; Neapolitan, 1990).

Readers, who would like to learn more about Bayesian inference and Bayesian networks, will find a list of recommended sources at the end of this chapter.

THE HEART RATE ESTIMATION ALGORITHM

In this section we will describe the derivation, implementation and testing of the proposed HR estimation algorithm. First, we will formulate the HR estimation as a problem of Bayesian inference, using a Bayesian network to describe the joint probability distribution of our random variables. Then, we will derive a recursive formula, which will allow the update of the HR estimate distribution after each QRS complex detection. Next, we will approximate this formula, creating a grid-based filter, which is suitable for a practical implementation. After, we will discuss how to express all the probabilities, which the grid-based filter contains. Last, our algorithm will be summarized and presented in a form of a pseudocode.

Problem Formulation

In the following text we will repeatedly use these symbols and notations:

- x_n will denote the HR during the n-th measurement. Note that x_n will be expressed in beats per minute (bpm); therefore, to convert it to the corresponding R-R interval, we have to compute $60 / x_n$.

- y_n will denote the estimate of the R-R interval between the n-th and $(n-1)$-th measurement, i.e. $y_n = R_n - R_{n-1}$, where R_n denotes the time index of the n-th detected QRS complex (note that if our QRS detector misses a heart beat in-between the n-th and $(n-1)$-th QRS detection, the value y_n will become the sum of several inter-beat intervals).

- $y_{1:n}$ and $x_{1:n}$ will denote vectors $[y_1, y_2, \ldots, y_n]$ and $[x_1, x_2, \ldots, x_n]$, respectively.

- w_n will denote the number of QRS complexes that were not detected immediately prior to the detection of the n-th QRS complex.

Also, we will often work with the following probability functions:

- $p\left(y_n \mid x_n, w_n\right)$ will denote the probability distribution of the R-R interval y_n, given we know the HR x_n, and we know that w_n QRS complexes were not detected immediately prior to the n-th measurement.

- $p\left(x_n \mid x_{1:n-1}\right)$ will denote the probability distribution of the HR estimate during the n-th measurement, given we know the HR for the first $n-1$ measurements.

- $p\left(x_n \mid y_{1:n}\right)$ will denote the probability distribution of the HR estimate during the n-th measurement, given we know all the

Figure 2. A Bayesian network representing the joint probability distribution of $x_{1:n+1}$, $y_{1:n+1}$ and $w_{1:n+1}$. The nodes x_n represent the HR, the nodes y_n represent the measured R-R intervals, and the nodes w_n represent the number of QRS complexes that were not detected immediately prior to the detection of the n-th QRS complex. Crossing indicates the nodes, the values of which are known after the detection of the n-th QRS complex.

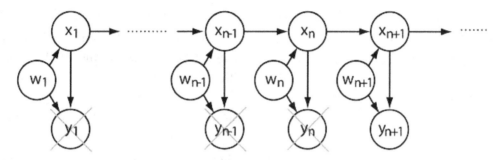

measured R-R intervals $y_{1:n}$. This probability distribution expresses our objective, which we will attempt to estimate.

Now, we will formulate our problem as a problem of inference in a Bayesian network. To construct our Bayesian network, we have to consider the following dependencies. Obviously, the length of the R-R interval y_n will depend on the HR x_n and the number of missed heart beat detections w_n immediately prior to the n-th measurement. Next, the HR x_n during the n-th measurement can generally depend on the HR during all the previous measurements $x_{1:n-1}$. However, to account for such dependence would require a Bayesian network too complex to trace; therefore, we opted for the following simplification: we will assume that the HR x_n depends only on its value during the previous measurement, i.e. x_{n-1}, and is independent of all its previous values $x_{1:n-2}$

$$\mathrm{p}\left(\mathrm{x}_n|\mathrm{x}_{1:n-1}\right)=\mathrm{p}\left(\mathrm{x}_n|\mathrm{x}_{n-1}\right). \qquad (1.3)$$

Further, we have to consider the following: it may be quite safe to assume that there is a single probability distribution $p\left(x_n \mid x_{n-1}\right)$ that describes

the distribution of x_n based on the knowledge of x_{n-1} sufficiently well, if x_n and x_{n-1} are the HR during two successive heart beats. However, if we missed some heart beat detections prior to the n-th measurement, more time passed since the last measurement, and the prediction of x_n based on x_{n-1} is less certain. Therefore, we have to take into account that the distribution of x_n is not dependent only on x_{n-1}, but also on w_n, the number of the missed beats prior to the n-th measurement.

When we consider the above-mentioned dependences, we can construct a Bayesian network that represents the joint probability of $x_{1:n+1}$, $y_{1:n+1}$ and $w_{1:n+1}$ as shown in Figure 2.

Now, we will use the this Bayesian network to express the probability $p\left(x_n \mid y_{1:n}\right)$ in a recursive form, i.e. as a function of $p\left(x_{1:n-1} \mid y_{1:n-1}\right)$ (which was obtained during the previous measurement) and the value of the last measurement y_n.

A simple application of Bayes' theorem gives

$$p(x_n \mid y_{1:n}) \propto p(y_n \mid x_n, y_{1:n-1})p(x_n \mid y_{1:n-1}), \qquad (1.4)$$

where $\propto$ denotes equality up to a multiplicative constant. Through the application of the law of

Box 1.

$$\sum_{w_n} p(y_n \mid x_n, y_{1:n-1}, w_n) \frac{p(x_n \mid w_n, y_{1:n-1})p(w_n \mid y_{1:n-1})}{p(x_n \mid y_{1:n-1})} p(x_n \mid y_{1:n-1}) \qquad (1.6)$$

total probability, the right hand side of (1.4) can be extended into

$$\sum_{w_n} p(y_n \mid x_n, y_{1:n-1}, w_n)p(w_n \mid x_n, y_{1:n-1})p(x_n \mid y_{1:n-1}). \qquad (1.5)$$

Application of Bayes' theorem to $p(w_n \mid x_n, y_{1:n-1})$ then gives (see Box 1 for Equation (1.6))

Now, thanks to the d-separation of sets $\{y_n\}$ and $\{y_{1:n-1}\}$ by the set $\{x_n, w_n\}$ it holds that

$$p(y_n \mid x_n, y_{1:n-1}, w_n) = p(y_n \mid x_n, w_n), \qquad (1.7)$$

and thanks to the d-separation of sets $\{y_{1:n-1}\}$ and $\{w_n\}$ by the empty set it holds that

$$p(w_n \mid y_{1:n-1}) = p(w_n). \qquad (1.8)$$

Thus, when we substitute (1.7) and (1.8) into (1.6) we obtain

$$p(x_n \mid y_{1:n}) \propto \sum_{w_n} p(y_n \mid x_n, w_n)p(x_n \mid w_n, y_{1:n-1})p(w_n). \qquad (1.9)$$

In (1.9) it is possible to recognize the following elements: a measurement model $p(y_n \mid x_n, w_n)$ (this probability distribution models the genesis of the measurement y_n based on the inner states x_n and w_n) and so called prediction $p(x_n \mid w_n, y_{1:n-1})$, which is the probability distribution of the sought HR x_n, based on the knowledge of all the previous $n-1$ measurements $y_{1:n-1}$ and the knowledge of w_n. Using the law of total probability, the prediction $p(x_n \mid w_n, y_{1:n-1})$ can be further expressed in Box 2, where (1.11) holds thanks to the d-separation of sets $\{x_n\}$ and $\{y_{1:n-1}\}$ by set $\{x_{n-1}, w_n\}$ and thanks to the d-separation of sets $\{x_{n-1}\}$ and $\{w_n\}$ by set $\{y_{1:n-1}\}$. The substitution of (1.11) into (1.9) finally gives Equations (1.12) in Box 3.

This expression serves as a recursive formula for the computation of $p(x_n \mid y_{1:n})$ using the result of the previous measurement, $p(x_{n-1} \mid y_{1:n-1})$ and the information about the latest measurement y_n. Thus, (1.12) allows a continuous updates of $p(x_n \mid y_{1:n})$ after each measurement of y_n.

Box 2.

$$p(x_n \mid w_n, y_{1:n-1}) = \int_{-\infty}^{\infty} p(x_n \mid x_{n-1}, w_n, y_{1:n-1})p(x_{n-1} \mid w_n, y_{1:n-1})dx_{n-1} \qquad (1.10)$$

$$= \int_{-\infty}^{\infty} p(x_n \mid x_{n-1}, w_n)p(x_{n-1} \mid y_{1:n-1})dx_{n-1}, \qquad (1.11)$$

Box 3.

$$p(x_n \mid y_{1:n}) \propto \sum_{w_n} p(y_n \mid x_n, w_n) \int_{-\infty}^{\infty} p(x_n \mid x_{n-1}, w_n) p(x_{n-1} \mid y_{1:n-1}) dx_{n-1} p(w_n).$$

(1.12)

Numerical Computation of Equation (1.12)

Unless the probabilities in (1.12) have a trivial form or belong to the family of exponential distributions (which, as we will discuss later, is not our case), the integrals in (1.12) have to be computed numerically. The most common approaches to the numerical computation of recursive formulas such as (1.12) are the application of the rectangle rule, or the Monte Carlo numerical integration (Arulampalam et al., 2002). The former approach leads to computational schemes termed as the *grid-based filters*, while the latter approach leads to computational schemes termed as the *particle filters*.

To decide which of these approaches is the most suitable for our application, we have to consider that the particle filters require temporally uneven load - after a certain runtime with relatively low computational load, they require so called regularization, which has to be performed in a short period of time, and so can represent a considerable computational load (Arulampalam et al., 2002; Liu & Chen, 1998). This behavior is unsuitable for implementation on devices with limited computational resources; therefore, we chose to implement (1.12) as a grid-based filter. Specifically, we can approximate $p\left(x_n \mid w_n, y_{1:n}\right)$ (which equals to the integral in (1.12)) as

$$p\left(x_n \mid w_n, y_{1:n-1}\right) \approx \Delta \cdot \sum_{m=1}^{M} p\left(x_n \mid x_{n-1}^{(m)}, w_n\right) p\left(x_{n-1}^{(m)} \mid y_{1:n-1}\right),$$

(1.13)

where $x_{\cdots}^{(m)}$, $m = 1, \ldots, M$ denotes an equally spaced sequence of values, i.e. the grid, with spacing $\Delta = x_{\cdots}^{(m+1)} - x_{\cdots}^{(m)}$. As Δ is merely a multiplicative constant, and it is sufficient for us to express $p\left(x_n \mid w_n, y_{1:n}\right)$ and $p\left(x_n \mid y_{1:n}\right)$ up to a multiplicative constant, Δ will be omitted in further computations.

Clearly the evaluation of (1.13) will be the most computationally demanding part of our HR estimation algorithm. Therefore, to ease the computational load, we have decided to approximate the predictions $p(x_n | w_n, y_{1:n-1})$ computed for various values of w_n, by a single probability distribution $p(x_n | w_n^*, y_{1:n-1})$, which is computed for the most probable value of w_n denoted as w_n^* (see Box 4), where the value of w_n^* is estimated as

$$w_n^* = \max\left\{R\left(y_n \; \tilde{x}_{n-1} \,/\, 60\right) - 1, 0\right\},$$

(1.15)

where $R(.)$ denotes rounding to the nearest integer, and $\tilde{x}_{n-1}$ denotes the HR estimated in the previous step $n-1$ (the estimation of $\tilde{x}_{n-1}$ from

Box 4.

$$p\left(x_n \mid w_n, y_{1:n-1}\right) \approx p\left(x_n \mid w_n^*, y_{1:n-1}\right) \approx \sum_{m=1}^{M} p\left(x_n \mid x_{n-1}^{(m)}, w_n^*\right) p\left(x_{n-1}^{(m)} \mid y_{1:n-1}\right)$$

(1.14)

$p(x_{n-1} \mid y_{1:n-1})$ will be given later by Equation (1.38)).

Once we use the approximations (1.14) and (1.13), expression (1.12) becomes

$$p\left(x_n \mid y_{1:n}\right) \approx \sum_{m=1}^{M} p\left(x_n \mid x_{n-1}^{(m)}, w_n^*\right) p\left(x_{n-1}^{(m)} \mid y_{1:n-1}\right) \cdot \sum_{w_n} p\left(y_n \mid x_n, w_n\right) p\left(w_n\right).$$

(1.16)

In this form, the probability distribution $p(x_n \mid y_{1:n})$ can be continually updated with acceptable computational load.

Specifications for Heart Rate Estimation

Now, that we have expressed $p\left(x_n \mid y_{1:n}\right)$ in a form suitable for implementation, we will concentrate on expressing the probabilities in (1.16). In this section we will discuss the form of $p\left(x_n \mid x_{n-1}, w_n\right)$, $p\left(w_n\right)$, and $p(y_n \mid x_n, w_n)$.

1. Expressing Probability Distribution $p\left(x_n \mid x_{n-1}, w_n\right)$

The probability distribution $p\left(x_n \mid x_{n-1}, w_n\right)$ describes how the HR changes in-between two successive detections of QRS complexes. More specifically, it gives the probability distribution of the HR x_n during the n-th QRS detection based on the knowledge of the HR x_{n-1} during the previous QRS detection and the number of missed QRS complexes immediately prior to the last (i.e. n-th) QRS detection.

Based on the characteristics discussed in the previous sections, we know that we have to consider at least two distinct types of HR behavior. The HR either changes relatively slowly (e.g. during rest, or sustained physical activity), or the HR changes relatively rapidly (e.g. immediately

after a highly stressful stimulus or after an onset of physical activity). Let us denote the type of HR behavior as q, where $q = 1$ will denote the relatively slow HR changes, while $q = 0$ will denote the rapid HR changes.

In the case of slow HR changes we will model $p\left(x_n \mid x_{n-1}, w_n\right)$ as

$$p(x_n \mid x_{n-1}, w_n, q = 1) = N(x_n, x_{n-1}, \sigma^2(w_n)),$$

(1.17)

where $N\left(x, \mu, \sigma^2\right)$ denotes the normal distribution with mean μ and variance σ^2. In the case of rapid HR changes we will model $p\left(x_n \mid x_{n-1}, w_n\right)$ as

$$p(x_n \mid x_{n-1}, w_n, q = 0) = U(x_n, x_{n-1}, \sigma_u^2), \quad (1.18)$$

where $U\left(x, \mu, \sigma^2\right)$ denotes the uniform distribution with mean μ and variance σ^2.

If we denote the probability of HR behavior as $p(q)$, and we denote $p(q = 1) = q_1$ and $p(q = 0) = q_0$, we can use the law of total probability to express $p\left(x_n \mid x_{n-1}, w_n\right)$ as

$$p(x_n \mid x_{n-1}, w_n) = p(x_n \mid x_{n-1}, w_n, q = 1)q_1 + p(x_n \mid x_{n-1}, w_n, q = 0)q_0.$$

(1.19)

The values of the parameters σ_u, $\sigma(w_n)$, q_0 and q_1 can be determined based on the following considerations.

σ_u describes how much the HR can change when it is changing rapidly. Examination of real ECG records shows that this rate of change can be quite substantial - it can reach tens of bpm within a few heart beats. Therefore, we have chosen $\sigma_u = 15$, which allows $p(x_n \mid x_{n-1}, w_n, q = 0)$ in (1.18) to account for HR changes as high as ± 26 bpm within one heart beat.

Box 5.

$$p(x_n \mid x_{n-2}, w_{1:n} = 0, q = 1) = \int_{-\infty}^{\infty} p(x_n \mid x_{n-1}, w_{1:n} = 0, q = 1) p(x_{n-1} \mid x_{n-2}, w_{1:n} = 0, q = 1) dx_{n-1} \tag{1.21}$$

$$= \int_{-\infty}^{\infty} p(x_n \mid x_{n-1}, w_n = 0, q = 1) p(x_{n-1} \mid x_{n-2}, w_{n-1} = 0, q = 1) dx_{n-1}. \tag{1.22}$$

Box 6.

$$p(x_n \mid x_{n-2}, w_n = 0, q = 1) = \int_{-\infty}^{\infty} N(x_n, x_{n-1}, \sigma_0^2) N(x_{n-1}, x_{n-2}, \sigma_0^2) dx_{n-1} = N(x_n, x_{n-2}, 2\sigma_0^2). \tag{1.23}$$

$\sigma(w_n)$ can be determined based on the following consideration. Let us assume that since the beginning of our measurement the HR manifested no rapid changes ($q = 1$), and there were no missed heart beat detections (i.e. $w_{1:n} = [0, 0, \dots, 0]$). In this case we can express $p(x_n \mid x_{n-1}, w_n = 0, q = 1)$ as

$$p(x_n \mid x_{n-1}, w_n = 0, q = 1) = p(x_n \mid x_{n-1}, w_{1:n} = 0, q = 1)$$
$$= N(x_n, x_{n-1}, \sigma_0^2), \tag{1.20}$$

where σ_0 is some chosen constant. Now, let us consider what would happen if we chose to ignore the $(n-1)$-th QRS detection, and attempted to predict x_n from the $(n-2)$-th measurement. Using the law of total probability we can write Equation (1.21) seen in Box 5, where (1.22) holds thanks to the d-separation of the sets $\{x_n\}$ and $\{w_{1:n-1}\}$ by the set $\{x_{n-1}\}$, thanks to the d-separation of the sets $\{x_{n-1}\}$ and $\{w_{1:n-2}\}$ by the set $\{x_{n-2}, w_{n-1}\}$, and thanks to the d-separation of $\{w_n\}$ and $\{x_{n-1}\}$ by the empty set. Substituting (1.20) into (1.22) then gives Equation (1.23) in Box 6.

So if we choose to ignore the information in the $(n-1)$-th measurement, and we predict the HR during the n-th measurement from the HR during the $(n-2)$-th measurement, the probability distribution of the predicted HR will have twice the variance. This is an expected result, and in similar fashion we could show that if we chose to ignore k previous measurements the probability distribution $p(x_n \mid x_{n-2}, w_n = 0, q = 1)$ will have its variance $(k+1)$-times greater. In reality, we will of course not ignore our measurements, but it is possible that some QRS detections will be missed. However, loosing the detection of k previous heart beats is essentially equivalent to a flawless detection and subsequent ignorance of k previous heart beats. Therefore, the probability $p(x_n \mid x_{n-1}, w_n, q = 1)$ can be modeled as

$$p(x_n \mid x_{n-1}, w_n, q = 1) = N(x_n, x_{n-1}, (w_n + 1)\sigma_0^2), \tag{1.24}$$

so the parameter $\sigma^2(w_n)$ in (1.17) can be expressed as

$$\sigma^2(w_n) = (w_n + 1)\sigma_0^2. \tag{1.25}$$

Table 1. Estimates of probability of missed QRS complex detections $p(w_n)$ for heavily corrupted ECG records

w_n	0	1	2	3	4
$p(w_n)$	0.6035	0.1087	0.0918	0.0740	0.0332

$, \sum\limits_{wn=5}^{\infty} p(w_n) = 0.0887$

The constant σ_0 can be adjusted during the fine tuning of the algorithm. In our trials, we have achieved good results with $\sigma_0 = 1$.

The last of the parameters to be determined are q_0 and q_1. The parameter q_0 corresponds to the frequency of occurrence of rapid HR changes, and can be obtained from the analysis of ECG. However, we chose a heuristic approach, and during the final tuning of our algorithm we set $q_0 = 0.001$. Consequently, $q_1 = 1 - q_0 = 0.999$. These parameters allowed to obtain stable HR estimates during show HR changes, as well as rapid tracking of fast HR changes without introduction of any lengthy transients.

2.   Expressing Probability $p(w_n)$

We determined $p(w_n)$ using a simple fixed point iteration algorithm. First, we initialized $p(w_n)$ as

$$p(w_n) = \begin{cases} 0.75, & w_n = 0, \\ 0.20, & w_n = 1, \\ 0.05, & w_n = 2, \\ 0, & otherwise. \end{cases} \qquad (1.26)$$

Then, we applied the HR estimation algorithm to real ECG data. After obtaining HR estimates $\tilde{x}_n$, we estimated w_n as

$$\tilde{w}_n = \max\left\{ R(y_n \tilde{x}_n / 60) - 1, 0 \right\}, \qquad (1.27)$$

where $\tilde{w}_n$ denotes the estimate of w_n. Next, we used $\tilde{w}_n$ to construct new values of $p(w_n)$

$$p(w_n = k) = \frac{\#\left\{ \tilde{w}_n = k \right\}}{\#\left\{ \tilde{w}_n \right\}}, \qquad (1.28)$$

where $\#\{\tilde{w}_n\}$ denotes the total number of estimates $\tilde{w}_n$, and $\#\left\{ \tilde{w}_n = k \right\}$ denotes the number of estimates $\tilde{w}_n$ with value k. Last, we used the newly constructed probability $p(w_n)$, and repeated the whole process again. After 20 iterations, $p(w_n)$ converged to the values shown in Table 1.

To account for the worst case scenario, we based the computation of $p(w_n)$ on ECG records, which were heavily corrupted by saturation, power noise interference and occasional electrode contact loss, but still contained sufficient number of recognizable QRS complexes to provide a reliable HR estimation.

3.   Expressing the Measurement Model $p(y_n \mid x_n, w_n)$

$p(y_n \mid x_n, w_n)$ expresses the probability distribution of the R-R interval measurements based on a known HR x_n and a known number of missed QRS complex detections. For $w_n < 5$ we chose to model this probability in the following way

$$p(y_n \mid x_n, w_n) = N(y_n, (w_n + 1)60 / x_n, (w_n + 1)\sigma_{mes,n}^2),$$
$$w_n < 5$$

$$(1.29)$$

Box 7.

$$\sum_{m=1}^{M} p\left(x_n \mid x_{n-1}^{(m)}, w_n^*\right) p\left(x_{n-1}^{(m)} \mid y_{1:n-1}\right) = \sum_{m=1}^{M} \left(p\left(x_n \mid x_{n-1}^{(m)}, w_n^*, q=1\right) q_1 + p\left(x_n \mid x_{n-1}^{(m)}, w_n^*, q=0\right) q_0 \right) p\left(x_{n-1}^{(m)} \mid y_{1:n-1}\right)$$

$$(1.31)$$

$$= q_1 \sum_{m=1}^{M} p(x_n \mid x_{n-1}^{(m)}, w_n^*, q=1) p(x_{n-1}^{(m)} \mid y_{1:n-1}) + q_0 \sum_{m=1}^{M} p(x_n \mid x_{n-1}^{(m)}, w_n^*, q=0) p(x_{n-1}^{(m)} \mid y_{1:n-1}).$$

$$(1.32)$$

where $\sigma_{mes,n}$ corresponds to the measurement precision, and this value can be either provided by a QRS detector, or it can be set to a fixed value during the fine tuning of this algorithm. The choice of the variance of the normal distribution in (1.29) is based on the same reasoning as the one leading to the choice of $\sigma^2(w_n)$ in (1.25). If the number of missed QRS detections is more or equal to 5, we chose to consider the information value of the last R-R interval measurement as negligible, and we modeled the measurement with a noninformative uniform distribution

$$p(y_n \mid x_n, w_n) = \alpha, y_n \in \left\langle \min\left\{x_{\cdots}^{(m)}\right\}, \max\left\{x_{\cdots}^{(m)}\right\}\right\rangle,$$
$$w_n \geq 5,$$

$$(1.30)$$

where $\min\left\{x_{\cdots}^{(m)}\right\}$ and $\max\left\{x_{\cdots}^{(m)}\right\}$ denote the minimal and maximal values of the grid $x_{\cdots}^{(m)}$, and α is a constant chosen so that

$$\int_{-\infty}^{\infty} p(y_n \mid x_n, w_n) dy_n = 1.$$

Final Algorithm

Now, that we have expressed the probabilities in (1.16) we can continue to express the final form of our algorithm.

First, let us substitute (1.19) into the first summation of (1.16) (see Box 7)

Now, we substitute (1.17), (1.18) and (1.25) into (1.32), and we get

$$q_1 \sum_{m=1}^{M} N\left(x_n, x_{n-1}^{(m)}, (w_n^* + 1)\sigma_0\right) p\left(x_{n-1}^{(m)} \mid y_{1:n-1}\right)$$
$$+ q_0 \sum_{m=1}^{M} U\left(x_n, x_{n-1}^{(m)}, \sigma_u\right) p\left(x_{n-1}^{(m)} \mid y_{1:n-1}\right).$$

$$(1.33)$$

Next, we can use the fact that
$N\left(x, \mu, \sigma^2\right) = N\left(x - \mu, 0, \sigma^2\right)$ and
$U\left(x, \mu, \sigma^2\right) = U\left(x - \mu, 0, \sigma^2\right)$, and rewrite (1.33) as

$$q_1 \sum_{m=1}^{M} N\left(x_n - x_{n-1}^{(m)}, 0, (w_n^* + 1)\sigma_0\right) p\left(x_{n-1}^{(m)} \mid y_{1:n-1}\right)$$
$$+ q_0 \sum_{m=1}^{M} U\left(x_n - x_{n-1}^{(m)}, 0, \sigma_u\right) p\left(x_{n-1}^{(m)} \mid y_{1:n-1}\right).$$

$$(1.34)$$

At this point we can recognize that the both sums can be expressed as convolutions; therefore, we can write Equation (1.35) seen in Box 8, where $*$ denotes the convolution.

Now, let us substitute (1.29) and (1.30) into the second sum of (1.16)

Box 8.

$$\sum_{m=1}^{M} p\left(x_n \mid x_{n-1}^{(m)}, w_n^*\right) p\left(x_{n-1}^{(m)} \mid y_{1:n-1}\right) = q_1 N(x_n, 0, (w_n^* + 1)\sigma_0) * p(x_n \mid y_{1:n-1}) + q_0 U(x_n, 0, \sigma_u) * p(x_n \mid y_{1:n-1}),$$

$$(1.35)$$

Box 9.

$$p\left(x_n \mid y_{1:n}\right) \approx \left(q_1 N(x_n, 0, (w_n^* + 1)\sigma_0) * p(x_n \mid y_{1:n-1}) + q_0 U(x_n, 0, \sigma_u) * p(x_n \mid y_{1:n-1})\right)$$

$$\cdot \left(\sum_{w_n=0}^{4} N(y_n, (w_n + 1)60 / x_n, (w_n + 1)\sigma_{mes,n}^2)p(w_n) + \alpha_m \sum_{w_n=5}^{\infty} p(w_n)\right).$$

$$(1.37)$$

$$\sum_{w_n} p(y_n \mid x_n, w_n)p(w_n) =$$

$$\sum_{w_n=0}^{4} N(y_n, (w_n + 1)60 / x_n, (w_n + 1)\sigma_{mes,n}^2)p(w_n) + \alpha_m \sum_{w_n=5}^{\infty} p(w_n)$$

$$(1.36)$$

When we use expressions (1.35) and (1.36), and substitute them into (1.16), we will get Equation (1.37) in Box 9.

To simplify the computation, and because the numerical integration in the $(n+1)$-th step will require discretization of x_n into the values $x_n^{(m)}$, $m = 1, \ldots, M$, we will compute $p(x_n \mid y_{1:n})$ only in these discrete values, i.e. we will compute $p\left(x_n^{(m)} \mid y_{1:n}\right)$. In this way, once $p\left(x_n^{(m)} \mid y_{1:n}\right)$ is obtained, the HR estimate $\tilde{x}_n$ can be computed as

$$\tilde{x}_n = \sum_{m=1}^{M} x_n^{(m)} p(x_n^{(m)} \mid y_{1:n}),$$

$$(1.38)$$

and its variance can be estimated as

$$\tilde{\sigma}_{x_n}^2 = \sum_{m=1}^{M} \left(x_n^{(m)} - \tilde{x}_n\right)^2 p(x_n^{(m)} \mid y_{1:n}).$$

$$(1.39)$$

Note, that if $p\left(x_n^{(m)}, y_{1:n}\right)$ was approximated using (1.37) it has to be normalized so that $\sum_{m=1}^{M} p\left(x_n^{(m)}, y_{1:n}\right) = 1$ prior to the computation of (1.38) and (1.39).

Before we continue with summarizing our algorithm, we will make a brief note about efficient computation of convolutions in (1.37). Note, that $U(x_n, 0, \sigma_u)$ in (1.37) is either zero or equal to a constant $a = U(0, 0, \sigma_u)$. Thus, the second convolution in (1.37) performs a rudimentary moving average filtering, which for $x_n = x_n^{(m)}$ can be more efficiently implemented as a recursive filter

$$z[m] = z[m-1] + a \cdot p(x_{n-1}^{(m)} \mid y_{1:n-1}) - a \cdot p(x_{n-1}^{(m-u)} \mid y_{1:n-1}),$$

$$(1.40)$$

where $z[m] = U(x_n^{(m)}, 0, \sigma_u) * p(x_n^{(m)} \mid y_{1:n-1})$, and u is the number of nonzero values of $U(x_n^{(m)}, 0, \sigma_u)$.

Additionally, in the first convolution in (1.37) it is not necessary to consider all the values of $N(x_n, 0, (w_n^* + 1)\sigma)$. To save computational resources, we suggest to use the following approximation in Box 10.

Box 10.

$$N\left(x_n, 0, (w_n^* + 1)\sigma_0\right) \approx \begin{cases} N\left(x_n, 0, (w_n^* + 1)\sigma_0\right), & |x_n| < 2(w_n^* + 1)\sigma_0, \\ 0, & otherwise. \end{cases} \quad (1.41)$$

Figure 3. The upper plot shows an almost complete reconstruction of the HR from an ECG signal (lower plot) that manifested a great amount of saturation (mostly in its second half). A detailed view is shown in Figure 4.

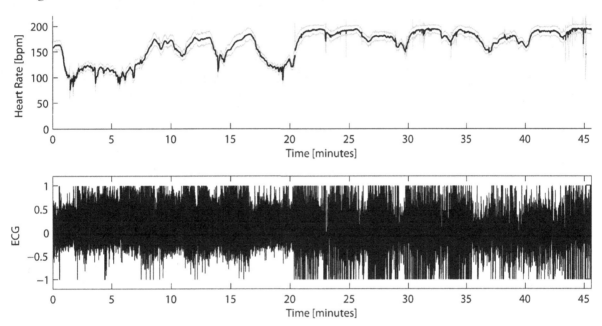

Algorithm Implementation

A pseudocode to facilitate the use of our algorithm is provided in Appendix A at the end of the chapter.

Algorithm Testing

We applied the algorithm described in the previous section on data records that captured ECG of subjects performing bouts of vigorous physical exercises separated by periods of rest. While the data contained a fair amount of well recorded ECG, there was also a number of intervals corrupted by substantial baseline wander, saturation, power noise interference and occasional contact loss (despite high physical load of the subjects, we observed a relatively small amount of muscular artifacts). The HR estimates of some of the ECG data sets, which we chose as representative, are shown in Figures 3, 4, 5, 6, 7, 8 and 9.

In each of these figures, the upper plot shows the HR estimate, and its confidence intervals (the confidence intervals were constructed using the 'two-sigma' rule, i.e. the confidence intervals were found as $\left\langle \tilde{x}_n - 2\tilde{\sigma}_{x_n}, \tilde{x}_n + 2\tilde{\sigma}_{x_n} \right\rangle$). In moments where the confidence intervals exceeded ± 30 bpm, the HR estimate was no longer considered as reliable, and was not plotted.

Figure 4. *A detailed view on a short part of the signal shown in Figure 3. Despite repeated saturation and considerable loss of ECG signal, the HR is well reconstructed.*

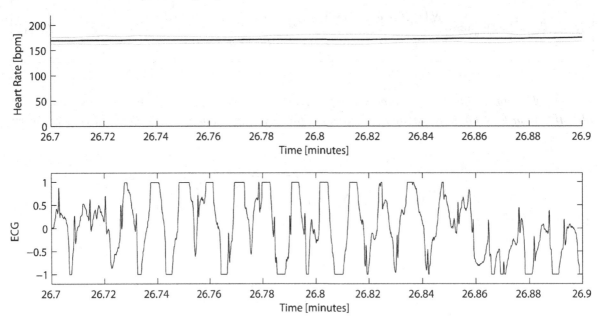

The bottom plot of each figure shows the original ECG signal. In the case of longer ECG records (with the length of several tens of minutes) it is not possible to plot the entire ECG signal, and still recognize the individual QRS complexes. In these plots only an 'envelope' of the signals can be recognized. Still, we have decided to plot these signals at their whole length, because the examination of their 'envelope' indicates the time intervals where the signal was often saturated (signals are scaled so that their lower and upper saturation bounds are -1 and 1, respectively; the saturation was often caused by a substantial baseline wander, and/or strong presence of the power noise interference). To allow a more detailed examination, the figures showing longer ECG records are supplemented by figures that show a detailed view on some shorter part of the longer signal.

Figure 3 shows a signal which has its second half corrupted by a frequent presence of saturation caused by a strong baseline wander. In this signal many QRS complexes are corrupted beyond recognition. A detailed view on a short part of this

signal is shown in Figure 4. Note that despite all the corruption and QRS complex losses the HR is well reconstructed.

Figure 5 shows a signal with several intervals, during which the electrode-skin contact was completely lost, and no ECG signal was recorded. The algorithm reacted to this situation correctly by increasing the width of the confidence intervals, which exceeded the amount beyond which the HR estimate is no longer considered as reliable. Consequently, in these intervals the HR is not plotted. A detailed view of the ECG signal and the respective HR estimate during a contact loss is shown in Figure 6.

Figure 7 presents an ECG record with a rapid HR change (specifically, it was a rapid decrease of the HR measured after a completion of a bout of physical exercise on a physically fit subject). The reaction of the algorithm was swift, without any lengthy transition. The lower HR was tracked promptly.

Figure 8 shows another ECG record that contains several intervals with strong interference

Figure 5. An example of an ECG signal with intervals where the electrode-skin contact was completely lost, and no ECG signal was recorded. In these intervals the algorithm indicates en excessive variance of HR estimates, which means that the corresponding HR estimate is not reliable (and therefore is not plotted). A detailed view of this signal is shown in Figure 6.

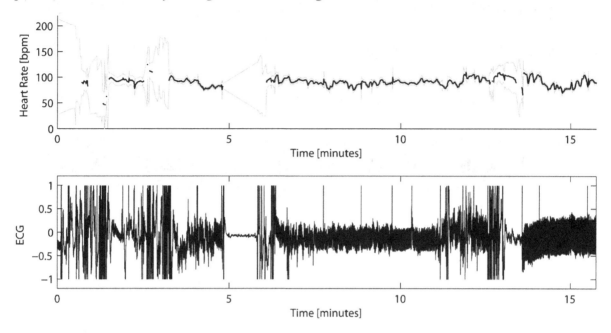

Figure 6. A detailed view on a short part of the signal shown in Figure 5. In time 4.83 min, the ECG signal is lost.

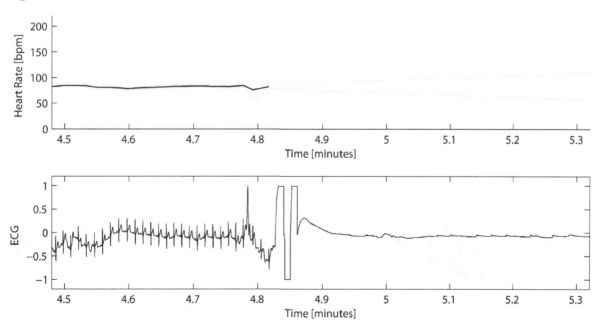

Figure 7. An example of an ECG signal with a rapid decrease of HR. Note that the algorithm reacts to the HR change promptly, without a lengthy transient.

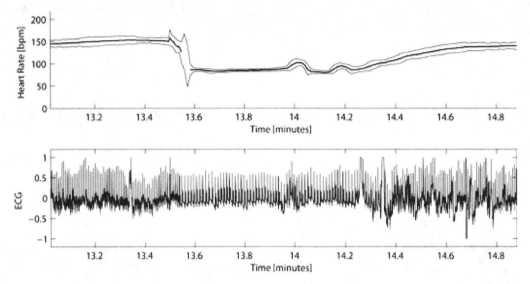

Figure 8. Another example of HR estimation. This ECG record contained intervals, where a complete loss of ECG signal prevented any HR estimation, and intervals, where despite a considerable loss of ECG signal the HR was reliably estimated. A detailed view of this signal is shown in Figure 9.

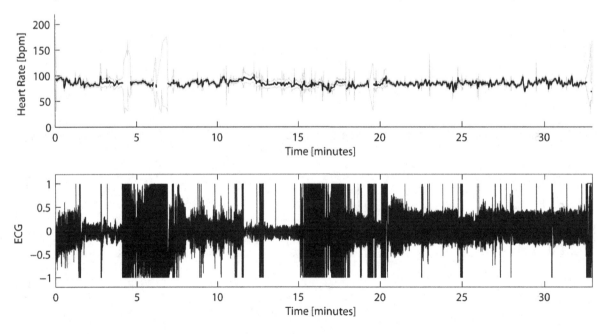

Figure 9. A detailed view on a short part of the signal shown in Figure 8

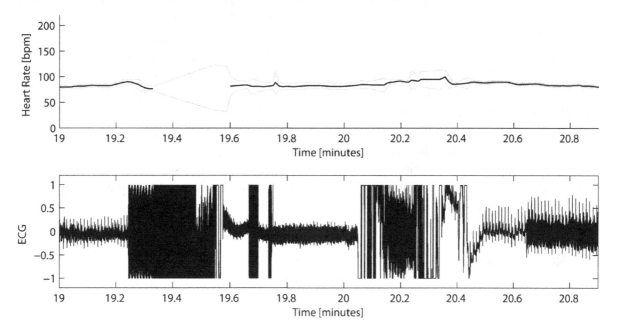

and signal corruption. There are intervals where the interference repeatedly prevented detection of many QRS complexes; nevertheless, the algorithm reliably reconstructed the HR. Also, there are intervals, where the ECG was temporarily lost, and the reconstruction was not possible. A detailed view on one of these intervals is shown in Figure 9.

Last, we would like to mention that besides the abovementioned tests, the algorithm was also implemented in HR monitors that are currently being developed for NATO soldiers. The algorithm performs very well on a small PDA.

FUTURE RESEARCH DIRECTIONS

Even though the presented algorithm is designed for the use in real-time, it would be interesting to expand its abilities for off-line ECG processing. In such case, the integrals in the recursive formula (1.12) could be computed through a Monte Carlo method, which would lead to the use of particle filters. Also, during the offline processing,

we could estimate $p\left(x_n \mid y_{1:n+k}\right)$, i.e. the probability distribution of HR during the n-th QRS detection, given all the previous and next k QRS detections. The addition of the next k QRS detections could further improve HR estimates in the intervals, where the QRS detections are frequently lost.

CONCLUSION

This chapter presented an algorithm for a real-time robust heart rate estimation. We formulated our problem in the framework of Bayesian networks, and used statistical inference to derive a formula for recursive heart rate estimation. This formula was subsequently implemented as a grid filter, which was further streamlined to allow its implementation on a device with limited computational resources.

The final algorithm was tested on ECG data recorded on subjects performing bouts of vigorous physical exercise. The testing showed that our algorithm manifests robust performance in the presence of strong interference and ECG data corruption. The algorithm can well withstand repeated loss of individual QRS complexes, and when an ECG signal was lost completely, the algorithm reacted correctly by widening the confidence intervals, and thus indicating the unreliability of the heart rate estimate. Also, the ability to track fast HR changes was confirmed. Therefore, we conclude that the suggested algorithm seems to be able to provide a robust real-time estimation of heart rate of subjects performing in highly stressful and harsh environments.

ACKNOWLEDGMENT

This work was supported by the research program Transdisciplinary Research in Biomedical Engineering II, MSM6840770012 of the Czech Technical University in Prague.

REFERENCES

Afonso, V.X., Tompkins, W., Nguyen, T., & Luo, S. (1999). ECG beat detection using filter banks. *IEEE Transactions on Bio-Medical Engineering, 46*(2), 192–202. doi:10.1109/10.740882

Afonso, V.X., Tompkins, W., Nguyen, T., Trautmann, S., & Luo, S. (1995). Filter bank-based processing of the stress ECG. In *IEEE 17th Annual Conference of the Engineering in Medicine and Biology Society,* (Vol. 2, pp. 887–888).

Andreassi, J. (2000). *Psychophysiology: Human behavior and physiological response*. Lawrence Erlabaum Associates, Inc.

Arulampalam, M., Maskell, S., Gordon, N., & Clapp, T. (2002). A tutorial on particle filters of online nonlinear/non-Gaussian Bayesian tracking. *IEEE Transactions on Signal Processing, 50*(2), 174–188. doi:10.1109/78.978374

Barro, S., Fernandez-Delgado, M., Vila-Sobrino, J. A., & Sanchez, E. (1998). Classifying multichannel ECG patterns with an adaptive neural network. *IEEE Engineering in Medicine and Biology, 17,* 45–55. doi:10.1109/51.646221

Cacioppo, J., Tassinary, L. G., & Berntson, G. G. (Eds.). (2007). *Handbook of psychophysiology*. Cambridge University Press.

Cheng, J.-L., Jeng, J.-R., & Chiang, Z.-W. (2006). Heart rate measurement in the presence of noises. In *Pervasive Health Conference and Workshops, 2006* (pp. 1-4).

Coast, A., Stern, R., Cano, G., & Briller, S. (1990). An approach to cardiac arrhythmia analysis using hidden Markov models. *IEEE Transactions on Bio-Medical Engineering, 37*(9), 826–835. doi:10.1109/10.58593

Dokur, Z., Olmez, T., Yazgan, E., & Ersoy, O. (1997). Detection of ECG waveforms by neural networks. *Medical Engineering & Physics, 19,* 738–741. doi:10.1016/S1350-4533(97)00029-5

Fiersen, G., Jannett, T., Jadallah, M., Yates, S., Quint, S., & Nagle, H. (1990). A comparison of the noise sensitivity of nine QRS detection algorithms. *IEEE Transactions on Bio-Medical Engineering, 37*(1), 85–98. doi:10.1109/10.43620

Hamilton, P., & Tompkins, W. (1988). Adaptive matched filtering for QRS detection. In *IEEE 10th Annual International Conference Engineering in Medicine and Biology Society,* (pp. 147–148).

Kohler, B., Hennig, C., & Orglmeister, R. (2002). The principles of software QRS detection. *IEEE Engineering in Medicine and Biology Magazine, 21*(1), 42–57. doi:10.1109/51.993193

Liu, J. S., & Chen, R. (1998). Sequential Monte Carlo methods for dynamical systems. *Journal of the American Statistical Association, 93,* 1032–1044. doi:10.2307/2669847

Neapolitan, R. (1990). *Probabilistic reasoning in expert systems.* New York, NY: Wiley & Sons Ltd.

Neapolitan, R. (2004). *Learning Bayesian networks.* New Jersey: Prentice Hall.

Pan, J., & Tomkins, W. (1985). A real-time QRS detection algorithm. *IEEE Transactions on Bio-Medical Engineering, BME-32*(3), 230–236. doi:10.1109/TBME.1985.325532

Piotrowski, Z., & Rozanowski, K. (2010). Robust algorithm for heart rate (HR) detection and heart rate variability (HRV) estimation. *Acta Physica Polonica A, 118.*

Ruha, A., Sallinen, S., & Nissila, S. (1997). A real-time microprocessor QRS detector system with a 1-ms timing accuracy for the measurement of ambulatory HRV. *IEEE Transactions on Bio-Medical Engineering, 44*(3). doi:10.1109/10.554762

Stegle, O., Fallert, V., MacKay, D., & Brage, S. (2008). Gaussian process robust regression for noisy heart rate data. *IEEE Transactions on Bio-Medical Engineering, 55*(9), 2143–2151. doi:10.1109/TBME.2008.923118

Verma, T., & Pearl, J. (1991). Equivalence and synthesis of causal models. In P. Bonissone & M. Henrion (Eds.), *Proceedings of Seventh Conference Uncertainty in Artificial Intelligence.* Amsterdam, The Netherlands: North Holland.

ADDITIONAL READING

Andreassi, J. (2000). *Psychophysiology: Human behavior and physiological response.* Mahwah, NJ: Lawrence Erlbaum Associates, Inc.

Arulampalam, M., Maskell, S., Gordon, N., & Clapp, T. (2002). A tutorial on particle filters of online nonlinear/non-Gaussian Bayesian tracking. *IEEE Transactions on Signal Processing, 50*(2), 174–188. doi:10.1109/78.978374

Bernado, J., & Smith, A. (1994). *Bayesian theory.* New York, NY: Wiley & Sons Ltd.

Berry, D. A. (1996). *Statistics: A Bayesian perspective.* Wadsworth, CA: Belmont.

Bruce, E. N. (2001). *Biomedical signal processing and signal modeling.* Wiley & Sons Ltd.

Castillo, E., Gutiérrez, J. M., & Hadi, A. S. (1997). *Expert systems and probabilistic network models.* New York, NY: Springer-Verlag.

Glymour, C. (2001). *The mind's arrows: Bayes nets and graphical causal models in psychology.* Cambridge, MA: MIT Press.

Gregory, P. C. (2005). *Bayesian logical data analysis for the physical sciences. A comparative approach with Mathematica™ support.* Cambridge, UK: Cambridge University Press. doi:10.1017/CBO9780511791277

Holmes, D. E., & Jain, L. C. (Eds.). (2008). *Innovations in Bayesian networks: Theory and applications.* Berlin, Germany: Springer-Verlag. doi:10.1007/978-3-540-85066-3

Jensen, F. V. (1996). *An introduction to Bayesian networks.* New York, NY: Springer-Verlag.

Jensen, F. V., & Nielsen, T. D. (2007). *Bayesian networks and decision graphs.* New York, NY: Springer.

Kjaerulff, U. B., & Madsen, L. A. (2007). *Bayesian networks and influence diagrams: A guide to construction and analysis.* New York, NY: Springer.

Koski, T., & Noble, J. M. (2009). *Bayesian networks: An introduction.* Chichester, UK: Wiley & Sons Ltd. doi:10.1002/9780470684023

Malmivuo, J., & Plonsey, R. (1995). *Bioelectromagnetism: Principles and applications of bioelectric and biomagnetic fields.* New York, NY: Oxford University Press. doi:10.1093/acprof:oso/9780195058239.001.0001

McLachlan, G. J., & Krishnan, T. (1997). *The EM algorithm and its extensions*. New York, NY: Wiley.

Naït-Ali, A. (2009). *Advanced biosignal processing*. Berlin, Germany: Springer-Verlag. doi:10.1007/978-3-540-89506-0

Neapolitan, R. E. (1990). *Probabilistic reasoning in expert systems*. New York, NY: Wiley & Sons Ltd.

Neapolitan, R. E. (2004). *Learning Bayesian networks*. New Jersey: Prentice Hall.

Neapolitan, R. E., & Morris, S. (2002). Probabilistic modeling using Bayesian networks. In Kaplan, D. (Ed.), *Handbook of quantitative methodology in the social sciences*. Thousand Oaks, CA: Sage.

Pearl, J. (1995). Bayesian networks. In Arbib, M. (Ed.), *Handbook of brain theory and neural networks*. Cambridge, MA: MIT Press.

Pourret, O., Naim, P., & Marcot, B. (2008). *Bayesian networks: A practical guide to applications*. Chichester, UK: Wiley & Sons Ltd.

Rangayyan, R. M. (2002). *Biomedical signal analysis*. IEEE Press.

Reddy, D. C. (2005). *Biomedical signal processing: Principles and techniques*. McGraw-Hill.

Rowe, D. B. (2003). *Multivariate Bayesian statistics: Models for source separation and signal unmixing*. Chapman & Hall/CRC.

Sörnmo, L., & Laguna, P. (2005). *Bioelectrical signal processing in cardiac and neurological applications*. Elsevier Academic Press.

Tompkins, W. J. (Ed.). (1993). *Biomedical digital signal processing*. New Jersey: Prentice Hall.

van der Heijden, F., Duin, R. P. W., de Ridder, D., & Tax, D. M. J. (2004). *Classification, parameter estimation and state estimation*. Chichester, UK: Wiley & Sons Ltd. doi:10.1002/0470090154

Webster, J. G. (Ed.). (1998). *Medical instrumentation*. Wiley & Sons Ltd.

KEY TERMS AND DEFINITIONS

Baseline Wander: A movement of ECG baseline often caused by changing properties of electrode-skin contact.

Bayesian Network: A graphical representation of joint probability distribution of a set of random variables, that represents the random variables as nodes, and their dependences as oriented edges between these nodes.

Electrocardiogram (ECG): A record of the electrical activity of a heart.

Grid-Based Filter: A structure used for Bayesian inference, which represents probabilities on a chosen (often equally spaced) discrete grid, thus facilitating the computation of otherwise untraceable integrals.

Heart Rate: Frequency of heart contractions, often expressed in beats per minute (bpm).

Missed QRS Detection: A QRS complex that is missed by a QRS detector.

QRS Complex: A complex of three waves (Q wave, R wave and S wave) in an electrocardiogram, which are generated by ventricular depolarization.

QRS Detector: An algorithm for detecting QRS complexes in ECG.

APPENDIX A: ALGORITHM IMPLEMENTATION

To facilitate the use of our algorithm, in this appendix we will now provide a pseudocode of its implementation.

Inputs

$y_{1:n}$ - values of R-R intervals estimated from the detection of QRS complexes ($y_n = R_n - R_{n-1}$, where R_n, is the position of the n - th QRS complex)

$\sigma_{mes,n}$ - standard deviation of the measurement of the position of the n - th QRS complex. If this value is not provided by the QRS detector, it can be set as a constant, and adjusted to fine tune the algorithm.

Outputs

$p\left(x_n \mid y_{1:n}\right)$ - the probability distribution of the HR after the detection of the n-th QRS complex, based on the knowledge of all previously measured R-R intervals,

$\tilde{x}_n$ - the estimate of the HR during the detection of the n-th QRS complex,

$\tilde{\sigma}^2_{x_n}$ - the estimate of the variance of the HR estimate.

Variables

$p\left(x_n^{(m)} \mid y_{1:n}\right), m = 1,\ldots,M$ will be represented by a vector variable $\mathbf{p}$;

$\sum_{m=1}^{M} p\left(x_n \mid x_{n-1}^{(m)}, w_n^*\right) p\left(x_{n-1}^{(m)} \mid y_{1:n-1}\right), m = 1,\ldots,M$ will be represented by a vector variable $\mathbf{p}_p$;

$\sum_{w_n} p(y_n \mid x_n^{(m)}, w_n) p(w_n), m = 1,\ldots,M$ will be represented by a vector variable $\mathbf{p}_{mes}$;

$z[m], m = 1,\ldots,M$, will be represented by a vector variable $\mathbf{z}$;

$\mathbf{p}[n]$ will denote the n-th element of the vector $\mathbf{p}$;

$\mathbf{p}[n_1 : n_2]$ will denote the vector $[\mathbf{p}[n_1], \mathbf{p}[n_1 + 1],\ldots,\mathbf{p}[n_2]]$;

$\tilde{x}_n$ will denote the HR estimate;

$\tilde{\sigma}^2_{x_n}$ will denote the estimate of the variance of the HR estimate;

$x_{\ldots}^{(m)}$ will denote the grid of M equally spaced points used in numerical integrations.

Computation

i. *Initialization*

$\sigma_0 = 1, \quad \sigma_u = 15, \quad q_0 = 0.001, \quad q_1 = 1 - q_0$ *// initialization of constants*

$\mathbf{p} = [1, 1, \ldots, 1]$ *// initialization of the sought probability by*

   // a noninformative prior

$\left[x_{\ldots}^{(m)} \right]_{m=1\ldots M} = [40, 41, \ldots, 230]$ *// initialization of the grid*

ii. *Measurement. At this Point y_n and $\sigma_{mes,n}$ have been obtained from the QRS Detector.*

$$\mathbf{p}_{mes}[m] = \sum_{w_n=0}^{4} N(y_n, (w_n + 1)60 / \mathbf{x}_n^{(m)}, (w_n + 1)\sigma_{mes,n}^2)p(w_n) + \alpha \sum_{w_n=5}^{\infty} p(w_n), \text{ for } m = 1, \ldots, M$$

   // computation of (1.36)

iii. *Prediction*

$\mathbf{z}[0] = 0$ *// initialization of temporary variable $\mathbf{z}$*

$\mathbf{z}[m] = \mathbf{z}[m-1] + a \cdot \mathbf{p}[m] - a \cdot \mathbf{p}[m-u], \quad m = 1 \ldots M + u - 1$ *// computation of the second convolution in*

   // (1.35) using (1.40)

$w_n^* = \max \left\{ R\left(y_n \tilde{x}_{n-1} / 60 \right) - 1, 0 \right\}$ *// computation of (1.15)*

$\mathbf{g}[m] = \sum_{k=1}^{M} N\left(x_n^{(m)} - x_n^{(k)}, 0, (w_n^* + 1)\sigma_0 \right) \mathbf{p}[k], \ m = 1, \ldots, M$ *// computation of*

   // the first convolution in (1.35);
   // $\mathbf{g}$ is an auxiliary variable;
   // for the sake of clarity,
   // this step does not include
   // possible simplification (1.41)

$\mathbf{p}_p = q_1 \cdot \mathbf{z}[1 + N_g / 2 : M - N_g / 2] + q_0 \cdot \mathbf{g}$ *// computation of (1.35)*

iv. *Combination of Measurement and Prediction (corresponds to the Computation of (1.37))*

$\mathbf{p}[m] = \mathbf{p}_{mes}[m] \cdot \mathbf{p}_p[m], \text{ for } m = 1, \ldots, M$

$\mathbf{p}[m] = \mathbf{p}[m] / \sum_{k=1}^{M} \mathbf{p}[m], \text{ for } m = 1, \ldots, M$ *//normalization*

v. *Estimation of Heart Rate $\tilde{x}_n$ and its Variance $\tilde{\sigma}_{x_n}^2$*

$\tilde{x}_n = \sum_{m=1}^{M} x_n^{(m)} \mathbf{p}[m]$ *// corresponds to (1.38)*

$\tilde{\sigma}_{x_n}^2 = \sum_{m=1}^{M} (x_n^{(m)} - \tilde{x}_n)^2 \mathbf{p}[m]$ *// corresponds to (1.39)*

vi. *Increment $n = n + 1$, and Continue the Algorithm with Step 2*

Chapter 6
Automated Diagnostics of Coronary Artery Disease:
Long-Term Results and Recent Advancements

Matjaž Kukar
University of Ljubljana, Slovenia

Igor Kononenko
University of Ljubljana, Slovenia

Ciril Grošelj
University Medical Centre Ljubljana, Slovenia

ABSTRACT

The authors present results and the latest advancement in their long-term study on using image processing and data mining methods in medical image analysis in general, and in clinical diagnostics of coronary artery disease in particular. Since the evaluation of modern medical images is often difficult and time-consuming, authors integrate advanced analytical and decision support tools in diagnostic process. Partial diagnostic results, frequently obtained from tests with substantial imperfections, can be thus integrated in ultimate diagnostic conclusion about the probability of disease for a given patient. Authors study various topics, such as improving the predictive power of clinical tests by utilizing pre-test and post-test probabilities, texture representation, multi-resolution feature extraction, feature construction and data mining algorithms that significantly outperform the medical practice. During their long-term study (1995-2011) authors achieved, among other minor results, two really significant milestones. The first was achieved by using machine learning to significantly increase post-test diagnostic probabilities with respect to expert physicians. The second, even more significant result utilizes various advanced data analysis techniques, such as automatic multi-resolution image parameterization combined with feature extraction and machine learning methods to significantly improve on all aspects of diagnostic performance. With the proposed approach clinical results are significantly as well as fully automatically, improved throughout the study. Overall, the most significant result of the work is an improvement in the diagnostic power of the whole diagnostic process. The approach supports, but does not replace, physicians' diagnostic process, and can assist in decisions on the cost-effectiveness of diagnostic tests.

DOI: 10.4018/978-1-4666-1803-9.ch006

INTRODUCTION

Internal medicine in general and cardiovascular medicine in particular utilize various diagnostic imaging tests to help physicians identify various problems and abnormalities. Such diagnostic tests produce structural and functional images of the insides of the human body. The choice of imaging technology depends on exhibited symptoms, the part of the body being examined, its cost and availability. X-rays, computer tomography (CT) scans, nuclear medicine scans (including scintigraphy), magnetic resonance imaging (MRI) scans and ultrasound are all types of diagnostic imaging.

Many imaging tests are painless and non-invasive. Some are slightly uncomfortable, as they require the patient to stay still for a long time inside a machine. Certain tests involve radiation, but these are generally considered safe because the dosage is very low. In some imaging tests, an implement (a tiny camera or other sensing device) is attached to a long, thin tube and inserted in the body. These procedures are quite unpleasant and often require anesthesia. If possible, such procedures should preferably be substituted with less invasive ones.

Cardiovascular diseases, specifically coronary artery disease (CAD), are among the developed world's premier causes of mortality. Currently, cardiovascular disease diagnostics rely on diagnostic imaging tests that require expensive, specialized equipment and trained personnel (both technicians and physicians) for efficient operation.

The aim of our long-term research is to improve the diagnostics of CAD from a computational perspective. Our early research on this topic, conducted between 1995 and 1998 (Kukar et al., 1999) showed that machine learning methods may enable objective interpretation of available diagnostic images and, as a result, increase the accuracy and reliability of the diagnostic process. Experiments conducted with various machine learning algorithms showed that these were able to exceed performance levels of clinicians.

The algorithms were also extended to deal with non-uniform misclassification costs in order to perform ROC analysis and control the trade-off between sensitivity and specificity. ROC analysis showed significant improvements of sensitivity and specificity of machine learning algorithms compared to the performance of clinicians. The predictive power of standard tests was therefore significantly improved using machine learning techniques. The major bottleneck of this study was that all data, including evaluation of diagnostic images, had to be provided by expert physicians; this caused long delays in data acquisition and a certain reluctance to accept the procedure in everyday practice.

In the present study (2006-2011), we alleviate the data acquisition problem by introducing algorithms for completely automatic evaluation (parameterization) of diagnostic images and for suggesting the most useful (informative) resolutions (Kukar et al., 2007). We also utilize a feature extraction method (principal component analysis) and machine learning/data mining techniques on extracted features that both aid in achieving excellent result. We describe the methodology used, relate results of both studies, and evaluate our contributions.

BACKGROUND

Coronary Artery Disease

Coronary artery disease is usually a consequence of the accumulation of atheromatous plaques within the walls of the coronary arteries that supply the myocardium with oxygen. While the symptoms and signs of coronary artery disease are easily observable in advanced stages of disease, most individuals with coronary artery disease show no evidence of disease until the first onset of symptoms finally arises, often as a sudden heart attack. As the coronary artery disease progresses, it may cause a near-complete obstruction of the coronary

Figure 1. Coronary angiography showing visible occlusions in coronary vessels (marked by black arrows). Accumulation of radiopaque materials in coronary artery shows defects caused by arteriosclerotic plaque.

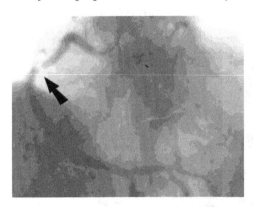 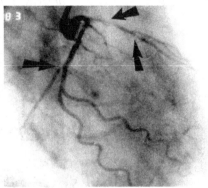

artery, severely restricting the flow of oxygen-carrying blood to the myocardium. Individuals with this degree of coronary artery disease typically have suffered from one or more myocardial infarctions, and may have signs and symptoms of chronic coronary ischemia, including symptoms of angina at rest and flash pulmonary edema.

The usual clinical process of coronary artery disease diagnostics consists of four steps:

1. Evaluation of signs and symptoms of the disease and electrocardiogram (ECG) at rest
2. ECG testing during controlled exercise
3. Myocardial scintigraphy
4. Coronary angiography

In this process, the fourth diagnostic level (coronary angiography, Figure 1) is by many physicians considered to be the ultimate reference method. Given that this diagnostic procedure is invasive and unpleasant for patients, as well as relatively expensive, there is an incentive to improve diagnostic performance of earlier diagnostic levels, especially of myocardial scintigraphy, in order to produce more reliable diagnoses at this step (Kukar & Grošelj, 1999; Kukar et al., 1999). Approaches previously used in this problem include neural networks (Allison et al., 2005; Mobley et al., 2000; Ohlsson, 2004), expert systems (Gar-

cia et al., 2001), subgroup mining (Gamberger et al., 2003), various statistical techniques (Slomka et al., 2005), and rule-based approaches (Kurgan et al., 2001).

In our studies we focus on various aspects of improving the diagnostic performance of the third diagnostic level. Myocardial perfusion scintigraphy consists of acquiring a series of medical images using an inexpensive and non-invasive procedure when the patient is at rest and during a controlled physical exercise. In clinical practice expert physicians use their medical knowledge and experience to manually describe (parameterize) and evaluate the images, often with the help of vendor-supplied image processing software tools.

Our first (past) study was based on patients' data compiled entirely by physicians – either by extracting data from medical records, or from test results (ECGs and scintigraphic images, Figure 2). Using these data, our machine learning algorithms showed excellent diagnostic accuracy and reliability in the diagnostics of coronary artery disease (Kukar & Grošelj, 1999).

Our second (present) study utilizes an automatic method as an alternative to manual image evaluation. The method consists of automatic multi-resolution image parameterization, based on texture description with specialized association

Figure 2. Myocardial scintigraphy with the older SPECT camera and software. Manually placed white arrows mark insufficiently perfused parts of the heart muscle (visible only for specially trained expert physicians). Scintigraphic defect seen at stress (upper series) fills at rest (lower series).

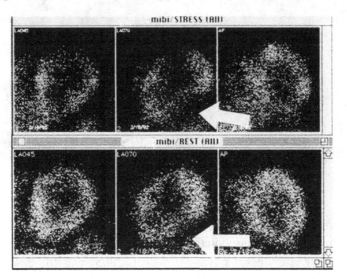

rules, coupled with image evaluation with machine learning methods. Since this approach yields a large number of relatively low-level features (though much more informative than simple pixel intensity values), we also apply additional dimensionality reduction techniques, either by throwing away some features (feature selection), or combining them into more informative, high-level features (feature construction). Our results show that this completely automated approach equals or even outperforms physicians in terms of the quality of image parameters and diagnostic performance.

Image Parameterization

Image parameterization is a technique for describing bitmapped images with numerical parameters - features or attributes. Traditionally, popular image features are first- and second-order statistics, structural and spectral properties, and several others. Image parameterization is used in quality control, identification, image grouping, surveillance, image storage and retrieval, and image querying.

Over the past few decades, image parameterization has been extensively applied to medical domains where texture classification is closely related to diagnostic process (Fitzpatrick & Sonka, 2000). This complements medical practice, where manual image parameterization (evaluation of medical images by expert physicians) frequently plays an important role in diagnostic process.

Digital images are usually described with spatial data matrices that are not suitable for distinguishing between the predefined image classes. Determining image features that can discriminate between observed image classes is a difficult task for which several algorithms exist (Nixon & Aguado, 2008). They transform the image from the matrix form into a set of numeric or discrete features (parameters) that convey useful high-level (compared to simple pixel intensities) information for discriminating between classes.

For the purpose of diagnostics from medical images, structural description are more appropriate (Šajn & Kononenko, 2009). Structural representations possess several desirable properties like invariance to global brightness and invariance to rotation. To obtain structural descriptions, we utilize spatial association rules (the ArTex algorithm, described later in the chapter). Association rules algorithms can be used for describing textures if appropriate texture representation formalism is used. They capture structural and statistical information and conveniently identify spatial configurations that occur frequently and possess considerable descriptive characteristics.

ArTex and ARes Algorithms

For efficient automatic image classification we need an appropriate image parameterization tool. The present study introduces the ArTex (**As**sociation **r**ules for **Tex**tures - ArTex) (Bevk & Kononenko, 2006) algorithm for parameterizing textures with association rules belonging to structural parameterization algorithms. The ArTex algorithm produces a structural representation based upon association rules. Such representation has several good properties like invariance to global brightness and invariance to rotation. Association rules capture structural and statistical information and conveniently identify frequently occurring descriptive and discriminative structures. Initially, the ArTex algorithm was used for texture classification. We later discovered that it also performs well in scintigraphic images despite the fact that they seemingly do not exhibit a pattern.

The obtained high quality image parameters can be used to describe images with relatively strong, but numerous features, which allows their use in machine learning process. Images of patients with known confirmed diagnosis can be used as learning data that, in conjunction with the applied machine learning methods, produces reliable decision support tools (classifiers) for the diagnostic problem at hand. In order to justify the use of the ArTex algorithm, its performance was compared to the performance of three other image parameterization algorithms, such as Haar wavelets (Chui, 1992), Laws filters (Laws, 1980) and

Gabor filters (Grigorescu et al., 2002), and found that it performs better in our particular problem.

The present study also combines parameterization with a multi-resolution approach. From experiments with synthetic data, it was observed that using parameterization-produced features at several different resolutions usually improves the classification accuracy of machine learning classifiers (Šajn & Kononenko, 2008). This parameterization approach is very effective in analyzing myocardial scintigraphy. The algorithm ARes (ArTex with resolutions - ARes) for selecting the resolution set yields more informative parameterization attributes when combining the parameters from the proposed resolutions. The idea of the ARes algorithm derives from the SIFT (Scale Invariant Feature Transform) algorithm (Lowe, 2004). ARes was designed especially for structural image parameterization algorithms, specifically for the ArTex algorithm. ArTex and ARes are independent of the applied machine learning algorithm.

A detailed presentation of both ArTex and ARes algorithms is given in (Šajn & Kononenko, 2008). The obtained texture parameters are subsequently used for image classification with machine learning methods (Kononenko & Kukar, 2007).

Image Classification with Machine Learning Methods

Provided that medical images are described with informative numerical attributes, various machine learning algorithms can be used (Kononenko & Kukar, 2007) to generate a classification system (classifier) for patient diagnosis. Among many available machine learning methods, we decided to use decision trees, naive Bayes classifiers, Bayesian networks, K-nearest neighbors, and support vector machines based on our previous experience with medical diagnostics (Kukar et al., 1999) and their use in other studies (Katsis et al., 2006; Peng et al., 2006).

Both our early work as well as recent results in the problem of diagnosing the coronary artery disease from myocardial scintigraphy images (Kukar et al., 1999; Kukar et al., 2007) indicate that the naive Bayes classifier gives the best results. Our results are consistent with several other studies (Kononenko, 1993; Kononenko, 2001) that also find that the naive Bayes classifier frequently outperforms other, often much more complex, classifiers in medical diagnoses. In addition, many authors have established feature subset selection as a necessary step before decision tree induction (Jelonek & Stefanowski, 1997; Yang & Honavar, 1998), therefore this must be taken into account when classifying images.

As usual in medical studies, we compare our results with some baseline approach; this is in our case an established approach of expert physicians whose diagnostic results were available. To compare the performance of their utilization of a certain diagnostic test we assess diagnostic accuracy, sensitivity, and specificity:

$$accuracy = \frac{\#\ true\ positives + \#\ true\ negatives}{\#\ all\ patients}$$

$$sensitivity = \frac{\#\ true\ positives}{\#\ all\ patients\ eith\ the\ disease}$$

$$specificity = \frac{\#\ true\ negatives}{\#\ all\ patients\ without\ the\ disease}$$

The *true positives* are all patients with the disease and a positive test result, whereas the true negatives are all patients without the disease and negative test result.

Dimensionality Reduction with Principal Component Analysis

Dimensionality reduction is a mapping from a multidimensional space into a space of fewer dimensions. It is often the case that data analysis can be carried out in the reduced space more accurately than in the original space. More formally, the dimensionality reduction problem can be stated as follows: given the a-dimensional random variable $x=(x_1, x_2, ..., x_d)$ find a lower dimensional representation of it, $s=(s_1, s_2, ..., s_k)$ with $k<a$, that captures the content in the original data, according to some criterion.

Principal components analysis (PCA) is a linear transformation that chooses a new coordinate system for the data such that the greatest variance by any projection of the data set lies on the first axis (called the first principal component), the second greatest variance on the second axis, and so on (Pearson, 1901). PCA can be used for reducing dimensionality in a dataset while retaining those characteristics of the dataset that contribute most to its variance by eliminating the lesser principal components (by a more or less heuristic decision).

PCA is sometimes used to extract features directly from images in matrix form, where pixel intensity values are used as primary features. Our experiments with using PCA directly on CAD images produced such dismal results of machine learning (on par with a simple majority classifier) that we were discouraged to further pursue in this direction. So in the case of CAD diagnostics from scintigraphic images, several thousands of ArTex/ARes-generated image features are used as an input for PCA.

In our present study, we use PCA to reduce the high number of ArTex/ARes-generated image features (several thousand), to more manageable levels (a few tens of compound attributes that explain most of data variance).

MATERIALS

The Two CAD Studies

In our early (1994) study, we used a dataset of 327 patients (250 males, 77 females, average age 55 years) selected from a population of approximately

Table 1: Past (1994) and present (2006) CAD data for different diagnostic levels. Of the attributes belonging to the coronary angiography diagnostic level, in the new study only the final diagnosis – the two-valued class – was used in experiments.

	Diagnostic level	Study	Number of attributes		
			Nominal	Numeric	Total
1.	Signs and symptoms	1994	23	7	30
		2006	22	5	27
2.	Exercise ECG	1994	7	9	16
		2006	11	7	18
3.	Myocardial scintigraphy	1994	22	9	31
	(+9 image series in 2006 study)	2006	8	2	10
4.	Coronary angiography	1994	1	6	7
		2006	1	6	7
	Class distribution	1994	98 (29.97%)		CAD negative
			229 (70.03%)		CAD positive
		2006	129 (46.40%)		CAD negative
			149 (53.60%)		CAD positive

4000 patients examined at the Nuclear Medicine Department between 1991 and 1994. All selected patients had complete diagnostic procedures (all four levels) (Kukar et al., 1997), consisting of clinical and laboratory examinations, exercise ECG, myocardial scintigraphy, and coronary angiograph. The features from the ECG and scintigraphy data were extracted manually by clinicians. Angiography confirmed the disease in 229 cases and excluded it in 98 cases. 162 patients had suffered a recent myocardial infarction. Our experiments were conducted on four problems. They differ in the amount of clinical and laboratory data (attributes) available for learning, corresponding to different diagnostic levels (Table 1).

In our present (2006) CAD study we use a newer dataset of 288 patients who completed clinical and laboratory examinations, exercise ECG, myocardial scintigraphy (including complete image sets) and coronary angiography because of suspected CAD. The features from the ECG an scintigraphy data were extracted manually by the clinicians. Ten patients were later

excluded for data pre-processing and calibration required by ArTex/ARes, so only 278 patients (66 females, 212 males, average age 60 years) were used in actual experiments. In 149 cases the disease was angiographically confirmed and in 129 cases it was excluded. The patients were selected from a population of several thousands patients who were examined at the Nuclear Medicine Department between 2001 and 2006. Again we selected only the patients with complete diagnostic procedures (all four levels), and for whom the imaging data was readily accessible. Some characteristics of the dataset are shown in Table 1. Although both data sets were collected in exactly the same way, there is a significant difference in class distributions between the two sets (see Table 1, bottom row). Due to improved diagnostic clinical capabilities as well as ageing population (average age increased by 5 years), the patients included in our present (2006) study are much more difficult to diagnose. Although the total number of patients examined for CAD is increasing, an increasing number of patients is being reliably diagnosed with less invasive diagnostic tests. The population in our present (2006) study therefore consists of patients that defy reliable diagnostics on lower diagnostic levels, and thus represent a challenge even for expert physicians.

Several patients in our 2006 dataset had already undergone cardiac surgery or dilatation of coronary vessels. This clearly reflects the situation in Central Europe with its ageing population. Our results are therefore not applicable to the general population: also, general findings only partially apply to our population.

The myocardial scintigraphy group of attributes consists of evaluation of myocardial defects (no defect, mild defect, well defined defect, serious defect) that could be observed in images either while resting or during a controlled exercise. They are assessed for four different myocardial regions: LAD (left anterior descending), LCx (left circumflex), and RCA (right coronary artery) vascular territories, as well as ventricular apex. Additional two attributes concern effective blood flow and volumes in myocardium: left ventricular ejection fraction (LVEF) and end-diastolic volume (EDV).

In our clinical practice, four expert physicians regularly assess myocardial scintigraphy images. They estimate the level of coronary artery congestion and produce attribute values for different myocardial regions. The final diagnosis summarizes the obtained attribute values. It is difficult to precisely describe how the attribute values are determined, as it is based on years of experience and medical knowledge of the myocardium. As an important step in data pre-processing, and to insure reliability, an additional expert physician re-evaluated all images. Only images whose original and retrospective diagnoses were in accord were retained for the experiments.

Scintigraphic Images

In the present (2006) study scintigraphic images were obtained from General Electric eNTEGRA SPECT camera, producing grayscale images with a 64 × 64 8-bit pixel resolution. Images were obtained while the patient was at rest and following a controlled exercise, producing a total of 64 images. Due to patient's movements and partial obscuring of the heart muscle by other internal organs, these images were not suitable for further use without heavy pre-processing. For this purpose, the ECToolbox workstation software (General Electric, 2001) was used to generate a series of 9 polar map images for each patient. Polar maps were chosen because previous work in this field (Lindahl et al., 1998) had shown that they have useful diagnostic value. Polar images, usually referred to as a bull's-eye plot, present the short axis section as rings of increasing diameter, with the apex at the center and the base of the heart at the periphery. This allows quick assessment of the number and the area of any defects at stress and rest. Comparison with a database of reference images highlights areas of reduced activity which meet a predefined criterion for significance, and subtraction images are produced to illustrate the extent of reversibility. The 9 polar map images for each patient consist of the following images produced by ECToolbox:

- Three raw images (the stress image, and the rest image, and the reversibility image, calculated as a difference between normalized rest and stress images);
- Three blackout (defect extent) images (the stress image and the rest image, both compared to the respective database of normal images, and suitably processed). Again the reversibility image is calculated as a difference between normalized rest and stress blackout images;
- Three standard deviation images that show relative perfusion variance when compared to the respective database of normal images.

An example of polar map images for three patients is shown in Figure 3. The first patient

Figure 3. Bull's eye images (polar maps) taken after exercise, at rest, and their difference for three patients exhibiting severe (1), moderate (2) and atypical (3) manifestation of CAD. The first three rows show raw images, the second three show blackout images, and the last three show standard deviation images. Black regions indicate insufficient perfusion of cardiac tissue (a potential defect).

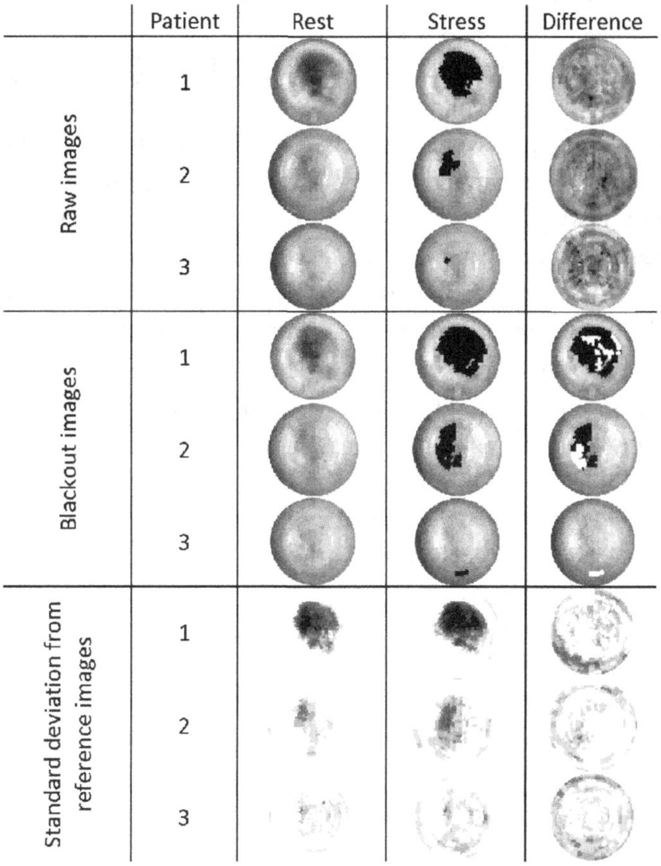

(1) exhibits very clear manifestation of CAD. The second patient (2) represents a moderate manifestation of CAD whereas the third patient (3) exhibits fairly atypical signs of the disease. Interpretation and evaluation of scintigraphic images therefore requires considerable knowledge and experience of expert physicians. Although specialized tools such as the ECToolbox software can aid in this process, they still require a lot of training and in-depth medical knowledge for reliable and replicable evaluation of results.

RESULTS

Experimental Methodology

For diagnostic support, expert physicians compare either raw images (our past study) or polar maps (our present study) taken after exercise, with that taken at rest, and assess the differences. For each type the raw image, the blackout image, and the standard deviation image is used 3×3=9 images). To objectively evaluate the proposed methodology, experiments were performed in the following manner. First, ten learning examples (images or sets of nine images for CAD) were excluded for data preprocessing and calibration of ArTex/ARes. Images from the remaining examples were parameterized and only the obtained parameters were subsequently used for evaluation. Further testing was performed in the ten-fold cross-validation setting: at each step 90% of examples were used for building a classifier and the remaining 10% of examples were used for testing.

For CAD diagnostics, the set of parameters generated from the set of nine polar map images for each patient were reduced by extracting the ten most informative parameters using either feature extraction or feature selection methods. Feature extraction consisted of applying PCA to the full set of parameters and retaining the 10 best principal components that together accounted for not less than 70% of data variance. Feature selection consisted of applying ReliefF (Robnik-Šikonja & Kononenko, 2003) attribute quality estimation and retaining only 10 best ArTex/ARes generated attributes. In addition, ten of the best attributes provided by physicians were also used, again as estimated by ReliefF.

In each cross-validation step the real-valued attributes were discretized in advance using the (Fayyad, 1993) algorithm if the applied method (such as the naive Bayes classifier) required only discrete attributes.

We applied four popular machine learning algorithms: naive Bayes classifier, tree-augmented Bayesian network, support vector machine (SMO using RBF kernel), and J4.8 (C4.5) decision tree, and two neural network algorithms (multilayered perceptron – MLP, and radial basis function network – RBFN). We performed experiments and analysis of experimental results with both Weka (Witten & Frank, 2005) and Orange (Demšar et al., 2004) machine learning toolkits. For CAD diagnostics, aggregated results of the coronary angiography (CAD negative/CAD positive) were used as the class variable. The results of clinical practice were validated by careful blind evaluation of images by an independent expert physician. Differences between physician and machine learning results were evaluated for statistical significance by using McNemar's test (Demšar, 2006).

Results in CAD Diagnostics

As described before, out of the 288 patients, 10 were excluded for data preprocessing and calibration required by ArTex/ARes. These patients were not used in further experiments. The remaining 278 patients with 9 images each were parameterized for three resolutions in advance. ARes proposed three resolutions: $0.95\times$, $0.80\times$, and $0.30\times$ of the original resolution (a resolution $0.30\times$ means using $0.30\cdot64\times0.30\cdot64$ pixels instead of 64×64 pixels). This produces 2944 additional attributes (features, parameters). Since this number is by far too large for most practical purposes, it was reduced either by applying feature selection (with ReliefF) or by feature extraction (with PCA).

The ReliefF algorithm was used to evaluate all 2944 features by assigning each a numerical value. Features were ranked according to their relevance, and only the best (most relevant) 10 features were used in subsequent experiments.

Experimental results were compared with diagnostic accuracy, specificity and sensitivity of expert physicians after evaluation of scintigraphic images (Table 2). Results of clinical practice were validated by careful blind evaluation of images by an expert physician.

For machine learning experiments we considered five different settings that are described in more detail in subsequent sections:

1. Evaluation of machine learning methods only on physician-provided attributes (Table 2),
2. Evaluation of all ArTex/ARres-generated attributes (the first half of Table 3),
3. Evaluation of all ArTex/ARres-generated attributes together with all attributes provided by physicians, (the second half of Table 3),

Table 2. Diagnostic results (in %) of physicians compared with results of machine learning classifiers obtained from the original attributes, as extracted by physicians. Results (classification accuracies) that are significantly (p<0.05) different (better or worse) from clinical results are emphasized.

	All attributes provided by physicians		
	Accuracy	Specificity	Sensitivity
Clinical	64.00	71.10	55.80
Naive Bayes	**68.34**	69.80	67.10
Bayes Net	**67.14**	68.20	66.70
SMO (RBF)	65.10	62.80	67.10
J4.8	**57.19**	53.50	60.40
MLP	**66.89**	64.87	68.68
RBFN	64.21	63.56	64.86

4. Evaluation of 10 best attributes (accounting for 70% of data variance) extracted by either ReliefF (the first half of Table 4) or PCA (the first half of Table 5) from ArTex/ARres-generated attributes,
5. Evaluation of the same 10 best attributes extracted by either ReliefF (the second half of Table 4) or PCA (the second half of Table 5) in conjunction with 10 best attributes provided by physicians, as estimated by the ReliefF algorithm.

Evaluation of Machine Learning Methods on Original Attributes Provided by Physicians

In this setup, only attributes provided by physicians were used for learning classifiers and subsequent classification in 10-fold cross validation setting. Thus we evaluate the contribution of machine learning methods alone. From Table 2 we can see that machine learning algorithms perform approximately on the level of expert physicians when evaluating the original data, as collected by physicians. The Naive Bayes classifier achieves significantly higher classification ($p<0.05$) accuracy and slightly (insignificantly) lower sensitivity than physicians, while the J4.8 decision tree achieves significantly lower classification accuracy. However, for physicians, improvements of specificity are more important than improvements of sensitivity or overall classification accuracy, since increased specificity decreases the number of unnecessarily performed higher-level diagnostic tests, and consequently shortens waiting times for truly ill patients. Unfortunately, no applied machine learning method attained this goal at this stage.

Evaluation of All ArTex/ARres-Generated Attributes

Let us first examine results obtained by using all the parameters provided by ArTex/ARes (Table 3). Results show only a slight improvement of classification accuracy with respect to machine learning on clinical data in both experimental setups (image attributes only, and both image and physicians' attributes).

When only image attributes are used (upper half of Table 3) we have a truly automated approach where diagnosis is proposed without any physician involvement. While the experimental result by itself look very nice, as they significantly improve diagnostic accuracy with respect to physicians, they do not improve in all three criteria (diagnostic accuracy, specificity, and sensitivity).

Table 3. Experimental results (in %) of machine learning classifiers on parameterized images obtained by using all available ArTex/ARes attributes as well those provided by physicians. Results in diagnostic accuracy that significantly (p<0.05) differ from clinical results are emphasized.

	All image attributes (ArTex/ARes)		
	Accuracy	Specificity	Sensitivity
Naive Bayes	70.14	68.50	72.10
Bayes Net	69.20	68.10	70.30
SMO (RBF)	61.15	58.10	63.80
J4.8	59.71	63.80	55.00
MLP	69.90	67.72	71.80
RBFN	67.13	66.45	67.81
Clinical	64.00	71.10	55.80
	All image and physicians' attributes		
	Accuracy	Specificity	Sensitivity
Naive Bayes	70.50	69.10	72.10
Bayes Net	69.80	68.30	71.40
SMO (RBF)	69.40	69.80	69.10
J4.8	65.10	60.50	69.10
MLP	70.92	69.00	72.58
RBFN	68.86	67.00	70.47

From the upper half of Table 3 we can also see that some machine learning algorithms — notably decision trees and surprisingly SMO have some trouble handling a huge number (2944) of additional attributes with only 278 learning examples (support vector machines are supposed to perform well on high-dimensional data). This leads to overfitting the learning data and reduction of diagnostic performance. When using all 2944 attributes, the naive Bayes classifier produced best results – significantly better than physicians as well as other tested machine learning algorithms. Using these 2944 attributes together with the physician-provided attributes again slightly improves the classification results. This improvement was significant in two of three cases. Especially notable is the improvement in the previously low-performing J4.8 (decision trees) and SMO, as they clearly cannot extract all the available knowledge from a large set of individual, possibly correlated attributes.

It is reasonable to assume that physicians' attributes are considerably more complex and much more informative than simple numerical features provided by ArTex/ARes. From machine learning and data mining theory (Kononenko & Kukar, 2007) we know that machine learning algorithms benefit considerably by using dimensionality reduction techniques. Specifically, extraction of new, less numerous possibly uncorrelated and more informative composite features usually contribute to more successful machine learning (in terms of higher classification accuracy and larger area under ROC curve – AUC).

Evaluation of Best ArTex/ARres-Generated or Extracted Attributes

In this setting, we either extracted 10 best principal components (linear combinations of original ArTex/ARes attributes) by PCA, or selected 10 best original attributes with ReliefF from the set

Table 4. Experimental results (in %) of machine learning classifiers on parameterized images obtained by selecting only the best 10 attributes from either ArTex/ARes (also combined with 10 best attributes provided by physicians). Classification accuracy results that are significantly better (p<0.05) than clinical results are emphasized.

	Best 10 attributes (ArTex/ARes)		
	Accuracy	**Specificity**	**Sensitivity**
Naive Bayes	**69.40**	58.90	78.50
Bayes Net	**69.40**	58.90	78.50
SMO (RBF kernel)	**71.90**	65.10	77.90
J4.8	**70.90**	61.20	79.20
MLP	**70.30**	68.10	72.20
RBFN	67.50	66.80	68.20
Clinical	64.00	71.10	55.80
	Best 10 attributes (ArTex/ARes)+physicians		
	Accuracy	Specificity	Sensitivity
Naive Bayes	**74.80**	70.50	78.50
Bayes Net	**74.40**	69.80	78.50
SMO (RBF kernel)	**73.40**	65.90	79.90
J4.8	**68.00**	63.60	71.80
MLP	**74.00**	72.00	75.70
RBFN	**72.00**	71.10	73.20

of 2944 ArTex/ARes attributes. We also enriched the data representation by using the same number (10) of best physicians' attributes as evaluated by ReliefF and compared with the results of machine learning.

Table 4 and Table 5 as well as Figure 4 and Figure 5 depict the results. We see that without any special tuning of learning parameters, the results are in all cases significantly better than the results of physicians in terms of classification (diagnostic) accuracy. Especially good results are that of the naive Bayes classifier (Table 5), that improve in all three criteria: diagnostic accuracy (by 17.3%), sensitivity (by 23.4%) and specificity (by 12.6%). Another interesting issue is that including the best physician-provided attributes does not necessarily improve diagnostic performance (SMO, J4.8 in Table 5). It seems that there is some level of redundancy between physicians' and principal components generated from ArTex/

ARes attributes that bothers some methods more than the others. Consequently, it seems that some of automatically generated attributes are (from the diagnostic performance point of view) at least as good as the physician-provided ones, and may therefore represent new knowledge about CAD diagnostics.

Explaining the Meaning of the New Attributes

Since the diagnostic performance of machine learning methods turned out to be significantly better than that of expert physicians, a question whether some new knowledge had been induced from images is imminent. To gain some insight into the new attributes, we performed an analysis of associations between best physician-provided and Artex/ARes-generated attributes.

Table 5. Experimental results (in %) of machine learning classifiers on parameterized images obtained by selecting only the best 10 attributes from PCA on ArTex/ARes (also combined with 10 best attributes provided by physicians). Classification accuracy results that are significantly better (p<0.05) than clinical results are emphasized.

	PCA on ArTex/ARes		
	Accuracy	**Specificity**	**Sensitivity**
Naive Bayes	**81.30**	83.70	79.20
Bayes Net	**71.90**	69.00	74.50
SMO (RBF kernel)	**78.40**	76.00	80.10
J4.8	**75.20**	78.30	72.50
MLP	**82.40**	79.80	84.60
RBFN	**79.10**	78.30	79.90
Clinical	64.00	71.10	55.80
	PCA on ArTex/ARes+physicians		
	Accuracy	Specificity	Sensitivity
Naive Bayes	**79.10**	82.90	75.80
Bayes Net	**79.10**	83.70	75.20
SMO (RBF)	**76.60**	77.50	75.80
J4.8	**74.10**	73.60	74.50
MLP	**81.30**	79.10	83.20
RBFN	**79.10**	79.10	79.10

Figure 4. Comparison of clinical results and results of machine learning classifiers on parameterized images from Table 5

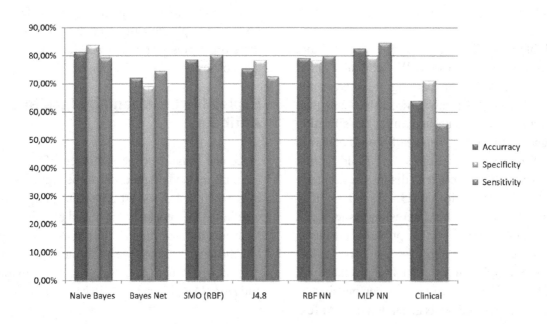

Figure 5. Improvements of machine learning classifiers on parameterized images from Table 5 relative to clinical results (baseline 0%)

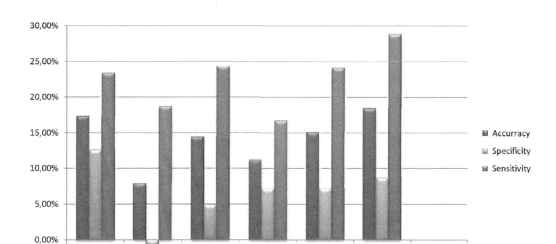

- When reviewing associations between in ARES-generated and physicians' attributes, several highly confident (more than 99%) rules of shape *"IF sex=Male AND value of ARES attribute is high THEN lbbb is absent"* surfaced. Left bundle branch block (lbbb) is a cardiac conduction abnormality seen on the electrocardiogram (ECG) and if present, may cause false readings of scintigrams. It seems that some generated attributes describe the absence of this anomaly in male patients. Another interesting type of rules associates (although with lower confidence about 70%) values of some ARES attributes with results of scintigraphy during rest and controlled exercise, and thus supports (or even improves on) physicians' findings. An example of such a rule is *"IF no anomalous reading at rest AND value of ARES attribute is high THEN no anomalous reading during exercise"*.

- When reviewing associations between principal components and physicians' attributes, we found two rules associating two PCA components with low HDL level and diabetes with confidence of about 90%. There were also a few rules relating PCA attributes with scintigraphic results in LCx territory (both during rest and stress), also with confidence over 90%.

In graphical representation of causal networks induced from learning data by the TAN algorithm (Sahami, 1996)(Figure 7, results shown for PCA+physicians only), causal relations are indicated by edges in the graph between scintigraphic attributes describing test results in RCA and LCx territories during rest and stress, for both ARES- and PCA-on-ARES- generated attributes. Although there are some similarities between physicians and association rules or causal networks, it seems that the new attributes convey considerably different diagnostic information and may therefore contribute new medical knowledge.

Figure 7. A causal network of best physician-provided and PCA-generated attributes. Arrows represent cause-effect relations, as induced from learning data by the TAN algorithm. Bold black line represents strong positive causality, whereas bold gray line represents negative causality.

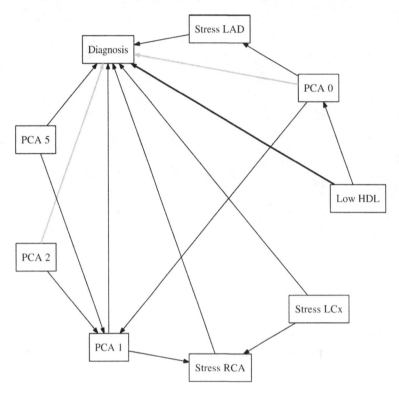

Assessing the Diagnostic Power

In order to assess the diagnostic power of our compound approach, we applied the post-test probability calculation method as described in (Olona-Cabases, 1994) for assessing reliability (probability of a correct diagnosis) of machine learning classifications in stepwise diagnostic process, To determine the pre-test probability we applied tabulated values (Table 6) as given in (Pollock, 1983). For each patient, the table was indexed by a subset of "signs and symptoms" attributes (age, sex, type of chest pain).

For both physicians and machine learning methods we calculated the post-test probabilities in the stepwise manner, starting from the pre-test probability and proceeding with evaluation of signs and symptoms, exercise ECG, and myocardial scintigraphy. For myocardial scintigraphy,

physicians achieved 64% diagnostic accuracy, 71.1% specificity, and 55.8% sensitivity. For the reliability threshold of 90%, 52% of diagnoses could be considered as reliable (their post-test probability was higher than 90% for positive, or lower than 10% for negative diagnoses). On the other hand, naive Bayes classifier achieved for myocardial scintigraphy 81.3% diagnostic accuracy, 83.7% specificity, and 79.2% sensitivity. For the reliability threshold of 90%, 69% of diagnoses could be considered as reliable. Improvement in 17% of reliable diagnostic accuracy is a result of 19% improvement for reliable positive diagnoses, and 16% for reliable negative diagnoses.

We also depict results automatic approach in ROC curves, obtained by varying reliability threshold between 0 and 1 (Figure 6), and compare it with physicians. A fully automatic approach

Table 6. Pre-test probabilities for the presence of CAD

Sex	Age	Asymptomatic patients	Nonang. chest pain	Atypical angina	Typical angina
Female	35-44	0.007	0.027	0.155	0.454
	45-54	0.021	0.069	0.317	0.677
	55-64	0.054	0.127	0.465	0.839
	65-74	0.115	0.171	0.541	0.947
Male	35-44	0.037	0.105	0.428	0.809
	45-54	0.077	0.206	0.601	0.907
	55-64	0.111	0.282	0.690	0.939
	65-74	0.113	0.282	0.700	0.943

Figure 6. ROC curves for automatically generated attributes (ArTex/ARes + PCA, Figures a and b) and automatically generated attributes with included best physicians' attributes (ArTex/ARes + PCA+physicians, Figures c and d). In each figure, x-axis values represents false positive rate (1-Specificity), whereas y-axis values represent true positive rate (Sensitivity).

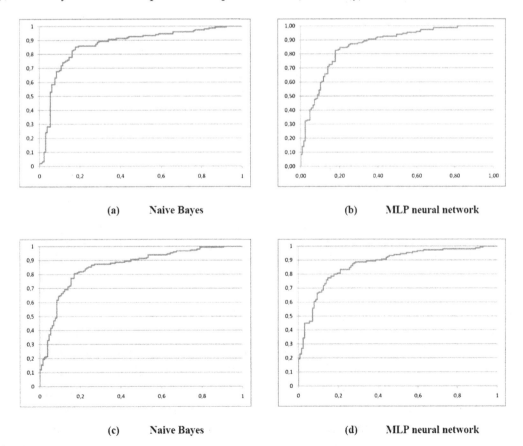

(a)   **Naive Bayes**

(b)   **MLP neural network**

(c)   **Naive Bayes**

(d)   **MLP neural network**

(Naive Bayes and MLP on parameterized images) has considerably higher ROC curve than physicians, both for reliable positive (AUC=0.90 vs. 0.82) and reliable negative patients (AUC=0.91 vs. 0.83). Of improvements in positive and negative reliable diagnoses, by far the more important is the 16% improvement for reliable negative diagnoses. The reason for this is that positive patients undergo further pre-operative diagnostic tests in any case, while for negative patients diagnostic process can reliably be finished on the myocardial scintigraphy level.

Summary of the Results Achieved through the Study

In Table 7 we summarize experimental results of our past (1994) study (Kukar & Grošelj, 1999). Compared to our present study, both diagnostic accuracy and sensitivity were considerably higher, whereas specificity was about the same. According to expert physicians' explanation this is a direct consequence of aging population and improved early diagnostic tests. Namely, our present study comprises a population that is much more difficult to diagnose reliably.

In Table 8 we summarize computational results of our present (2006) study and compare them with results from clinical practice (Table 8, first row). We notice that machine learning algorithms have some trouble when handling a huge number (2944) of attributes, with only 278 learning examples (Table 8, second and third row). This can lead to overfitting the learning data and diminished diagnostic performance. Only naive Bayes classifier is significantly better than physicians when using all attributes. However, using these 2944 attributes together with the original attributes invariably improves upon physicians' results, in two of three cases even significantly.

Most utilized learning algorithms benefit considerably from attribute filtering. In all cases the results are significantly better than the results of physicians. Especially good results are that of

naive Bayes classifier, which improves diagnostic accuracy, sensitivity and specificity (Table 8, fourth row). Attributes were filtered with the ReliefF algorithm. However, even better results are achieved by extracting higher-level, compound attributes with principal component analysis (Table 8, fifth row).

FUTURE RESEARCH DIRECTIONS

The utilized combination of machine learning and image parameterization algorithms opens a new research area of multi-resolution image parameterization and could be utilized in several medical, industrial and other domains where textures or texture-like surfaces are classified. The resolution selection algorithm ARes can be improved with additional domain-specific resolution search refinements, and with heuristic methods for controlling selection of resolutions.

In our case study – the CAD diagnostics problem – we intend to concentrate even more on improving the diagnostic performance of the myocardial perfusion scintigraphy and assess problem-dependent criteria for resolution quality. We will study in-depth relations between automatically generated and physician-provided attributes and try to establish the possible correspondence between them. Potential improvements of the parameterization and classification scheme will be used in the post-test probability estimation setting (Olona-Cabases, 1994) for evaluating the reliability of machine-generated diagnoses.

CONCLUSION

A major bottleneck in clinical evaluation of medical imaging test results is that usually expert physicians need to be involved – by using their medical knowledge and experience as well as image processing capabilities provided by various imaging software – to manually describe (parameterize) and

Table 7. Experimental results (in %) of our past (1994) CAD study compared to respective expert physicians' results

Results of past (1994) study	Accuracy	Specificity	Sensitivity
Physicians	83%	85%	83%
Naive Bayes (scintigraphy)	90%	81%	94%
Naive Bayes (all attributes)	91%	81%	96%

Table 8. Diagnostic performance (in %) of best machine learning classifiers achieved over the study. Results (classification accuracies) that are significantly (p<0.05) better than clinical results are emphasized.

Results of present (2006) study	Accuracy	Specificity	Sensitivity
1. Clinical results	**64.00**	**71.10**	**55.80**
2. Machine learning results on the original attributes as extracted by physicians.	All attributes provided by physicians		
	68.34	69.80	67.10
3. Results of machine learning on parameterized images obtained by using all available attributes.	All image (2944) and physicians' attributes		
	70.50	69.10	72.10
	All image attributes (2944)		
	70.14	68.50	72.10
4. Results of machine learning on parameterized images obtained by selecting only the best 10 attributes.	10 best image and physicians' attributes		
	74.80	70.50	78.50
	10 best image attributes		
	71.90	65.10	77.90
5. Results on parameterized images obtained by selecting the best 10 attributes from PCA on ArTex / ARes parameters	PCA on ArTex/ARes		
	81.30	83.70	79.20
	PCA on ArTex/ARes +		
	10 best physicians' attributes		
	79.10	82.90	75.80

evaluate the images. We describe an automatized alternative to manual image evaluation - multi-resolution image parameterization based on spatial association rules (ArTex/ARes) supplemented with feature selection or (preferably) feature extraction. Our results significantly improve upon physicians in terms of diagnostic quality of image parameters. By using these parameters for building machine learning classifiers, diagnostic performance can be significantly improved with respect to the results of clinical practice. We also explore relations between newly generated image attributes and physicians' description of images.

Our findings indicate that ArTex/ARes with PCA is likely to extract more useful information from images than the physicians do, as it significantly outperforms them in terms of diagnostic accuracy, specificity and sensitivity.

Utilizing automated image classification methods can help interns or inexperienced physicians to more reliably evaluate medical images and thus improve their diagnostic accuracy, sensitivity and specificity. From the practical use of described approaches two-fold improvements of the diagnostic procedure can be expected. In our experiments, higher diagnostic accuracy (up to 17.3%) and sensitivity (up to 23.4%) represent a very considerable gain. Due to higher specificity of tests (up to 12.6%), fewer patients without the disease would have to be examined with the invasive and possibly dangerous coronary angiography. Together with higher sensitivity this would save money and shorten the waiting times of the truly ill patients. Also, new attributes generated by ArTex/ARes with PCA are invoking considerable interest from expert physicians, since they significantly contribute to increased diagnostic performance and may therefore convey some novel medical knowledge of the CAD diagnostics problem.

Finally, we need to emphasize again that the results of our studies are based on data from a significantly restricted population and therefore may not be generally applicable to the normal population or to all the patients coming to the Nuclear Medicine Department, University Clinical Centre Ljubljana, Slovenia.

ACKNOWLEDGMENT

This work was partly supported by the Slovenian Ministry of Higher Education, Science, and Technology.

REFERENCES

Allison, J. S., Heo, J., & Iskandrian, A. E. (2005). Artificial neural network modeling of stress single-photon emission computed tomographic imaging for detecting extensive coronary artery disease. *The American Journal of Cardiology*, *95*(2), 178–181. doi:10.1016/j.amjcard.2004.09.003

Bevk, M., & Kononenko, I. (2006). Towards symbolic mining of images with association rules: Preliminary results on textures. *Intelligent Data Analysis*, *10*(4), 379–393.

Brodatz, P. (1966). *Textures - A photographic album for artists and designers*. Reinhold.

Chui, C. (1992). *An introduction to wavelets*. San Diego, CA: Academic Press.

Demšar, J. (2006). Statistical comparisons of classifiers over multiple data sets. *Journal of Machine Learning Research*, *7*, 1–30.

Demšar, J., Zupan, B., & Leban, G. (2004). *Orange: From experimental machine learning to interactive data mining*. White paper. Retrieved August 16, 2009, from http://www.ailab.si/orange

Fayyad, U. M. (1993). Multi-interval discretization of continuous-valued attributes for classification learning. In R. Bajcsy (Ed.), *Proceedings of the International Joint Conferences on Artificial Intelligence*, (pp. 1022–1027). San Mateo, CA: Morgan Kaufmann.

Fitzpatrick, J., & Sonka, M. (2000). *Handbook of medical imaging, medical image processing and analysis* (*Vol. 2*). Bellingham, WA: SPIE.

Gamberger, D., Lavrac, N., & Krstacic, G. (2003). Active subgroup mining: A case study in coronary heart disease risk group detection. *Artificial Intelligence in Medicine*, *28*(1), 27–57. doi:10.1016/S0933-3657(03)00034-4

Garcia, E. V., Cooke, C. D., Folks, R. D., Santana, C. A., Krawczynska, E. G., Braal, L. D., & Ezquerra, N. F. (2001). Diagnostic performance of an expert system for the interpretation of myocardial perfusion aspect studies. *Journal of Nuclear Medicine*, *42*(8), 1185–1191.

General Electric. (2001). *ECToolbox protocol operators guide*.

Grigorescu, S., Petkov, N., & Kruizinga, P. (2002). Comparison of texture features based on gabor filters. *IEEE Transactions on Image Processing*, *11*(10), 1160–1167. doi:10.1109/TIP.2002.804262

Jelonek, J., & Stefanowski, J. (1997). Feature subset selection for classification of histological images. *Artificial Intelligence in Medicine*, *9*(3), 227–239. doi:10.1016/S0933-3657(96)00375-2

Katsis, C.D., Goletsis, Y., Likas, A., Fotiadis, D., & Sarmas, I. (2006). A novel method for automated EMG decomposition and MUAP classification. *Artificial Intelligence in Medicine*, *37*(1), 55–64. doi:10.1016/j.artmed.2005.09.002

Kira, K., & Rendell, L. (1992). A practical approach to feature selection. In D. Sleeman & P. Edwards, (Eds.), *Proceedings of the International Conference on Machine Learning*, (pp. 249–256). Aberdeen, UK: Morgan Kaufmann.

Kononenko, I. (1993). Inductive and Bayesian learning in medical diagnosis. *Applied Artificial Intelligence*, *7*, 317–337. doi:10.1080/08839519308949993

Kononenko, I. (2001). Machine learning for medical diagnosis: History, state of the art and perspective. *Artificial Intelligence in Medicine*, *3*, 89–109. doi:10.1016/S0933-3657(01)00077-X

Kononenko, I., & Kukar, M. (2007). *Machine learning and data mining: Introduction to principles and algorithms*. Chichester, UK: Horwood Publishing.

Kukar, M., & Grošelj, C. (1999). Machine learning in stepwise diagnostic process. In W. Horn, Y. Shahar, G. Lindberg, S. Andreassen & J. Wyatt (Eds.), *Proceedings of the Joint European Conference on Artificial Intelligence in Medicine and Medical Decision Making*, (pp. 315–325). Aalborg, Denmark: Springer.

Kukar, M., Grošelj, C., Kononenko, I., & Fettich, J. (1997). An application of machine learning in the diagnosis of ischaemic heart disease. In *Proceedings of the Sixth European Conference of AI in Medicine Europe AIME97*, Grenoble, France, (pp. 461–464).

Kukar, M., Kononenko, I., Grošelj, C., Kralj, K., & Fettich, J. (1999). Analysing and improving the diagnosis of ischaemic heart disease with machine learning. *Artificial Intelligence in Medicine*, *16*(1), 25–50. doi:10.1016/S0933-3657(98)00063-3

Kukar, M., & Šajn, L. (2009). Improving probabilistic interpretation of medical diagnoses with multi-resolution image parameterization: A case study. In C. Combi, Y. Shahar & A. Abu-Hanna (Eds.), *12th Conference on Artificial Intelligence in Medicine*, (pp. 136–145). Springer.

Kukar, M., Šajn, L., Grošelj, C., & Grošelj, J. (2007). Multi-resolution image parametrization in sequential diagnostics of coronary artery disease. In Bellazzi, R., Abu-Hanna, A., & Hunter, J. (Eds.), *Artificial intelligence in medicine* (pp. 119–129). Berlin, Germany: Springer. doi:10.1007/978-3-540-73599-1_13

Kurgan, L. A., Cios, K. J., & Tadeusiewicz, R. (2001). Knowledge discovery approach to automated cardiac spect diagnosis. *Artificial Intelligence in Medicine*, *23*(2), 149–169. doi:10.1016/S0933-3657(01)00082-3

Laws, K. I. (1980). *Textured image segmentation*. PhD thesis, Dept. Electrical Engineering, University of Southern California, Los Angeles, California, USA.

Lindahl, D., Palmer, J., Pettersson, J., White, T., Lundin, A., & Edenbrandt, L. (1998). Scintigraphic diagnosis of coronary artery disease: Myocardial bulls-eye images contain the important information. *Clinical Physiology (Oxford, England)*, *6*(18).

Lowe, D. G. (2004). Distinctive image features from scale-invariant keypoints. *International Journal of Computer Vision*, *60*(2), 91–110. doi:10.1023/B:VISI.0000029664.99615.94

Mobley, B. A., Schechter, E., & Moore, W. E. (2000). Predictions of coronary artery stenosis by artificial neural network. *Artificial Intelligence in Medicine*, *18*(3), 187–203. doi:10.1016/S0933-3657(99)00040-8

Nixon, M., & Aguado, A. (2008). *Feature extraction and image processing* (2nd ed.). Amsterdam, The Netherlands: Elsevier.

Ohlsson, M. (2004). WeAidU–A decision support system for myocardial perfusion images using artificial neural networks. *Artificial Intelligence in Medicine*, *30*, 49–60. doi:10.1016/S0933-3657(03)00050-2

Ojala, T., Mäenpää, T., Pietikäinen, M., Viertola, J., Kyllönen, J., & Huovinen, S. (2002). Outex - New framework for empirical evaluation of texture analysis algorithms. In *International Conference on Pattern Recognition,* Vol. 1, (p. 10701). Los Alamitos, CA: IEEE Computer Society.

Olona-Cabases, M. (1994). The probability of a correct diagnosis. In Candell-Riera, J., & Ortega-Alcalde, D. (Eds.), *Nuclear cardiology in everyday practice* (pp. 348–357). Dordrecht, The Netherlands: Kluwer Academic Publishers. doi:10.1007/978-94-011-1984-9_19

Pearson, K. (1901). Principal components analysis. *The London, Edinburgh, and Dublin Philosophical Magazine and Journal of Science*, 559.

Peng, Y., Yao, B., & Jiang, J. (2006). Knowledge-discovery incorporated evolutionary search for microcalcification detection in breast cancer diagnosis. *Artificial Intelligence in Medicine*, *37*(1), 43–53. doi:10.1016/j.artmed.2005.09.001

Pollock, B. H. (1983). Computer-assisted interpretation of noninvasive tests for diagnosis of coronary artery disease. *Cardiovascular Reviews & Reports*, *4*, 367–375.

Robnik-Šikonja, M., & Kononenko, I. (2003). Theoretical and empirical analysis of ReliefF and RReliefF. *Machine Learning*, *53*, 23–69. doi:10.1023/A:1025667309714

Sahami, M. (1996). Learning limited dependence Bayesian classifiers. In *KDD-96: Proceedings of the Second International Conference on Knowledge Discovery and Data Mining*, (pp. 335–338). AAAI Press.

Šajn, L., & Kononenko, I. (2008). Multiresolution image parametrization for improving texture classification. *EURASIP Journal on Advances in Signal Processing*, (1): 1–13. doi:10.1155/2008/617457

Šajn, L., & Kononenko, I. (2009). Image segmentation and parametrization for automatic diagnostics of whole-body scintigrams. In *Computational intelligence in medical imaging: Techniques & applications* (pp. 347–377). Boca Raton, FL: CRC Press. doi:10.1201/9781420060614.ch12

Slomka, P. J., Nishina, H., Berman, D. S., Akincioglu, C., Abidov, A., & Friedman, J. D. (2005). Automated quantification of myocardial perfusion spect using simplified normal limits. *Journal of Nuclear Cardiology*, *12*(1), 66–77. doi:10.1016/j.nuclcard.2004.10.006

Witten, I. H., & Frank, E. (2005). *Data mining: Practical machine learning tools and techniques* (2nd ed.). San Francisco, CA: Morgan Kaufmann.

Yang, J., & Honavar, V. (1998). Feature subset selection using a genetic algorithm. In *IEEE Intelligent Systems*, (pp. 380–385).

Chapter 7
The Use of Prediction Reliability Estimates on Imbalanced Datasets:
A Case Study of Wall Shear Stress in the Human Carotid Artery Bifurcation

Domen Košir
University of Ljubljana, Slovenia & Httpool Ltd., Slovenia

Zoran Bosnić
University of Ljubljana, Slovenia

Igor Kononenko
University of Ljubljana, Slovenia

ABSTRACT

Data mining techniques are extensively used on medical data, which is typically composed of many normal examples and few interesting ones. When presented with highly imbalanced data, some standard classifiers tend to ignore the minority class which leads to poor performance. Various solutions have been proposed to counter this problem. Random undersampling, random oversampling, and SMOTE (Synthetic Minority Oversampling Technique) are the most well-known approaches. In recent years several approaches to evaluate the reliability of single predictions have been developed. Most recently a simple and efficient approach, based on the classifier's class probability estimates was shown to out-perform the other reliability estimates. The authors propose to use this reliability estimate to improve the SMOTE algorithm. In this study, they demonstrate the positive effects of using the proposed algorithms on artificial datasets. The authors then apply the developed methodology on the problem of predicting the maximal wall shear stress (MWSS) in the human carotid artery bifurcation. The results indicate that it is feasible to improve the classifier's performance by balancing the data with their versions of the SMOTE algorithm.

DOI: 10.4018/978-1-4666-1803-9.ch007

INTRODUCTION

Increase of the stroke risk is induced by many factors: age, systolic and diastolic hypertension, diabetes, cigarette smoking, high levels of cholesterol, arrhythmia, etc. Changes of the geometrical vessel dimensions in the region of the carotid artery bifurcation certainly affect the blood flow and may lead to stenosis process (Schulz & Rothwell, 2001).

The stenosis is a narrowing of the inner surface (lumen) of the blood vessel. Carotid artery stenosis is usually caused by the cholesterol plaque buildup. The plaque makes the blood flow to become faster and more turbulent. Irregular blood flow can cause pieces of plaque to break off and block smaller arteries in the brain. The pieces of plaque can partially or completely restrict blood flow to parts of the brain which that vessel supplies. The risk of this happening is especially high in patients with arrhythmia.

The common carotid artery supplies the neck, head and brain with oxygenated blood. In the neck it bifurcates into the internal and external carotid artery. The blood flow in this section was simulated using a 3D model in order to analyze the influence of geometric parameters on maximum wall shear stress (MWSS) in the human carotid artery bifurcation (Radović & Filipović, 2010).

We transformed the regression problem of predicting the MWSS value into two classification problems by setting two thresholds for wall shear stress values. We try to predict the levels MWSS using the 3D model's geometric parameters, but both classification datasets (mwss95 and mwss99) suffer from the class imbalance problem.

Big imbalance in data can cause some classifiers to perform poorly. Imbalanced data is common in real world problems, such as image analysis (Kubat, Holte & Matwin, 1998), fraud detection (Fawcett & Provost, 1996), text classification (Zheng, Wu & Srihari, 2004) and medicine (Mac Namee, Cunningham, Byrne & Corrigan, 2002; Cohen, Hilario, Sax, Hugonnet & Geissbuhler, 2006). When the majority examples heavily out-number the minority examples some classifiers tend to ignore the minority class. Classification accuracy measure, however, does not consider this. For instance, a simple classifier that always predicts the majority class would show a 99% classification accuracy when presented with a dataset that consists of 99% majority examples and 1% minority examples. This classifier would of course be useless. In this study, we focus more on the informative AUC value (Area Under the ROC Curve) instead of relying on classification accuracy.

Several already existant approaches enable even the imbalance-sensitive classifiers to be able to successfully predict minority examples. Some of the proposed solutions focus on the algorithmic level – they modify existing classifiers and present new algorithms that are not sensitive to imbalanced learning data. Other approaches focus on the data. They modify the data itself in order to soften the ratio between the numbers of majority and minority examples.

The imbalance in data can be, for example, countered by reducing the number of majority examples by randomly removing majority examples from the dataset (random undersampling) or by replicating minority examples (random oversampling). Random undersampling and random oversampling are very straightforward algorithms that can be used to change the numbers of majority and minority examples. The effects of data undersampling and oversampling were extensively studied in the last decade (Estabrooks & Japkowitz, 2001; Chawla, Japkowitz & Koltz, 2004).

A new algorithm called SMOTE (Chawla, Bowyer, Hall & Kegelmeyer, 2002) was introduced in 2002 (see Algorithm 1). Instead of deleting or duplicating random examples in the dataset, this algorithm generates synthetic examples using the existing minority examples. For every synthetic example a minority example and one of its nearest neighbors are used to generate a new minority example. Several researchers used this algorithm in their research and developed new variations of the SMOTE algorithm (Chavla, Lazarevic, Hall

& Bowyer, 2003; Akbani, Kwek & Japkowitz, 2004; Han, Wang & Mao, 2005).

Algorithm 1. Algorithm SMOTE

```
Until enough synthetic examples are
 generated do:
    Select a minority example A.
    Select one of the example's
     nearest neighbors B.
    Select a random weight W
     between 0 and 1.
    Create a new synthetic example C.
    For every attribute do:
    attValue_C = attValue_A
     + (attValue_B - attValue_A) * W
```

The area of prediction reliability estimation is relatively new. Estimates of a single prediction's reliability enable the users of the model to know how much they can trust the prediction before making a decision based on it. There are several approaches to the evaluation of the single prediction reliability (Kukar, 2001; Kukar & Kononenko 2002; Bosnić & Kononenko, 2009). Most recently, a simple and efficient approach, based on the classifiers' own class probability estimates, was shown to outperform the other reliability estimates (Pevec, Štrumbelj & Kononenko, 2011).

SMOTE uses all minority examples to generate new examples. Many research papers show that good classification performance can be achieved by balancing the learning data using SMOTE before building a model. The basic idea of SMOTE is to randomly select a minority instance and construct from it a new instance by modifying it in a direction towards its nearest neighbor from the same class. We believe that better results can be achieved by using a modified algorithm that uses prediction reliability estimates. This way we can be more selective when choosing the source minority examples to be used to generate new ones. In this chapter we propose two new algorithms: SMOTERAND-ASC and SMOTERAND-DESC, each focusing on the other part of minority ex-

amples' population in terms of prediction reliability estimates values. Both algorithms use the reliability estimates to choose the source minority examples. SMOTERAND-ASC is more likely to choose examples with lower prediction reliability estimates and SMOTERAND-DESC those with higher prediction reliability estimates. Both approaches can be useful in different situations which are demonstrated in this chapter.

We use all the mentioned algorithms on previously described medical datasets and measure improvements of AUC values and classification accuracies when predicting wall shear stress in human carotid artery bifurcation using artificial neural networks and support vector machines for classification (Kononenko & Kukar, 2007).

USING PREDICTION RELIABILITY ESTIMATES IN SMOTE

Algorithm SMOTERAND-ASC and SMOTERAND-DESC

In this section we describe two new algorithms for reducing imbalance in data. Both algorithms are based on the SMOTE algorithm. They differ from SMOTE in the way they choose the source minority examples that are used as a basis for generating synthetic examples. SMOTE has no preference regarding the choice of source examples. It uses all minority examples one after another until enough synthetic examples are generated. Our proposed algorithms are more selective.

SMOTERAND-ASC and SMOTERAND-DESC both use the leave-one-out method to calculate predictions for all minority examples (see Algorithm 2). The prediction reliability estimate (Pevec et al., 2011) is calculated from the model's predicted class probability *prob* using the formula: *reliability = 1 – (2 × prob × (1 – prob))* . By using the model's predicted class, the example's true class and *reliability* we can focus only on correctly classified minority examples with high or low prediction reliability estimates, depending on our needs. From *reliability* we derive the *preference* for ordering the training examples. For ordering the examples from the minority class in SMOTERAND-DESC we use *preference = reliability*. The formula for *preference* used in SMOTERAND-ASC is modified so that examples with lower prediction reliability estimates are preferred: *preference = 1.5 - reliability = 0.5 + (2 × prob × (1 − prob))*. In both algorithms the variable *preference* is confined to values between *0.5* and *1*. Both SMOTERAND-ASC and SMOTERAND-DESC use weighted random to choose the source minority examples from which new examples are synthesized. In order to increase the selectiveness of both algorithms *preference* to the power of four (*preference⁴*) is used in the weighted random. The exponent was chosen heuristically. The exponentiation step is needed to increase the difference between the lowest and the highest weight used and therefore to increase the chance for SMOTERAND-ASC to choose a minority example with a low prediction reliability estimate and for SMOTERAND-DESC to choose an example with a high prediction reliability estimate.

Algorithm 2. Algorithms SMOTERAND-ASC and SMOTERAND-DESC

```
Calculate the prediction reliability
  estimates for all minority examples
  in the dataset.
Until enough synthetic examples are
  generated do:
    Use weighted random to select
    a minority example
    (weight = preference⁴).
  Select one of the example's
    nearest neighbors.
  Select a random weight
    between 0 and 1.
  Calculate attribute values for
    the new synthetic example
    the same way as in SMOTE.
```

Test Framework

In order to be able to compare the data imbalance reducing algorithms among themselves, we developed a simple framework. We modified the standard 10-fold cross-validation technique and added a preprocessing stage for the training set. In the preprocessing stage the training set is modified by one of the imbalance reducing algorithms and then used to build a model. The test data is left unmodified. This way the balancing algorithms can only influence the model training and have no direct influence on test examples' predictions.

We then use the modified 10-fold cross-validation to measure classification accuracy and AUC values.

Classification accuracy is added only for completeness as AUC is a much more important measure in classification, especially for imbalanced datasets where extremely high classification accuracy can be achieved by trivial (default) majority classifiers.

Illustrative Experiments for SMOTERAND-ASC

In this section we show how algorithm SMOTERAND-ASC works on a simple artificial dataset. The dataset, which was generated randomly purely for the purpose of this illustration, is shown in Figure 1. The majority class (x) heavily outnumbers the minority class (o). In addition, the border between classes is quite clear to the human eye, but there very few minority examples along the border. We use SMOTERAND-ASC to generate synthetic examples close to the class' border in order to strengthen the border and increase the prediction reliability estimates in this area.

We used a SVM classifier with a polynomial kernel with our test framework—modified 10-fold cross-validation. Minority class of every training set was expanded to 50% of the majority class size. This test was run five times (to average the influence of stochastic parts of the SMOTE* al-

Figure 1. An illustration of the workings of the algorithm SMOTERAND-ASC on an artificial dataset. On the left is the original dataset and on the right the same dataset with new minority examples that were generated with SMOTERAND-ASC. The algorithm used the borderline minority examples more frequently and strengthened the border between the classes.

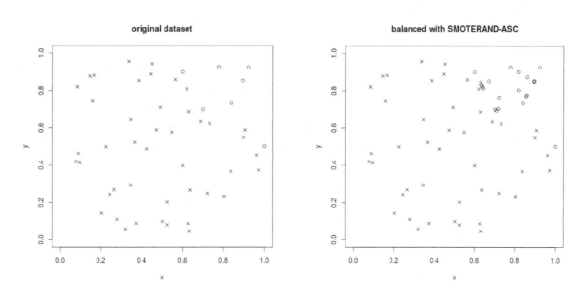

Table 1. AUC values and classification accuracies for the artificial dataset that illustrates the workings of algorithm SMOTERAND-ASC

results	no preprocessing	SMOTE	SMOTERAND-ASC	SMOTERAND-DESC
AUC	0.874	0.915	**0.940**	0.897
CA	0.920	0.908	0.908	0.908

gorithms) and we measured the AUC values. The averages in Table 1 show a significant AUC increase for SMOTERAND-ASC.

Illustrative Experiment for SMOTERAND-DESC

We generated another artificial dataset (see Figure 2) to illustrate a situation where SMOTERAND-ASC does not perform well and SMOTERAND-DESC does. In this example the border between the majority and minority class is much fuzzier. There are a few minority examples deep inside the majority class. When new examples are generated, those examples should not be used to generate

new examples as they are obviously noisy and will distort the model by increasing the entropy with newly generated examples. Instead, only the reliable minority examples in the top-right corner should be used as the source for synthetic examples. This is shown on Figure 2 where most of the synthetic examples are also located in the top-right corner. There are a few synthetic examples that were obviously generated using the minority examples located in the middle of the majority class – this is the price we pay for using weighted random when selecting the source examples. We ran the test in the same way as in the previous subsection and results in Table 2 show that using SMOTERAND-DESC on the learning set can increase the AUC value of a model.

Table 2. AUC values and classification accuracies for the artificial dataset that illustrates the workings of algorithm SMOTERAND-DESC

results	no preprocessing	SMOTE	SMOTERAND-ASC	SMOTERAND-DESC
AUC	0.744	0.745	0.740	**0.767**
CA	0.935	0.935	0.935	0.935

Figure 2. An illustration of the workings of the algorithm SMOTERAND-DESC on an artificial dataset. On the left we have the original dataset and on the right the same dataset with new minority examples that were generated with SMOTERAND-DESC. The border between the two classes in the original dataset is very fuzzy as there are a few minority examples deep inside the majority class. Most of the new examples were generated using the minority examples with higher prediction reliability estimates and are located in the top-right corner.

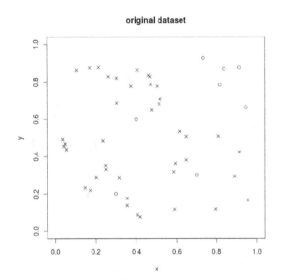
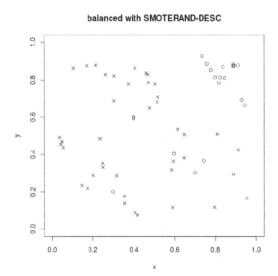

Predicting Wall Shear Stress

For evaluation of the stenosis process, a set of candidate geometries was randomly created for steady state three dimensional flow analyses. 12 geometric parameters were used for the generation of the blood vessel internal surfaces (see Figure 3), which are the boundaries for the blood flow domain. With the use of these geometric parameters, a 3D finite element model for the blood flow domain was generated. Steady state simulations for 1886 geometries were afterwards undertaken and MWSS for each geometry was computed.

The generated data were used to construct various models which approximated the MWSS as a function of geometric variables.

The simulation results were saved into a relational form, appropriate for applying machine learning algorithms. Since the MWSS study focuses on detecting vessels with high MWSS values, the MWSS variable was discretized into two classes ('high' and 'low') and was used as a class variable. In our experiments, two experimental MWSS thresholds were used for discretization into the two classes, corresponding to 95 and 99 percentile of MWSS. Such values were

Figure 3. Geometrical data for the carotid artery model. The abbreviations here are: CCA –common carotid artery, CBR – carotid bifurcation region, CBRE – carotid bifurcation region external, ECA- external carotid artery, CBRI- carotid bifurcation region internal, ICA- internal carotid artery, ICB- internal carotid bulbus. The axes denote the coordinate system in which the position of the MWSS is measured.

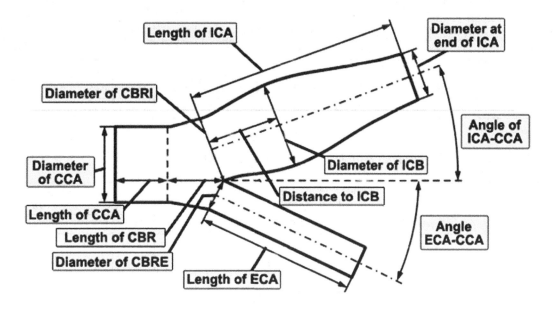

chosen in order to allow the discretized problem to concur with the main motivation of the study (i.e. to detect outstandingly high MWSS values which correlate with the level of danger to the cardiovascular system).

Our experiments include two datasets. With each of the datasets we used the artificial neural network and SVM to build a model that should be able to reliably predict high MWSS values. The following attributes were used:

- Diameter of common carotid artery,
- Length of common carotid artery,
- Length of carotid bifurcation region,
- Diameter of carotid bifurcation region internal,
- Diameter of carotid bifurcation region external,
- Angle between internal carotid artery and common carotid artery,
- Angle between external carotid artery and common carotid artery,
- Length of internal carotid artery,
- Length of external carotid artery,
- Distance to internal carotid bulbus,
- Diameter of internal carotid bulbus and
- Diameter at end of internal carotid artery.

All the attributes are continuous. In order to prevent the class imbalance to impair the predictor's performance we preprocessed the training data with various algorithms (as described earlier in this chapter).

Results

We used the previously described modified 10-fold cross validation and averaged the results. Random undersampling, random oversampling, SMOTE and the proposed algorithms SMOTERAND-ASC and SMOTERAND-DESC were used in the

Table 3. Average classification accuracies and AUC values using artificial neural networks

DATA SET, balancing %	original		random undersampl.		random oversampling		SMOTE		SMOTERAND-ASC		SMOTERAND-DESC	
	AUC	CA	AUC	CA	AUC	CA	AUC	CA	AUC	CA	AUC	CA
mwss95, 50%	0.621	0.953	0.646	0.884	0.690	0.917	0.669	0.906	**0.704**	0.928	0.670	0.902
mwss95, 33%	0.616	0.953	0.665	0.927	0.659	0.943	0.658	0.944	**0.695**	0.941	0.652	0.935
mwss95, 25%	0.615	0.954	0.634	0.943	**0.657**	0.949	0.629	0.949	0.627	0.949	0.611	0.945
mwss99, 50%	0.508	0.989	0.552	0.804	0.556	0.882	0.541	0.870	**0.570**	0.854	0.561	0.865
mwss99, 33%	0.529	0.989	0.526	0.915	0.567	0.948	0.561	0.926	**0.620**	0.950	0.566	0.946
mwss99, 25%	0.503	0.989	0.527	0.928	**0.581**	0.968	0.573	0.961	0.514	0.969	0.568	0.968

Table 4. Classification accuracies and AUC values using a SVM classifier

DATA SET, balancing %	original		random undersampl.		random oversampling		SMOTE		SMOTERAND-ASC		SMOTERAND-DESC	
	AUC	CA	AUC	CA	AUC	CA	AUC	CA	AUC	CA	AUC	CA
mwss95, 50%	**0.743**	0.957	0.671	0.930	0.673	0.901	0.670	0.889	0.675	0.920	0.658	0.885
mwss95, 33%	**0.743**	0.957	0.674	0.946	0.704	0.924	0.704	0.934	0.698	0.941	0.678	0.915
mwss95, 25%	**0.742**	0.957	0.726	0.950	0.698	0.935	0.713	0.941	0.705	0.946	0.705	0.936
mwss99, 50%	0.558	0.990	0.499	0.970	0.618	0.980	0.616	0.931	**0.638**	0.934	0.627	0.931
mwss99, 33%	0.562	0.990	0.537	0.982	0.597	0.980	**0.633**	0.945	0.624	0.941	0.629	0.938
mwss99, 25%	0.555	0.990	0.530	0.986	0.607	0.981	0.590	0.953	**0.624**	0.935	0.595	0.935

preprocessing stage to reduce the class imbalance in the training data. All the balancing algorithms were run on the same training datasets.

In our first experiment we used the neural network classifier which is widely used in medical problems. The neural network classifier often gives unstable results (due to random initialization of weights). That is why we decided to run the 10-fold cross-validation procedure 10 times and average the results. We kept the same starting training and test folds for all 10 tests. The results for neural network are presented in Table 3 and for SVM in Table 4.

For SVM classifiers we used polynomial kernels. The same modified 10-fold cross-validation procedure was used to measure the classifiers' performance when predicting the MWSS level. Because the SVM classifiers always give stable results we ran the procedure only once. Table 4 shows AUC values and classification accuracies for SVM classifiers.

In our initial experiments with the artificial neural networks we saw very poor results on both medical datasets (Table 3). We used various balancing algorithms to increase the number of minority examples to 25% of the size of the majority class random. This resulted in an increase of AUC values, especially when we used random oversampling. When we further increased the size of the minority class we saw the best results when we used SMOTERAND-ASC. AUC values increased for up to 0.08.

We then replaced the neural networks with a SVM classifier with a polynomial kernel and we saw a whole different picture. The results on original datasets were somewhat better than when we used neural networks. But when we applied the balancing algorithms to dataset mwss95 (5%

minority class share), all the AUC values dropped. The AUC values increased however (up to 0.12), when we used the balancing algorithm on dataset mwss99 (only 1% minority class share). The reason for this behavior could be that SVM classifiers are not as sensitive to imbalanced data as are neural networks.

FUTURE RESEARCH DIRECTIONS

Our proposed algorithms were briefly illustrated on two small artificial datasets using only one classifier. A comprehensive analysis including more classification algorithms, commonly used datasets and artificially generated datasets would probably show in detail which dataset characteristics can be associated with increased classifier's performance when using specific data balancing algorithms.

The selectiveness of both proposed algorithms can be further increased by eliminating certain subpopulations of the minority class from the source pool of examples that are used for the synthesis of new examples.

CONCLUSION

In this chapter we describe our approach when we were presented with the problem of predicting the level of wall shear stress in the human carotid artery bifurcation. As it is common in medical problems, we were confronted with a dataset where the interesting examples (examples with high wall shear stress values) were heavily outnumbered by normal examples. We converted this regression problem into two classification problems by setting two thresholds for wall shear stress values. The new mwss95 dataset has 5% minority class share and dataset mwss99 has a 1% minority class share. The threshold used for mwss99 is higher which means that predictions for high wall shear stress based on this dataset are even more important than those based on mwss95.

Our approach to measuring the success of predicting wall shear stress is based on the 10-fold cross-validation and measuring the AUC values. Our initial experiments with the artificial neural networks (Table 3) show very poor classificatory performance – AUC value of 0.62 on dataset mwss95 and 0.51 on mwss99. This indicates that the prediction of wall shear stress in the human carotid artery bifurcation is a difficult problem.

We decided to add a preprocessing stage to the 10-fold cross-validation in which we use various balancing algorithms to reduce the imbalance in training sets. We used random undersampling, random oversampling and SMOTE. In addition we developed two new variations of the SMOTE algorithm that incorporate prediction reliability estimates in the process of selecting the source minority examples from which new examples are synthesized. SMOTERAND-ASC generates new examples using minority examples with lower prediction reliability estimates and SMOTER-AND-DESC uses those with higher prediction reliability estimates.

As can be seen in Table 3 using balancing algorithms on training sets can significantly increase AUC values. In this case using the SMOTERAND-ASC algorithm gave highest AUC values, increasing the values from initial test for up to 0.08.

The results from our experiments on dataset mwss95 using SVM classifiers (Table 4) however show relatively high AUC values when no preprocessing was done and a decrease in AUC values from use of balancing algorithms. Experiments on mwss99 on the other hand show that a 1% minority class share in the training data represents a difficult problem for a SVM classifier and that the imbalanced should be reduced before building a model. The highest AUC values were again achieved when we used SMOTERAND-ASC to balance the data.

Our results show that using balancing algorithms on training data can significantly increase the AUC value of the model when we are dealing with an imbalanced dataset. The best results were obtained when we used SMOTERAND-ASC to balance the training sets but we expect tests on other datasets to also show usefulness of SMOTERAND-DESC.

Despite the significant improvements in the AUC values they are still very low. We can safely assume that there is still room for improvement.

ACKNOWLEDGMENT

We thank Prof. Dr. Nenad Filipović of the Faculty of Mechanical Engineering, University of Kragujevac, Serbia, for providing the original MWSS dataset. Operation part financed by the European Union, European Social Fund. Operation implemented in the framework of the Operational Programme for Human Resources Development for the Period 2007-2013, Priority axis 1: Promoting entrepreneurship and adaptability, Main type of activity 1.1.: Experts and researchers for competitive enterprises.

REFERENCES

Akbani, R., Kwek, S., & Japkowitz, N. (2004). Applying support vector machines to imbalanced datasets. In Boulicaut, J. F., Esposito, F., Giannotti, F., & Pedreschi, D. (Eds.), *Machine Learning: ECML 2004* (*Vol. 3201*, pp. 39–50). Lecture Notes in Computer Science Berlin, Germany: Springer-Verlag. doi:10.1007/978-3-540-30115-8_7

Bosnić, Z., & Kononenko, I. (2009). An overview of advances in reliability estimation of individual predictions in machine learning. *Intelligent Data Analysis*, *13*(2), 385–401. doi:doi:10.3233/IDA-2009-0371

Chawla, N. V., Bowyer, K. W., Hall, L. O., & Kegelmeyer, W. P. (2002). SMOTE: Synthetic minority over-sampling technique. *Journal of Artificial Intelligence Research*, *16*(1), 321–357. Retrieved from http://www.jair.org/media/953/live-953-2037-jair.pdf

Chawla, N. V., Japkowitz, N., & Koltz, A. (2004). Editorial: Special issue on learning from imbalanced data sets. *SIGKDD Explorations Newsletter – Special Issue on Learning from Imbalanced Datasets*, *6*(1), 1-6. doi: 10.1145/1007730.1007733

Chawla, N. V., Lazarevic, A., Hall, L. O., & Bowyer, K. W. (2003). SMOTEBoost: Improving prediction of the minority class in boosting. In Lavrac, N., Gamberger, D., Todorovski, L., & Blockeel, H. (Eds.), *Knowledge Discovery in Databases: PKDD 2003* (*Vol. 2838*, pp. 107–119). Lecture Notes in Computer Science Berlin, Germany: Springer-Verlag. doi:10.1007/978-3-540-39804-2_12

Cohen, G., Hilario, M., Sax, H., Hugonnet, S., & Geissbuhler, A. (2006). Learning from imbalanced data in surveillance of nosocomial infection. *Artificial Intelligence in Medicine*, *37*(1), 7–18. doi:10.1016/j.artmed.2005.03.002

Estabrooks, A., & Japkowitz, N. (2001). A mixture-of-experts framework for learning from imbalanced data sets. In Hoffmann, F., Hand, D. J., Adams, N., Fisher, D., & Guimaraes, G. (Eds.), *Advances in Intelligent Data Analysis* (*Vol. 2189*, pp. 34–43). Lecture Notes in Computer Science Berlin, Germany: Springer-Verlag. doi:10.1007/3-540-44816-0_4

Fawcett, T., & Provost, F. (1997). Adaptive fraud detection. *Data Mining and Knowledge Discovery*, *1*(3), 291–316. doi:10.1023/A:1009700419189

Han, H., Wang, W. Y., & Mao, B. H. (2005). Borderline-SMOTE: A new over-sampling method in imbalanced data sets learning. *Advances in Intelligent Computing, 3644*, 878–887. doi:10.1007/11538059_91

Kononenko, I., & Kukar, M. (2007). *Machine learning and data mining: Introduction to principles and algorithms*. Chichester, UK: Horwood Publishing.

Kubat, M., Holte, R., & Matwin, S. (1998). Machine learning for the detection of oil spills in satellite radar images. *Machine Learning, 30*(2-3), 195–215. doi:10.1023/A:1007452223027

Kukar, M. (2001). *Estimating classifications' reliability and cost-sensitive combination of machine learning methods*. Doctoral dissertation, University of Ljubljana.

Kukar, M., & Kononenko, I. (2002). Reliable classifications with machine learning. In Elomaa, T., Mannila, H., & Toivonen, H. (Eds.), *Machine Learning: ECML 2002 (Vol. 2430*, pp. 1–8). Lecture Notes in Computer Science Berlin, Germany: Springer-Verlag. doi:10.1007/3-540-36755-1_19

MacNamee, B., Cunningham, P., Byrne, S., & Corrigan, O. (2002). The problem of bias in training data in regression problems in medical decision support. *Artificial Intelligence in Medicine, 24*(1), 51–70. doi:10.1016/S0933-3657(01)00092-6

Pevec, D., Štrumbelj, E., & Kononenko, I. (2011). Evaluating reliability of single classifications of neural networks. In Dobnikar, A., Lotrič, U., & Šter, B. (Eds.), *Adaptive and Natural Computing Algorithms (Vol. 5182*, pp. 22–30). Lecture Notes in Computer Science Berlin, Germany: Springer-Verlag. doi:10.1007/978-3-642-20282-7_3

Radović, M., & Filipović, N. (2010). Mining data from hemodynamic simulations via multilayer perceptron neural network. *Journal of Serbian Society for Computational Mechanics, 4*(1), 31–42. Retrieved from http://www.singipedia.com/attachment.php?attachmentid=2381

Schulz, U. G. R., & Rothwell, P. M. (2001). Sex differences in carotid bifurcation anatomy and the distribution of atherosclerotic plaque. *Stroke, 32*(7), 1525–1531. Retrieved from http://stroke.ahajournals.org/cgi/content/abstract/32/7/1525 doi:10.1161/01.STR.32.7.1525

Zheng, Z., Wu, X., & Srihari, R. (2004). Feature selection for text categorization on imbalanced data. *SIGKDD Explorations Newsletter, 6*(1), 80–89. doi:10.1145/1007730.1007741

ADDITIONAL READING

Cook, N. R. (2007). Use and misuse of the receiver operating characteristic curve in risk prediction. *Circulation, 115*, 928–935. Retrieved from http://circ.ahajournals.org/cgi/content/full/115/7/928 doi:10.1161/CIRCULATIONAHA.106.672402

Demšar, J. (2006). Statistical comparisons of classifiers over multiple data sets. *Journal of Machine Learning Research, 7*, 1–30. Retrieved from http://jmlr.csail.mit.edu/papers/v7/demsar06a.html

Dimitriadou, E., Hornik, K., Leisch, F., Meyer, D., & Weingessel, A. (2009). *e1071: Misc functions of the department of statistics* (Version 1.5-25) [R Library]. Retrieved February 4, 2011, from http://cran.r-project.org/web/packages/e1071/

Friedman, M. (1937). The use of ranks to avoid the assumption of normality implicit in the analysis of variance. *Journal of the American Statistical Association, 32*, 675–701. doi:10.2307/2279372

Friedman, M. (1940). A comparison of alternative tests of significance for the problem of m rankings. *Annals of Mathematical Statistics*, *11*, 86–92. doi:10.1214/aoms/1177731944

Japkowitz, N., & Stephen, S. (2002). The class imbalance problem: A systematic study. *Intelligent Data Analysis*, *6*(5), 429–449. Retrieved from http://iospress.metapress.com/content/mxug8cjkjylnk3n0/

Nemenyi, P. B. (1963). *Distribution-free multiple comparisons*. Doctoral dissertation, Princeton University.

Peek, N., Arts, D. G. T., Bosman, R. J., van der Voort, P. H. J., & de Keizer, N. F. (2007). External validation of prognostic models for critically ill patients required substantial sample sizes. *Journal of Clinical Epidemiology*, *60*(5), 491–501. doi:10.1016/j.jclinepi.2006.08.011

Provost, F. (2000). Machine learning from imbalanced data sets 101. *AAAI'2000 Workshop on Imbalanced Data Sets*, (pp. 1-3). Retrieved from http://hdl.handle.net/2451/27763

R Development Core Team. (2011). *R: A language and environment for statistical computing* (Version 2.11.1) [R Computer Language]. Vienna, Austria: R Foundation for Statistical Computing. Retrieved February 4, 2011, from http://www.r-project.org/

Stefanowski, J., & Wilk, S. (2008). Selective pre-processing of imbalanced data for improving classification performance. In Song, I. Y., Eder, J., & Nguyen, T. M. (Eds.), *Data Warehousing and Knowledge Discovery* (*Vol. 5182*, pp. 283–292). Lecture Notes in Computer Science Berlin, Germany: Springer-Verlag. doi:10.1007/978-3-540-85836-2_27

Zar, J. H. (1998). *Biostatical analysis* (4th ed.). New Jersey: Prentice-Hall Press.

KEY TERMS AND DEFINITIONS

Carotid Artery Bifurcation: The left and right common carotid arteries transport oxygenated blood to the head and neck. In the neck they bifurcate into the internal and external carotid arteries.

Carotid Artery Stenosis: The stenosis is a narrowing of the inner surface (lumen) of the blood vessel. Carotid artery stenosis is usually caused by the cholesterol plaque buildup.

Classification Performance: The correctness of classification results is usually evaluated using measures like classification accuracy, precision, sensitivity, AUC (Area Under Curve) values or F1 scores.

Imbalanced Dataset: A dataset with an imbalanced class distribution. They are very common in real-world domains.

Single Prediction Reliability Estimate: Global measures such as classification accuracy and AUC values do not provide reliability estimates for single predictions. Single prediction reliability estimates play major role in risk-sensitive applications.

SMOTE: The SMOTE algorithm is used to reduce class imbalance in a dataset. It uses minority examples from the dataset to synthesize additional minority examples.

Synthetic Example: An example that is not part of the original dataset. The values of its attributes are calculated using attribute values of examples from the dataset.

Chapter 8
Pattern Mining for Outbreak Discovery Preparedness

Zalizah Awang Long
Malaysia Institute Information Technology, Universiti Kuala Lumpur, Malaysia

Abdul Razak Hamdan
Universiti Kebengsaan Malaysia, Malaysia

Azuraliza Abu Bakar
Universiti Kebengsaan Malaysia, Malaysia

Mazrura Sahani
Universiti Kebengsaan Malaysia, Malaysia

ABSTRACT

Today, the objective of public health surveillance system is to reduce the impact of outbreaks by enabling appropriate intervention. Commonly used techniques are based on the changes or aberration in health events when compared with normal history to detect an outbreak. The main problem encountered in outbreaks is high rates of false alarm. High false alarm rates can lead to unnecessary interventions, and falsely detected outbreaks will lead to costly investigation. In this chapter, the authors review data mining techniques focusing on frequent and outlier mining to develop generic outbreak detection process model, named as "Frequent-outlier" model. The process model was tested against the real dengue dataset obtained from FSK, UKM, and also tested on the synthetic respiratory dataset obtained from AUTON LAB. The ROC was run to analyze the overall performance of "frequent-outlier" with CUSUM and Moving Average (MA). The results were promising and were evaluated using detection rate, false positive rate, and overall performance. An important outcome of this study is the knowledge rules derived from the notification of the outbreak cases to be used in counter measure assessment for outbreak preparedness.

DOI: 10.4018/978-1-4666-1803-9.ch008

INTRODUCTION

The public health surveillance system caught the researcher's attention into developing the detection algorithm after 21 September for terrorist detection and also for H1N1 pandemic. WHO reported that earlier case reported for H1N1 was first noticed in North America in April 2009 and then the spread to the other part of the world. In June 2009 there were 74 countries affected by H1N1. Various data sources had been considered to detect the outbreak including data from emergency department, over the counter sales, medical image and also test-order for early detection of an outbreak case.

In detecting outbreak, the detection system identified the anomaly pattern when compared to previous pattern to detect an outbreak. In statistical analysis, it is known as aberration (Wong, 2004). The main problem indicated in most of the studies shows that high in false alarms will lead to unnecessary intervention resulting high in operation cost.

To solve the indicated problem there are few techniques that have been identified such as statistical-based, Bayesian-based, and also knowledge-based techniques. Those discussed techniques showed the improvement in terms of detection rate and also false-positive-rate. The techniques proposed are more toward the complement observation and not to replace any available techniques (G. F. Cooper, Dowling, Levander, & Sutovsky, 2007; Shen & Cooper, 2007). Statistical-based methods face problems in requiring long training time (Guthrie, Stacey, & Calvert, 2005) and validation for the error rate is not significant since the value is too small while Bayesian and knowledge-based suffered to provide more accurate results due to limited numbers of actual cases of true outbreaks to be tested on the approaches.

To reduce the false positive rate and high in detection rate are the objectives of most outbreak detection techniques. Our approach is to provide a new process model in detecting outbreak and provide rules for the preparedness awareness. These will lead towards prevention of the recurrent outbreaks.

BACKGROUND

There is no specific definition in defining outbreak. According to Lai & Kwong, (2010), from the epidemiology view, an outbreak occurs if individuals develop similar symptoms one after another and the disease incidence is higher than usual. The general definition from Center Disease Control (CDC) defined an outbreak as the occurrence of more cases of disease than what is expected in a given area over a particular period of time. Different diseases possess their own outbreak definition. Dengue outbreak, for example, is defined as increase of cases per week persisting for at least 3 successive weeks to a level at least three times above the mean of previous 3 weeks (Runge-Ranzinger, Horstick, Marx, & Kroeger, 2008). Another definition obtained for dengue outbreaks is an increase in 2 SD above the mean ((Carme, et al., 2003; Oum, Chandramohan, & Cairncross, 2005; Rigau-Pérez, et al., 1998; Talarmin, et al., 2000)). In this study, the focus concentrates on the Malaysia dengue environment. Based on the study conducted by Seng, Chong, & Moore, (2005) the dengue outbreak was defined according to Johor Health State Department, which is an occurrence of more than one case in the same locality, where the date of onset between the cases are greater than 14 days. The outbreak is clear when there is no new case reported within 14 days.

There are numbers of outbreak detection algorithm based on statistical analysis such as CuSUM focusing on detecting the outbreak with the same motivation to reduce numbers of false detection and at the same time to increase the detection rate. Outbreak detection required combination of clinical and non-clinical data source for better detecting outbreaks and also depending on the automatic analysis on the combination of data sources(Blind & Das, 2007; Brown & Gray, 2005; Buehler, et al., 2004b; D. L. Cooper, et al., 2005; German, Armstrong, Birkhead, Horan, & Herrera, 2001; Stoto, Schonlau, & Mariano, 2004). Surveillance system required definition of outbreak cases in determining the capabilities of the detection algorithm or detecting techniques in computing the outbreak. In general, outbreak can be defined as more than one case from the normal distribution in a given period of time with identified sources and causes of epidemic based on epidemiology investigation. Basically, surveillance systems focused on the detecting outbreak operating by viewing the abnormality within the dataset or the aberration. Looking at the vast possibilities of anomaly or aberration techniques being used in fraud detection and intrusion detection, it is an opportunity for the techniques in anomaly being applied into an outbreak detection (Chandola, Banerjee, & Kumar, 2007, 2009; Chandola, Mithal, & Kumar, 2008; Hodge & Austin, 2004). Many techniques employed detection outlier but describing the approach as novelty detection, noise detection, deviation detection, anomaly detection or exception detection but leading to the same approach to identify or observe the one appears to deviate markedly from other members of the sample(Ben-Gal, 2005; Hodge & Austin, 2004). The change in the occurrence of health events when compared to normal history is the same as the observation of the one that markedly deviates from the groups. This leads to the motivation in developing a proposed process model called Frequent-outlier with the objective- to generate the pattern derived from the rules based on detected outbreaks cases.

One of the objectives in achieving better health for Malaysian under Malaysia Plan is to improve the standard and sustainability of quality of life.

Towards achieving the direction, Ministry of health in Malaysia has guided some strategies in managing the health-related crisis and disaster effectively and also enhancing research and development for evidence-based decision making (MOH, 2009). Our approach is based on the use of frequent mining and outlier mining to detect outbreak cases or health crisis and disaster. The approach based on the aberration defined by Wong (2004) is the motivation in this research in developing the outbreak detection based on frequent and outlier mining. The interpretation of significant changes is then driven to the conclusion of the related techniques being used in outlier detection techniques. Basically the development of detection techniques is derived from various domains such as network intrusion, fraud detection, industrial damage, image processing and medical and public health application.

The penetrations of various supervision and data dimension and techniques are extensively conducted on the fraud and intrusion detection, while medical and public health requires more space to conduct research in various concentrations. Based on Table 1, the exploration on unsupervised data with high dimension data should be highlighted as the promising research areas. The current approach of the techniques is on the statistics and neural network-based (Chandola, et al., 2009; Hodge & Austin, 2004; Patcha & Park, 2007; Zhang, Meratnia, & Havinga, 2007). The exploration of various techniques in data mining should be considered as part of detecting diseases outbreaks particularly in dengue cases. The natures of surveillance data are high in dimension and reside the unsupervised data. High amount of data is added to the complexity of the dataset including clinical and non-clinical dataset (Blind & Das, 2007; Brown & Gray, 2005; Buehler, Hopkins, Overhage, Sosin, & Tong, 2004a; D. L. Cooper, et al., 2005; German, et al., 2001; Stoto, et al., 2004).

Table 1. Detection techniques for various domains

Detection Domain	Supervision			Data type		Techniques					
	A	B	C	1	2	CLB	CB	NNB	ST	IT	SP
Network Intrusion		√	√		√	√			√		
Banking Fraud	√	√		√	√	√	√	√	√	√	
Medical & Public Health		√			√	√		√	√		
Industry Damage		√	√	√	√	√			√		√
Image processing	√			√	√	√	√	√	√		

Note: A = full supervise, B=Semi Supervise,C=unsupervised; 1=High dimension, 2=Low dimension; CLB=Classification-based, CB=Cluster-based, NNB=Nearest Neighbor-based, ST=Statistic, IT=Information teoretic, SP=Spectral

FREQUENT- OUTLIER MODEL

Surveillance system is passive and outbreak detection requires rapid recognition toward identifying the outbreaks signal and these will need historical data and trend analysis for baseline comparison. Basically adopted definition of diseases outbreaks is obtained from CDC, which is the occurrence of more cases of disease than is expected in a given area over a particular period of time. (Anom, 2010) Viewing the definition of diseases outbreaks, analyzing the increase case patterns would help in identifying outbreak signal for the baseline comparison. The commonly used data mining tasks for pattern discovery is association rules. Frequent mining as part of association techniques applying market basket analysis would be adding advantages in designing outbreak detection process model (Agrawal, Imieli ski, & Swami, 1993; Agrawal & Srikant, 1994; Ceglar & Roddick, 2006; Han, Cheng, Xin, & Yan, 2007; Zhao & Bhowmick, 2006).

Based on the generic model in surveillance system(Buehler, et al., 2004a; German, et al., 2001), we propose to integrate data mining techniques in which focus on frequent mining as the baseline creation and outlier mining to detect the outbreak(A. R. H. Zalizah A. L, Norsuhaili S 2008; Zalizah A.L, 2009). The technique called *frequent-outlier* is based on the Apriori and outlier algorithm (Agrawal & Srikant, 1994; Brin, Motwani, Ullman, & Tsur, 1997; He, Xu, Huang,

& Deng, 2005; Koufakou, Ortiz, Georgiopoulos, Anagnostopoulos, & Reynolds, 2007). The proposed process model will consist of three main phases, which are learning phase, detecting phase and repository phase. We introduce the frequent mining analysis to retrieve normal behavior and outlier mining for calculating the outbreak.

Figure 1 indicates four stages involved in the process of detecting outbreaks. The stages consist of pre-processing; outbreak detection stage; field investigation and forensic stage. The output from the pre-processing stage is an input to the outbreak detection stage. Field investigation and forensic stage receiving input from the outbreak detection stage in form of certain value of rates and set of rules. The discussion focusing on the outbreak detection stage, which is consist of the proposed detection process model as shown in Figure 2.

As in the proposed detection process model, 3 main phases are involved:

1. **Learning:** Involving sub component frequent mining technique and outlier mining technique together with metric performance. The MAV function as in Figure 1 is to generate the frequent item for the FO analysis in detecting outlier. Based on the score computed, the baseline and threshold value will be stored in metric performance to be executed in detecting phase as in the Figure 2. Generally the sub component learning as in Figure 3.

Figure 1. Frequent-outlier detection process model

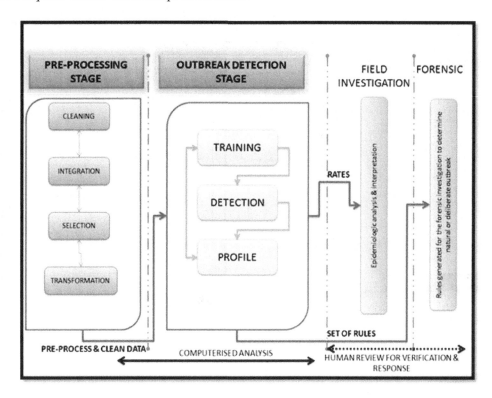

The sub-component of metric performance as in Figure 3, serve as summation for the creation of threshold and baseline. The input of metric performance is based on the frequent item generated by MAV and FO as in Figure 4.

2. **Detecting**: Those values that exceed the threshold value from the learning stage will be considered as potential outbreak and again will be calculated for the detection rate, false positive rate and overall accuracy.

3. **Repository**: The stored patterns are based on the outbreaks data for the rules generation. The patterns are designed for behavior pattern of the outbreak cases to be used as discovery preparedness. Learning processes from the interesting rules are generated. The interpretation of the generated rules is done by domain expert.

Data mining involves the process of discovering interesting knowledge from large amount of data and the extractions of implicit, previously unknown, and potentially useful information by observing datasets to find unexpected relationship within the dataset(Frank, 2005; Han & Kamber, 2001; Zhou, 2003). Looking at the possibilities of vast amount of data from the surveillance sources, more knowledge can be discovered based on the proposed detection process model using frequent and outlier mining.

EXPERIMENTAL RESULTS AND INTERPRETATION

The result is based on the proposed model using real dengue dataset obtained from vector control unit, hulu langat health center and faculty of allied health science ukm and synthetic dataset obtained

Figure 2. Outbreak detection process model

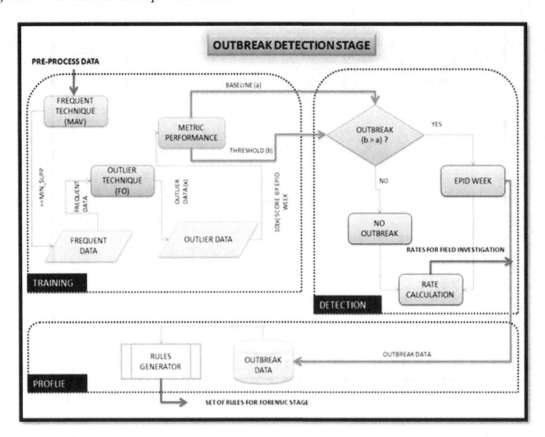

from autonlab for respiratory cases. The algorithm is analyzed with cusum in detecting outbreak. The calculation for the detection rate (dr), false positive rate (fr) and overall performance (op), are adopted from (German, et al., 2001; Mukhi, 2007) as in Table 2.

$$Detection\ rate\quad \frac{A}{(A+C)}\qquad \text{(Equation 3)}$$

$$False\ postive\ rate\quad \frac{B}{(B+D)}\qquad \text{(Equation 4)}$$

$$Overall\ Performance\quad \frac{(A+D)}{(A+B+C+D)}$$
$$\text{(Equation 5)}$$

The extensive experiment was conducted. In this experiment, non-clinical dataset was focused.

Dataset consists of information on year and epic week (week 1 to week 52), age, sex, races, address, nature of work, type of dengue, incubation period, epidemic type, recurrent cases and dead code. Demographic effect to the recurrent cases and incubation period from the onset onward to confirm diagnose was focused. Data respiratory which was obtained from AUTONLAB is the patient_of the status 72. The dataset consists of information on location, age, gender, flu intensity, day of week, weather, season, action, reported_symptom, and drug. Approximately 0.14% data was reduced through the pre-processing stage. We tried to maintain closely to the real sets of the original dataset in analyzing the real dataset.

The experiment result was plotted as in Table 3 below. The experiment was run using Cumulative SUM (CUSUM) as standard techniques to detect

Figure 3. Learning phase

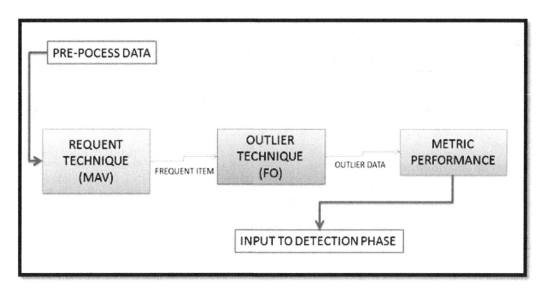

Figure 4. Metric performance

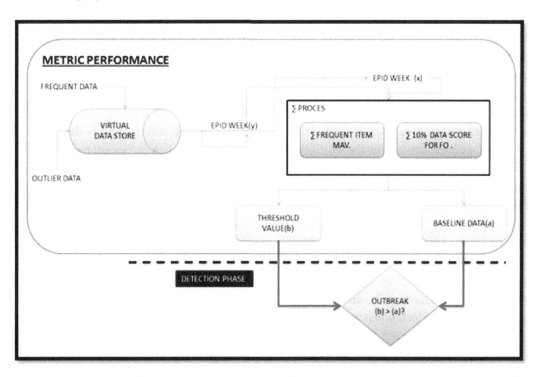

Table 2. Calculation matrix for detection rate (DR) False positive rate (FPR) and overall performance (OP)

Detected by algorithm	Actual outbreak cases		
	Outbreak	**No outbreak**	
Outbreak	True positive (A)	False positive (B)	A+B
No Outbreak	False negative (C)	True negative (D)	C+D
	A+C	B+D	TOTAL

Table 3. Dengue and respiratory results

Measurement	Dengue Dataset		Respiratory Dataset	
	CuSUM	**FO**	**CuSUM**	**FO**
Detection rate	70.8%	85.0%	76.5%	93.3%
False positive rate	28.0%	11.5%	27.3%	8.3%
Overall accuracy	67.3%	76.9%	74.0%	92.2%

outbreak in literature. To detect an outbreak, the process model using Frequent-Outlier (FO) technique was proposed. The previous experiment was run using the MAV and compared with CUSUM and Moving Average (MA), the result for MA is lower than CUSUM and MAV. The details on the experiment can be found in (A. R. H. Zalizah A. L, Azuraliza A.B, 2010). Therefore, in this experiment we are conducted without using MA.

Based on the result populated in Table 3, generally, we managed to outperform the CUSUM for both dataset. The performance for respiratory dataset reaches up to 93.3% due to the nature of dataset which has been prepared for the outbreak detection, while dengue dataset presents the real world dataset. Quoted from(German, et al., 2001) "False Positive rate reports can lead to unnecessary interventions, and falsely detected outbreaks can lead to costly investigations"(German et al., 2001, p.19).Therefore, the techniques were applied to real dataset to gain as much knowledge for further possible improvements. The definition of outbreak was noticed to be varied from one disease to another. The statistical analysis was also conducted to evaluate the method performance using ROC (Han & Kamber, 2001). ROC indicates that

MAV and FO outperform CUSUM, while FO produce more significance 0.01 as compared to MAV 0.04. The confidence intervals showed CUSUM is in lower and upper bound with 95% asymptotic confidence interval for MAV and FO. This indicates that MAV and FO are still leading as in Figure 5.

The dataset produced by the algorithm FO was executed to produce rules. The objective of the rules generated was to identify the knowledge of interesting cases from the outbreak dataset. Based on the real dengue dataset cases, the outbreaks consist of 236 instances with 10 attributes. Due to limited space only 5% of the generated rules were highlighted from each length out of 1027 rules generated. The results were classified into the length of the rules produced:

1. CASE=DD 234 ==> RECURRENT=NO 234 conf:(1)
2. SEX=FEMALE138==>RECURRENT=NO 138 conf:(1)
3. DEATH_CODE=NO 129 ==> CASE=DD 129 conf:(1)

Figure 5. ROC curve for the MAV, FO, and CUSUM

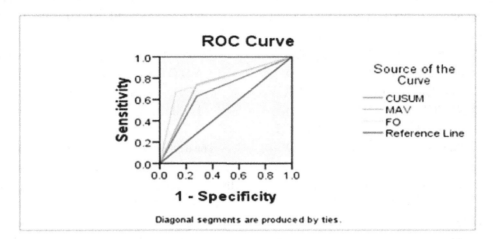

1. CASE=DD SEX=FEMALE 137 ==> RECURRENT=NO 137 conf:(1)
2. CASE=DD DEATH_CODE=NO 129 ==> RECURRENT=NO 129 conf:(1)
3. CASE=DD PLAGUE=DKW 118 ==> RECURRENT=NO 118 conf:(1)
4. CASE=DD PLAGUE=TKW 111 ==> RECURRENT=NO 111 conf:(1)
5. CASE=DD DEATH_CODE=YES 105 ==> RECURRENT=NO 105 conf:(1)
6. CASE=DD AGE=ADULT 102 ==> RECURRENT=NO 102 conf:(1)
7. CASE=DD SEX=MALE 97 ==> RECURRENT=NO 97 conf:(1)
8. CASE=DD ADDRESS=CHERAS 88 ==> RECURRENT=NO 88 conf:(1)
9. CASE=DD RACES=MELAYU 87 ==> RECURRENT=NO 87 conf:(1)
10. CASE=DD RACES=CINA 81 ==> RECURRENT=NO 81 conf:(1)
11. ADDRESS=KAJANG RECURRENT=NO 81 ==> CASE=DD 81 conf:(1)
12. DEATH_CODE=NO PLAGUE=DKW 79 ==> RECURRENT=NO 79 conf:(1)
13. SEX=FEMALE DEATH_CODE=NO 77 ==> RECURRENT=NO 77 conf:(1)
14. SEX=FEMALE PLAGUE=TKW 70 ==> RECURRENT=NO 70 conf:(1)

15. CASE=DD PROFESION=STUDENT 68 ==> RECURRENT=NO 68 conf:(1)

1. CASE=DD DEATH_CODE=NO PLAGUE=DKW79==>RECURRENT=NO 79 conf:(1)
2. CASE=DD SEX=FEMALE DEATH_CODE=NO 77 ==> RECURRENT=NO 77 conf:(1)
3. CASE=DD SEX=FEMALE PLAGUE=TKW70==>RECURRENT=NO 70 conf:(1)
4. CASE=DD SEX=FEMALE PLAGUE=DKW64==>RECURRENT=NO 64 conf:(1)
5. CASE=DD DEATH_CODE=YES PLAGUE=TKW63==>RECURRENT=NO 63 conf:(1)
6. CASE=DD SEX=FEMALE DEATH_CODE=YES 60 ==> RECURRENT=NO 60 conf:(1)
7. CASE=DD RACES=MELAYU DEATH_CODE=YES 60 ==> RECURRENT=NO 60 conf:(1)
8. CASE=DD AGE=ADULT SEX=FEMALE 59 ==> RECURRENT=NO 59 conf:(1)

9. CASE=DD AGE=ADULT DEATH_CODE=NO 56 ==> RECURRENT=NO 56 conf:(1)

10. CASE=DD AGE=ADULT PLAGUE=DKW 54 ==> RECURRENT=NO 54 conf:(1)

11. CASE=DD SEX=MALE PLAGUE=DKW 54 ==> RECURRENT=NO 54 conf:(1)

12. CASE=DD ADDRESS=CHERAS DEATH_CODE=NO 54 ==> RECURRENT=NO 54 conf:(1)

13. CASE=DD SEX=FEMALE RACES=MELAYU 53 ==> RECURRENT=NO 53 conf:(1)

14. CASE=DD RACES=CINA DEATH_CODE=NO 53 ==> RECURRENT=NO 53 conf:(1)

15. CASE=DD SEX=MALE DEATH_CODE=NO 52 ==> RECURRENT=NO 52 conf:(1)

16. CASE=DD RACES=CINA PLAGUE=TKW 51 ==> RECURRENT=NO 51 conf:(1)

17. CASE=DD ADDRESS=KAJANG DEATH_CODE=YES 50 ==> RECURRENT=NO 50 conf:(1)

18. CASE=DD SEX=FEMALE RACES=CINA 49 ==> RECURRENT=NO 49 conf:(1)

19. CASE=DD SEX=FEMALE ADDRESS=KAJANG 49 ==> RECURRENT=NO 49 conf:(1)

20. CASE=DD RACES=MELAYU PLAGUE=DKW 48 ==> RECURRENT=NO 48 conf:(1)

1. 246. CASE=DD SEX=FEMALE DEATH_CODE=NO PLAGUE=DKW 40 ==> RECURRENT=NO 40 conf:(1)

2. 257. CASE=DD SEX=MALE DEATH_CODE=NO PLAGUE=DKW 39 ==> RECURRENT=NO 39 conf:(1)

3. 297. CASE=DD AGE=ADULT DEATH_CODE=NO PLAGUE=DKW 37 ==> RECURRENT=NO 37 conf:(1)

4. 318. CASE=DD SEX=FEMALE DEATH_CODE=NO PLAGUE=TKW 36 ==> RECURRENT=NO 36 conf:(1)

5. 341. CASE=DD RACES=MELAYU ADDRESS=KAJANG DEATH_CODE=YES 35 ==> RECURRENT=NO 35 conf:(1)

The derived knowledge from the 1-length rules is directly implied to the situation, for example, the outbreak cases rarely happen toward females and it is not a recurrent case. In the 2-length rules the dengue cases were identified to occur rarely among men and also there were rarely dengue outbreak cases at Cheras areas. It was also found that dengue cases were the outlier cases for the Malays and it was normally non recurrent cases. The outlier pattern generated from the frequent pattern was also generated rules as females who stay in Kajang area and recurrent cases are rarely found. It was identified that the death cases due to dengue outbreak were rare among Malays in Kajang. Based on this knowledge produced from the rules generated based on the outbreak cases, the counter measure was managed to be analyzed for the actions of outbreaks preparedness such as awareness campaign to the identified areas.

REFERENCES

Agrawal, R., Imieli ski, T., & Swami, A. (1993). Mining association rules between sets of items in large databases. *SIGMOD Record*, *22*(2), 207–216. doi:10.1145/170036.170072

Agrawal, R., & Srikant, R. (1994). *Fast algorithms for mining association rules*.

Anom. (2010). Introduction to investigating an outbreak. Excellence in Curriculum Innovation through Teaching Epidemiology and the Science of Public Health. Retrieved from http://www.cdc.gov/excite/classroom/outbreak/objectives.htm

Ben-Gal, I. (2005). Outlier detection. In Maiman, O., & Rokach, L. (Eds.), *Data mining and knowledge discovery handbook: A complete guide for practitioners and researchers*. Kluwer Academic Publishers. doi:10.1007/0-387-25465-X_7

Blind, J., & Das, S. (2007). *Disease outbreak detection and tracking for biosurveillance: A data fusion approach*.

Brin, S., Motwani, R., Ullman, J. D., & Tsur, S. (1997). *Dynamic itemset counting and implication rules for market basket data*.

Brown, D., & Gray, G. A. (2005). *Implementation of a data fusion algorithm for RODS, a real-time outbreak and disease surveillance system. SAND2005-6007*. Sandia National Laboratories. doi:10.2172/876344

Buehler, J. W., Berkelman, R. L., Hartley, D. M., & Peters, C. J. (2003). Syndromic surveillance and bioterrorism-related epidemics. *Emerging Infectious Diseases*, *9*(10), 1197–1204.

Buehler, J. W., Hopkins, R. S., Overhage, J. M., Sosin, D. M., & Tong, V. (2004a). Framework for evaluating public health surveillance systems for early detection of outbreaks. *Morbidity and Mortality Weekly Report Recommendations and Reports*, *53*, 1–11.

Buehler, J. W., Hopkins, R. S., Overhage, J. M., Sosin, D. M., & Tong, V. (2004b). Framework for evaluating public health surveillance systems for early detection of outbreaks: Recommendations from the CDC Working Group. *Recommendations and Reports: Morbidity and Mortality Weekly Report*, *53*(RR-5), 1.

Carme, B., Sobesky, M., Biard, M., Cotellon, P., Aznar, C., & Fontanella, J. (2003). Non-specific alert system for dengue epidemic outbreaks in areas of endemic malaria. A hospital-based evaluation in Cayenne (French Guiana). *Epidemiology and Infection*, *130*(1), 93–100. doi:10.1017/S0950268802007641

Ceglar, A., & Roddick, J. F. (2006). Association mining. *ACM Computing Surveys*, *38*(2). doi:10.1145/1132956.1132958

Chandola, V., Banerjee, A., & Kumar, V. (2007). *Outlier detection: A survey*. USA: Technical Report. Univeristy of Minnesota.

Chandola, V., Banerjee, A., & Kumar, V. (2009). Anomaly detection: A survey. *ACM Computing Surveys*, *41*(3), 15. doi:10.1145/1541880.1541882

Chandola, V., Mithal, V., & Kumar, V. (2008). *A comparative evaluation of anomaly detection techniques for sequence data*.

Frank, I. H. W. E. (2005). *Data mining: Practical machine learning tools and techniques*. Morgan Kaufmann Publishers.

German, R. R., Armstrong, G., Birkhead, G. S., Horan, J. M., & Herrera, G. (2001). Updated guidelines for evaluating public health surveillance systems. *MMWR. Recommendations and Reports*, *50*, 1–35.

Guthrie, G., Stacey, D. A., & Calvert, D. (2005). *Detection of disease outbreaks in pharmaceutical sales: Neural networks and threshold algorithms*.

Han, J., Cheng, H., Xin, D., & Yan, X. (2007). Frequent pattern mining: current status and future directions. *Data Mining and Knowledge Discovery*, *15*(1), 55–86. doi:10.1007/s10618-006-0059-1

Han, J., & Kamber, M. (2001). *Data mining: Concepts and techniques*. Morgan Kaufmann.

He, Z., Xu, X., Huang, Z., & Deng, S. (2005). FP-outlier: Frequent pattern based outlier detection. *Computer Science and Information Systems/ ComSIS*, *2*(1), 103-118.

Hodge, V., & Austin, J. (2004). A survey of outlier detection methodologies. *Artificial Intelligence Review*, *22*(2), 85–126. doi:10.1023/B:AIRE.0000045502.10941.a9

Hutwagner, L., Thompson, W., Seeman, G. M., & Treadwell, T. (2003). The bioterrorism preparedness and response early aberration reporting system (EARS). *Journal of Urban Health: Bulletin of the New York Academy of Medicine, 80*(Supplement 1), i89–i96.

Koufakou, A., Ortiz, E., Georgiopoulos, M., Anagnostopoulos, G., & Reynolds, K. (2007). *A scalable and efficient outlier detection strategy for categorical data.*

Lai, P., & Kwong, K. (2010). Spatial analysis of the 2008 influenza outbreak of Hong Kong. *Computational Science and Its Applications–ICCSA, 2010*, 374–388.

MOH. (2009). *Health facts 2009.* Retrieved from http://www.moh.gov.my/images/gallery/stats/heal_fact/healthfact-P_2009.pdf

Mukhi, S. N. (2007). *Integrated approach to real-time biosurveillance in a federated data source environment.* Winnipeg, Manitoba, Canada: University of Manitoba.

Neill, D., Moore, A., & Cooper, G. (2006). A Bayesian spatial scan statistic. *Advances in Neural Information Processing Systems, 18*, 1003.

Neill, D. B., Moore, A. W., Sabhnani, M., & Daniel, K. (2005). *Detection of emerging space-time clusters.*

Neill, D. B., Moore, A. W., Sabhnani, M. R., & Daniel, K. (2006). An expectation-based scan statistic for detection of space-time clusters. *Advances in Disease Surveillance, 1*(1), 56.

Oum, S., Chandramohan, D., & Cairncross, S. (2005). Community based surveillance: A pilot study from rural Cambodia. *Tropical Medicine & International Health, 10*(7), 689–697. doi:10.1111/j.1365-3156.2005.01445.x

Patcha, A., & Park, J. M. (2007). An overview of anomaly detection techniques: Existing solutions and latest technological trends. *Computer Networks, 51*(12), 3448–3470. doi:10.1016/j.comnet.2007.02.001

Rigau-Pérez, J. G., Clark, G. G., Gubler, D. J., Reiter, P., Sanders, E. J., & Vance Vorndam, A. (1998). Dengue and dengue haemorrhagic fever. *Lancet, 352*(9132), 971–977. doi:10.1016/S0140-6736(97)12483-7

Runge-Ranzinger, S., Horstick, O., Marx, M., & Kroeger, A. (2008). What does dengue disease surveillance contribute to predicting and detecting outbreaks and describing trends? *Tropical Medicine & International Health, 13*(8), 1022–1041. doi:10.1111/j.1365-3156.2008.02112.x

Seng, S. B., Chong, A. K., & Moore, A. (2005). *Geostatistical modelling, analysis and mapping of epidemiology of Dengue fever in Johor State.* Malaysia.

Shen, Y., & Cooper, G. F. (2007). A Bayesian biosurveillance method that models unknown outbreak diseases. *Lecture Notes in Computer Science, 4506*, 209. doi:10.1007/978-3-540-72608-1_21

Stoto, M. A., Schonlau, M., & Mariano, L. T. (2004). Syndromic surveillance: Is it worth the effort. *Chance, 17*(1), 19–24.

Talarmin, A., Peneau, C., Dussart, P., Pfaff, F., Courcier, M., & de Rocca-Serra, B. (2000). Surveillance of dengue fever in French Guiana by monitoring the results of negative malaria diagnoses. *Epidemiology and Infection, 125*(1), 189–193. doi:10.1017/S0950268899004239

Wong, W., Moore, A., Cooper, G., & Wagner, M. (2003). *Bayesian network anomaly pattern detection for disease outbreaks.*

Wong, W. K. (2004). *Data mining for early disease outbreak detection.* Pittsburgh, PA: Carnegie Mellon University.

Wong, W. K., Moore, A., Cooper, G., & Wagner, M. (2002). *Rule-based anomaly pattern detection for detecting disease outbreaks.*

Wong, W. K., Moore, A., Cooper, G., & Wagner, M. (2003). WSARE: What's strange about recent events? *Journal of Urban Health: Bulletin of the New York Academy of Medicine, 80*(2 Supplement 1).

Zalizah, A. L., Abu Bakar, A., Hamdan, A. R., & Sahani, M. (2010). Multiple attribute frequent mining-based for dengue outbreak. *Proceedings of the 6ᵗʰ International Conference on Advanced Data Mining and Applications, Part 1.*

Zalizah, A. L., Hamdan, A. R., & Azuraliza, A. B. (2009 5-6 Jun 2009). *Framework on outlier sequential patterns for outbreak detection.* Paper presented at the International Conference Knowledge Discovery (ICKD) Manila

Zalizah, A. L., Hamdan, A. R., & Norsuhaili, S. (2008). *Outbreak detection techniques for public health surveillance: A preliminary study* Paper presented at the 2nd International Conference on Science & Technology (ICSTIE 2008).

Zhang, Y., Meratnia, N., & Havinga, P. J. M. (2007). *A taxonomy framework for unsupervised outlier detection techniques for multi-type data sets.*

Zhao, Q., & Bhowmick, S. S. (2006). *Association rule mining: A survey.* Singapore: Nanyang Technological University.

Zhou, Z. H. (2003). Three perspectives of data mining. *Artificial Intelligence, 143*(1), 139–146. doi:10.1016/S0004-3702(02)00357-0

Chapter 9
Development of Surrogate Models of Orthopedic Screws to Improve Biomechanical Performance:
Comparisons of Artificial Neural Networks and Multiple Linear Regressions

Ching-Chi Hsu
Graduate Institute of Applied Science and Technology, National Taiwan University of Science and Technology, Taiwan

ABSTRACT

An optimization approach was applied to improve the design of the lag screws used in double screw nails. However, finite element analyses with an optimal algorithm may take a long time to find the best design. Thus, surrogate methods, either artificial neural networks or multiple linear regressions, were used to substitute for the finite element models. The results showed that an artificial neural network method can accurately develop the objective functions of the lag screws for both the bending strength and the pullout strength. A multiple linear regression method can successfully develop the objective function of the lag screws for the pullout strength, but it failed to construct the objective function for the bending strength. The optimal design of the lag screws could be obtained using the artificial neural network method and genetic algorithms.

DOI: 10.4018/978-1-4666-1803-9.ch009

INTRODUCTION

This chapter investigates the design improvements of the lag screw used in double screw nails and evaluates the applicability of surrogate methods using finite element analyses, Taguchi robust design methods, artificial neural networks, multiple linear regressions, and genetic algorithms. First, two types of the finite element models, bending strength models and pullout strength models, were developed. Six design variables for the lag screws were selected and arranged using the L_{25} orthogonal array provided by the Taguchi robust design methods. Then, two types of surrogate methods, artificial neural network methods and multiple linear regression methods, were applied to reduce the computational time required for the design optimization process. Finally, the optimal designs of the lag screws were obtained using genetic algorithms. The purposes of this study were to evaluate the strengths and limitations of the surrogate methods in developing the objective functions of the lag screws and to search for the optimal design of the lag screws to improve their biomechanical performance.

BACKGROUND

Dynamic hip screws or gamma nails are used to treat patients with proximal femoral fractures (Bellabarba, Herscovici, Ricci, & Hudanich, 2003; Hartford, Patel, & Powell, 2005; Hesse & Gächter, 2004; Willoughby, 2005). A dynamic hip screw consists of a metal plate, a lag screw, and locking screws, and has the advantage of a sliding lag screw in the barrel of the side plate that facilitates fracture impaction and healing and prevents lag screw cut-out (Bucholz, Heckman, & Court-Brown, 2006; Lorich, Geller, & Nielson, 2004; Schipper, Steyerberg, & Castelein, 2004). A gamma nail consists of a nail, a proximal lag screw, distal locking screws, and a set screw, and has the

advantage of a lower risk of implant failure and prevents femoral shortening and hip deformity. These implants have been successfully applied to treat subtrochanteric fractures, intertrochanteric fractures, and basal neck fractures. However, a dynamic hip screw with excessive sliding of the lag screw may cause limb shortening and lag screw cut-out (Lin, 2006). In addition, gamma nails have the drawbacks of postoperative femoral shaft fracture via the nail tip due to stress concentration and intraoperative splintering because of the bulky proximal part (Pervez & Parker, 2001).

To solve the above problems, a double screw nail design, which consists of a nail, two proximal lag screws, and distal locking screws, is presented (Lin, 2006). Double screw nails can avoid postoperative femoral fracture and intraoperative splintering because of a long nail length and a small nail diameter on the proximal part, respectively. Although double screw nails have been demonstrated to have greater biomechanical performance than dynamic hip screws and gamma nails (C. C. Hsu, Lin, Amaritsakul, Antonius, & Chao, 2009), the failure of fracture fixation for double screw nails still exists (Banan, Al-Sabti, Jimulia, & Hart, 2002). Fatigue failure and screw loosening of the lag screws were the main problems found for double screw nails. Thus, improving the design of double screw nails might solve these two clinical problems.

Past research has evaluated and improved the design of double screw nails using clinical trials (Banan et al., 2002; Lin, 2006), mechanical testing (Kouvidis, Sommers, Giannoudis, Katonis, & Bottlang, 2009; Kubiak et al., 2004), and numerical simulations (C. C. Hsu et al., 2009; Wang, Brown, Yettram, & Procter, 2000). However, it is impossible to achieve an optimal design for double screw nails using either clinical trials or mechanical tests exclusively. Fortunately, numerical simulation with an optimal algorithm might decrease the efforts for designing new orthopedic implants or engineering products (Hernández, 2009; C C Hsu, Chao, Wang, & Lin, 2006; Lee

& Lee, 2004; Shokrieh & Rezaei, 2003). This optimization process requires a huge number of numerical calculations. In addition, even numerical simulations with an optimal algorithm may take a long time to find the best design if the objective value is calculated using a numerical model with a large number of degrees of freedom (Schmid, Hirschen, Meynen, & Schäfer, 2005; Schneider, Schneider, & Schwarz, 2002; Uysal, Gul, & Uzman, 2007). Past studies have developed surrogate models to substitute for numerical models or experimental tests including artificial neural networks (Gismondi, Almeida, & Infantosi, 2002; Schöllhorn, 2004), multiple linear regressions (Brown, 2001; Gatti et al., 2008; C C Hsu et al., 2006), and the Taguchi methods (Ajaal & Smith, 2009; Hwang, Lin, Liang, Yang, & Yeh, 2009). These surrogate methods can develop the relationship between the input factors and the output results while decreasing the computational time. Therefore, the purposes of this study were to evaluate the strengths and limitations of each surrogate method and to find the optimal design of a double screw nail.

MATERIALS AND METHODS

Finite Element Models

To analyze the design of the double screw nail, two types of finite element models were developed, namely the bending strength model and the pullout strength model, using ANSYS 12 Workbench (ANSYS, Inc. Canonsburg, PA, USA). The bending strength model consisted of the femur, the lag screws, and the nail. The femur model used in this study was developed by Viceconti et al. (Viceconti et al., 1996). This femur model was modified to create cancellous bone with the use of SolidWorks 2008 (SolidWorks Corporation, Concord, MA, USA). Thus, it consists of cortical bone and cancellous bone. The elastic moduli for the cortical bone and the cancellous bone were

17 GPa and 0.36 GPa, respectively. The Poisson's ratio of the bones was 0.3. The lag screws and the nail were made from 316L stainless steel. The elastic modulus and Poisson's ratio were 230 GPa and 0.3, respectively. The bending strength model was free-meshed with ten-node tetrahedral elements (SOLID 187). The interfaces between the nail and the femur were assumed to be in contact with surface-to-surface contact elements (CONTA 174 and TARGE 170). In addition, the contact condition was also applied to the lag screws and the femur, and the lag screws and the nail. For the loading and boundary conditions, a hip-joint force of 700 N was applied at the center of the femoral head and the degrees of freedom at the end of the proximal femur were fully constrained (Figure 1A). To investigate the bending strength of the double screw nail, the maximal tensile stress of the lag screws was calculated. The pullout strength model consisted of the bone and the lag screw. The bone was assumed to be a cylinder with a diameter of 30 mm. The elastic modulus and the Poisson's ratio of the bone were 137.5 MPa and 0.3, respectively. The bone compaction effects were considered by changing the elastic modulus of the bone surrounding the conical core according to the density change of the bone (C. C. Hsu et al., 2005). The material properties of the lag screw were the same as in the bending strength model. The pullout strength model was meshed using ten-node tetrahedral elements and high-order twenty-node hexahedral elements (SOLID 186). The interfaces between the lag screw and the bone were assumed to be in contact. For the loading and boundary conditions, an axial displacement of 0.01 mm was applied at the end surface of the lag screw and the degrees of freedom at the end of the bone were fully constrained (Figure 1B). The total reaction force was calculated to investigate the pullout strength of the double screw nail, which is defined as the summation of the axial force on the nodes with pre-applied displacement. The convergent studies were done by increasing

Figure 1. The finite element models: (A) the bending strength model, (B) the pullout strength model, (C) the maximal tensile stress distribution, and (D) the displacement distribution

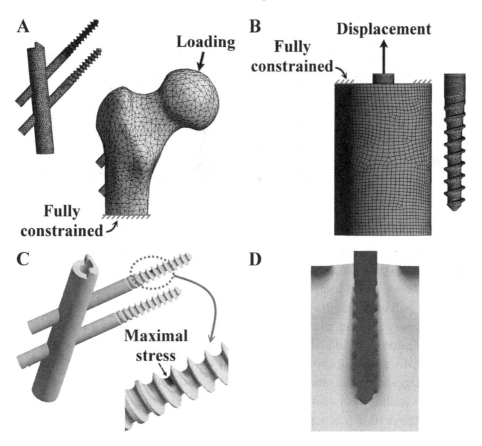

the mesh density for both the bending strength model and the pullout strength model.

Taguchi Robust Design Methods

The Taguchi robust design method is often applied to evaluate and conduct improvements in processes, products, and equipment (Fowlkes & Creveling, 1995). The benefits of this method include reducing the number of experiments or calculations according to the use of orthogonal arrays. Six design variables for the lag screws of the double screw nail were selected including the initial position of the conical angle (IP), the inner diameter (ID), the proximal root radius (RR_p), the pitch (P), the proximal half angle (HA_p),

and the thread width (TW) (Figure 2). In addition, the discrete values for each design variable were defined as follows: 0, 7, 14, 21, or 28 mm for IP; 3.30, 3.73, 4.15, 4.58, or 5.00 mm for ID; 0.40, 0.55, 0.70, 0.85, or 1.00 mm for RR_p; 2.60, 2.95, 3.30, 3.65, or 4.00 mm for P; 5.00, 8.75, 12.50, 16.25, or 20.00 degrees for HA_p; and 0.10, 0.15, 0.20, 0.25, or 0.30 mm for TW. An L_{25} orthogonal array, which can contain six design variables at five levels, was used in this study (Table 1). The other design variables of the lag screws were kept constant, such as the outer diameter (OD) of 6.5 mm, the distal root radius (RR_D) of 1.0 mm, and the distal half angle (HA_D) of 25 degrees. For the bending strength model, a smaller maximal tensile stress of the lag screws

Figure 2. Definition of design variables for the lag screw used in the double screw nail

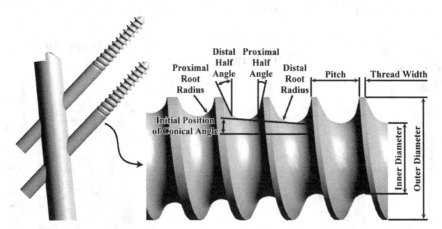

represented a lower risk of implant failure. Therefore, the maximal tensile stress was transformed into a the-lower-the-better signal-to-noise ratio (Equation 1). In the pullout strength model, a larger total reaction force of the lag screw represented better bone adhesion to the implant. Thus, the total reaction force was transformed into a the-larger-the-better signal-to-noise ratio (Equation 2). The optimal variable-level combination of the lag screw of the double screw nail was found based on the factor levels corresponding to the maximal signal-to-noise (S/N) ratio. The analysis of variance (ANOVA) statistical method was used to estimate the significance of the design variable of the lag screws. An ANOVA table consists of the total sum of squares, the degrees of freedom, the mean square, the F value, and the weight of contribution. The total sum of squares measures the overall variability of the data (Equation 3). The sum of squares for each variable measures the variability due to the variables (Equation 4). The sum of squares for the error measures the variability due to the error (Equation 5). The degree of freedom for each factor is defined by subtracting 1 from the number of discrete levels ($m-1$). Thus, there were twenty-four degrees of freedom in the L_{25} orthogonal array. The mean squares for the factor were calculated by dividing the sum of squares for each variable

by the respective degrees of freedom (Equation 6). The mean squares for the error were calculated by dividing the sum of squares for the error by the respective degrees of freedom (Equation 7). The F value for each variable was calculated by Equation 8, and the percentage contribution of each variable was calculated by Equation 9. The optimum combination of the design was conducted using the optimum parameter level settings and the additive model (Equation 10).

$$S/N = -10\log\left(y_i^2\right)$$

where y_i is the result of the ith run (1)

$$S/N = -10\log\left(1/y_i^2\right) \tag{2}$$

$$SS_T = \sum_{i=1}^{n}\left(S/N_i - \overline{S/N}\right)^2$$

where n = number of runs

S/N_i = the S/N of the ith run

$\overline{S/N}$ = overall mean of S/N. (3)

Table 1. The design combinations of the lag screws for the learning process (from L-01 to L-25), the verification process (from V-01 to V-05), and the optimal design (GA-O)

Run	Initial position of conical angle (mm)	Inner diameter (mm)	Proximal root radius (mm)	Pitch (mm)	Proximal half angle (°)	Thread width (mm)	Maximal tensile stress (MPa)	Total reaction force (N)
L-01	0	3.30	0.40	2.60	5.00	0.10	91.0	38.6
L-02	0	3.73	0.55	2.95	8.75	0.15	79.1	35.8
L-03	0	4.15	0.70	3.30	12.50	0.20	79.5	32.6
L-04	0	4.58	0.85	3.65	16.25	0.25	72.6	28.6
L-05	0	5.00	1.00	4.00	20.00	0.30	67.3	23.6
L-06	7	3.30	0.55	3.30	16.25	0.30	93.7	36.3
L-07	7	3.73	0.70	3.65	20.00	0.10	84.5	33.6
L-08	7	4.15	0.85	4.00	5.00	0.15	80.3	30.3
L-09	7	4.58	1.00	2.60	8.75	0.20	73.2	31.1
L-10	7	5.00	0.40	2.95	12.50	0.25	71.4	32.5
L-11	14	3.30	0.70	4.00	8.75	0.25	116.7	33.9
L-12	14	3.73	0.85	2.60	12.50	0.30	119.4	35.5
L-13	14	4.15	1.00	2.95	16.25	0.10	88.5	32.9
L-14	14	4.58	0.40	3.30	20.00	0.15	82.0	33.7
L-15	14	5.00	0.55	3.65	5.00	0.20	76.8	30.0
L-16	21	3.30	0.85	2.95	20.00	0.20	162.5	36.0
L-17	21	3.73	1.00	3.30	5.00	0.25	131.9	34.0
L-18	21	4.15	0.40	3.65	8.75	0.30	130.8	34.9
L-19	21	4.58	0.55	4.00	12.50	0.10	98.9	35.0
L-20	21	5.00	0.70	2.60	16.25	0.15	87.2	32.5
L-21	28	3.30	1.00	3.65	12.50	0.15	149.2	33.9
L-22	28	3.73	0.40	4.00	16.25	0.20	169.9	33.8
L-23	28	4.15	0.55	2.60	20.00	0.25	138.4	33.3
L-24	28	4.58	0.70	2.95	5.00	0.30	120.0	34.1
L-25	28	5.00	0.85	3.30	8.75	0.10	102.3	31.0
V-01	2.07	3.48	0.60	2.78	5.00	0.21	83.4	36.4
V-02	23.09	4.52	0.94	2.91	10.34	0.21	109.8	32.9
V-03	18.40	4.23	0.90	2.72	7.88	0.24	106.4	34.2
V-04	27.82	3.52	0.42	3.08	13.22	0.29	156.7	36.1
V-05	10.23	4.20	0.95	3.37	19.40	0.25	88.7	31.4
GA-O	0	3.90	0.40	2.60	20.00	0.10	73.88	36.68

$$SS_F = \sum_{i=1}^{m} N_{Fi} \left(\overline{S/N}_{Fi} - \overline{S/N} \right)^2$$

where F = the design factor from U to Z

m = the number of discrete levels

N_{Fi} = the number of runs at each level of each factor

$\overline{S/N}_{Fi}$ = the mean of S/N at each level of each factor.   (4)

$$SS_E = SS_T - SS_U - SS_V - SS_W - SS_X - SS_Y - SS_Z$$
(5)

$$MS_F = SS_F / DOF_F$$

where DOF_F = the degrees of freedom for the respective factor. (6)

$$MS_E = SS_E / DOF_E$$

where DOF_E = the degrees of freedom for the respective error. (7)

$$F = MS_F / MS_E \qquad (8)$$

$$C = SS_F / SS_T \times 100\% \qquad (9)$$

$$S/N_{add} = \overline{S/N} + \sum_{i=1}^{k} \left(\overline{S/N}_{OPTi} - \overline{S/N} \right)$$

where k = the number of design variables

$\overline{S/N}_{OPTi}$ = the mean S/N of each design factor at the optimal level   (10)

Artificial Neural Networks

A three-layered artificial neural network (ANN) architecture, which consists of an input layer, hidden layer, and output layer, was used in this study. To develop the best ANN models, the number of neurons in the hidden layer was varied from one to seven. The input variables were normalized to a range of -1 to 1, and the output performances were normalized to a range of 0 to 1. The learning cycles were varied from 5,000 to 20,000 for the ANN models with different numbers of neurons in the hidden layer. The learning rate and the coefficient of momentum term were 0.5 and 0.5, respectively. A sigmoid function was selected as the activation function for the neurons in the hidden layer. The iterations were stopped when the desired learning cycle was achieved. Twenty-five lag screw designs, which were selected according to the L_{25} orthogonal array, were prepared as the learning data set. Five lag screw designs, which were randomly selected, were used as the verification data set. Seven types of ANN models for the bending strength were developed: ANN-B1, ANN-B2, ANN-B3, ANN-B4, ANN-B5, ANN-B6, and ANN-B7. In addition, seven types of ANN models for the pullout strength were developed: ANN-P1, ANN-P2, ANN-P3, ANN-P4, ANN-P5, ANN-P6, and ANN-P7. One neuron in the hidden layer was used for ANN-B1 and ANN-P1 as shown in Equation 11, and there are nine unknown coefficients for ANN-B1 and ANN-P1. Two neurons in the hidden layer were used for ANN-B2 and ANN-P2 as shown in Equation 12, and there are seventeen unknown coefficients for ANN-B2 and ANN-P2. Three neurons in the hidden layer were used for ANN-B3 and ANN-P3 as shown in Equation 13, and there are twenty-five unknown coefficients for ANN-B3 and ANN-P3. Similarly, ANN-B7 and ANN-P7 used seven neurons in the hidden layer as shown in Equation 14, and there are fifty-seven unknown coefficients for ANN-B7 and ANN-P7. The unknown coefficients for each ANN model were determined using a computer package. This computer package was coded using Microsoft Visual Basic (Redmond, WA, USA) (Figure 3A). The mean percentage error, maximum percentage error, minimum percentage error, and the correlation coefficient were used to evaluate the relationship between the finite element models and the ANN models.

$$F = \left(1 + e^{-(C_1 \cdot H_1 + C_2)}\right)^{-1}$$

where

$$H_1 = \left(1 + e^{-(C_3 \cdot IP + C_4 \cdot ID + C_5 \cdot RR_P + C_6 \cdot P + C_7 \cdot HA_P + C_8 \cdot TW + C_9)}\right)^{-1}$$

$F =$ the predicted objective value

$C_i =$ the coefficients of the predicted equation

(11)

$$F = \left(1 + e^{-(C_1 \cdot H_1 + C_2 \cdot H_2 + C_3)}\right)^{-1}$$

where

$$H_1 = \left(1 + e^{-(C_4 \cdot IP + C_5 \cdot ID + C_6 \cdot RR_P + C_7 \cdot P + C_8 \cdot HA_P + C_9 \cdot TW + C_{10})}\right)^{-1}$$

$$H_2 = \left(1 + e^{-(C_{11} \cdot IP + C_{12} \cdot ID + C_{13} \cdot RR_P + C_{14} \cdot P + C_{15} \cdot HA_P + C_{16} \cdot TW + C_{17})}\right)^{-1}$$

(12)

$$F = \left(1 + e^{-(C_1 \cdot H_1 + C_2 \cdot H_2 + C_3 \cdot H_3 + C_4)}\right)^{-1}$$

where

$$H_1 = \left(1 + e^{-(C_5 \cdot IP + C_6 \cdot ID + C_7 \cdot RR_P + C_8 \cdot P + C_9 \cdot HA_P + C_{10} \cdot TW + C_{11})}\right)^{-1}$$

$$H_2 = \left(1 + e^{-(C_{12} \cdot IP + C_{13} \cdot ID + C_{14} \cdot RR_P + C_{15} \cdot P + C_{16} \cdot HA_P + C_{17} \cdot TW + C_{18})}\right)^{-1}$$

$$H_3 = \left(1 + e^{-(C_{19} \cdot IP + C_{20} \cdot ID + C_{21} \cdot RR_P + C_{22} \cdot P + C_{23} \cdot HA_P + C_{24} \cdot TW + C_{25})}\right)^{-1}$$

(13)

$$F = \left(1 + e^{-(C_1 \cdot H_1 + C_2 \cdot H_2 + C_3 \cdot H_3 + C_4 \cdot H_4 + C_5 \cdot H_5 + C_6 \cdot H_6 + C_7 \cdot H_7 + C_8)}\right)^{-1}$$

where

$$H_1 = \left(1 + e^{-(C_9 \cdot IP + C_{10} \cdot ID + C_{11} \cdot RR_P + C_{12} \cdot P + C_{13} \cdot HA_P + C_{14} \cdot TW + C_{15})}\right)^{-1}$$

$$H_2 = \left(1 + e^{-(C_{16} \cdot IP + C_{17} \cdot ID + C_{18} \cdot RR_P + C_{19} \cdot P + C_{20} \cdot HA_P + C_{21} \cdot TW + C_{22})}\right)^{-1}$$

$$H_3 = \left(1 + e^{-(C_{23} \cdot IP + C_{24} \cdot ID + C_{25} \cdot RR_P + C_{26} \cdot P + C_{27} \cdot HA_P + C_{28} \cdot TW + C_{29})}\right)^{-1}$$

$$H_4 = \left(1 + e^{-(C_{30} \cdot IP + C_{31} \cdot ID + C_{32} \cdot RR_P + C_{33} \cdot P + C_{34} \cdot HA_P + C_{35} \cdot TW + C_{36})}\right)^{-1}$$

$$H_5 = \left(1 + e^{-(C_{37} \cdot IP + C_{38} \cdot ID + C_{39} \cdot RR_P + C_{40} \cdot P + C_{41} \cdot HA_P + C_{42} \cdot TW + C_{43})}\right)^{-1}$$

$$H_6 = \left(1 + e^{-(C_{44} \cdot IP + C_{45} \cdot ID + C_{46} \cdot RR_P + C_{47} \cdot P + C_{48} \cdot HA_P + C_{49} \cdot TW + C_{50})}\right)^{-1}$$

$$H_7 = \left(1 + e^{-(C_{51} \cdot IP + C_{52} \cdot ID + C_{53} \cdot RR_P + C_{54} \cdot P + C_{55} \cdot HA_P + C_{56} \cdot TW + C_{57})}\right)^{-1}$$

(14)

Multiple Linear Regressions

Multiple linear regressions (MLRs) were used as another surrogate method to develop the relationship between two or more input factors and output performance by adapting a linear equation to the learning data set. As for the artificial neural networks, twenty-five lag screw designs were used to construct the MLR models. Five lag screw designs were used to validate their applicability. Four types of MLR models for the bending strength were created: MLR-B1, MLR-B2, MLR-B3, and MLR-B4. In addition, four types of MLR models for the pullout strength were created: MLR-P1, MLR-P2, MLR-P3, and MLR-P4. MLR-B1 and MLR-P1 were based on a first-order equation as shown in Equation 15, and there are seven unknown coefficients for MLR-B1 and MLR-P1. MLR-B2 and MLR-P2

Figure 3. The computer programs developed in this study: (A) the ANN program, (B) the GA program

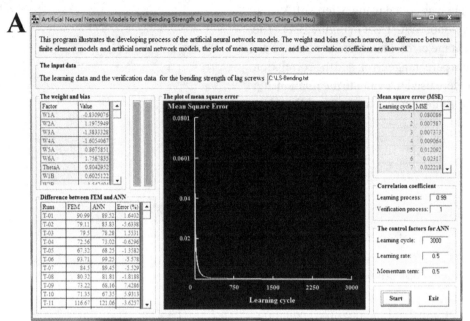

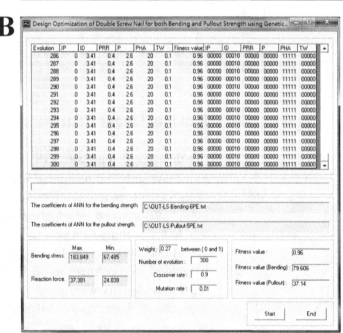

were based on a second-order equation as shown in Equation 16, and there are thirteen unknown coefficients for MLR-B2 and MLR-P2. MLR-B3 and MLR-P3 were based on a third-order equation as shown in Equation 17, and there are nineteen

unknown coefficients for MLR-B3 and MLR-P3. Similarly, MLR-B4 and MLR-P4 were based on a fourth-order equation as shown in Equation 18, and there are twenty-five unknown coefficients for MLR-B4 and MLR-P4. The unknown coefficients for each MLR model were determined using SPSS (Chicago, IL, USA). The mean error, the maximum error, the minimum error, and the correlation coefficient were also used to evaluate the feasibility of the MLR models.

$$F = C_1 \cdot IP + C_2 \cdot ID + C_3 \cdot RR_p + C_4 \\ \cdot P + C_5 \cdot HA_p + C_6 \cdot TW + C_7 \quad (15)$$

$$F = C_1 \cdot IP^2 + C_2 \cdot ID^2 + C_3 \cdot RR_p^2 \\ + C_4 \cdot P^2 + C_5 \cdot HA_p^2 + C_6 \cdot TW^2 \\ + C_7 \cdot IP + C_8 \cdot ID + C_9 \cdot RR_p \\ + C_{10} \cdot P + C_{11} \cdot HA_p + C_{12} \cdot TW + C_{13} \quad (16)$$

$$F = C_1 \cdot IP^3 + C_2 \cdot ID^3 + C_3 \cdot RR_p^3 \\ + C_4 \cdot P^3 + C_5 \cdot HA_p^3 + C_6 \cdot TW^3 \\ + C_7 \cdot IP^2 + C_8 \cdot ID^2 + C_9 \cdot RR_p^2 \\ + C_{10} \cdot P^2 + C_{11} \cdot HA_p^2 + C_{12} \cdot TW^2 \\ + C_{13} \cdot IP + C_{14} \cdot ID + C_{15} \cdot RR_p \\ + C_{16} \cdot P + C_{17} \cdot HA_p + C_{18} \cdot TW + C_{19} \quad (17)$$

$$F = C_1 \cdot IP^4 + C_2 \cdot ID^4 + C_3 \cdot RR_p^4 \\ + C_4 \cdot P^4 + C_5 \cdot HA_p^4 + C_6 \cdot TW^4 \\ + C_7 \cdot IP^3 + C_8 \cdot ID^3 + C_9 \cdot RR_p^3 \\ + C_{10} \cdot P^3 + C_{11} \cdot HA_p^3 + C_{12} \cdot TW^3 \\ + C_{13} \cdot IP^2 + C_{14} \cdot ID^2 + C_{15} \cdot RR_p^2 \\ + C_{16} \cdot P^2 + C_{17} \cdot HA_p^2 + C_{18} \cdot TW^2 \\ + C_{19} \cdot IP + C_{20} \cdot ID + C_{21} \cdot RR_p \\ + C_{22} \cdot P + C_{23} \cdot HA_p + C_{24} \cdot TW + C_{25}$$

$$(18)$$

Optimal Designs of Orthopedic Screws

To find the best design for the lag screws used in the double screw nail design, genetic algorithms (GAs) were used in this study. GAs, which were invented by John Holland in 1975, were inspired by Darwin's theory of evolution (Michalewicz, 1992; Mitchell, 1996). This algorithm can successfully search for a global optimum with the use of rules of probability. In this study, the lowest maximal tensile stress ("the smaller-the-better") and the highest total reaction force ("the larger-the-better") were expected. However, these two output metrics could not be combined directly because they had different scales and purposes. Thus, the maximal tensile stress and the total reaction force should be normalized and transformed into a "the larger-the-better" problem. In addition, this multi-objective problem was combined into a single-objective problem with use of a weighted-sum aggregating approach. The objective function for this problem was maximized as shown in Equation 19. The weight, w, was systematically changed (from 0 to 1) to investigate the different combinations of both the bending strength and the pullout strength. To eliminate infeasible designs for the lag screws, the geometric constraints were applied as shown in Equations. 20, 21, and 22 (C C Hsu et al., 2006). The parameters used in the GAs are described below. The crossover rate and the mutation rate were 90% and 1%, respectively. Each population had 10 lag screw designs, and each design factor had five strings. The design optimization strategy was stopped when 10,000 populations were produced. The Pareto front, which represents the best solution of the multi-objective optimization problem, was obtained after the optimization strategy. The computational software for the GAs was created using Microsoft Visual Basic (Figure 3B). To validate the results of the design optimization, three optimal designs for the lag screws were selected from the knee region, and they were confirmed using finite element simulations.

$$F = w \cdot F_{bending} + (1 - w) \cdot F_{pullout}$$

where F = the combined objective function (fitness function)

$F_{bending}$ = the normalized objective function of the bending strength

$F_{pullout}$ = the normalized objective function of the bone holding power

w = the assigned weighting of the fitness function (19)

$$RR_p \cdot \cos(90 - HA_p) < (\frac{OD - ID}{2}) \cdot \tan(HA_p) \cdot \tan(\frac{HA_p + 90}{2})$$

(20)

$$RR_D \cdot \cos(90 - HA_D) < (\frac{OD - ID}{2}) \cdot \tan(HA_D) \cdot \tan(\frac{HA_D + 90}{2})$$

(21)

$$P - TW - RR_p \cdot \cot(\frac{HA_p + 90}{2}) - RR_D \cdot \cot(\frac{HA_D + 90}{2}) > (\frac{OD - ID}{2}) \cdot [\tan(HA_p) + \tan(HA_D)]$$

(22)

RESULTS

Finite Element Models

Both types of models, the bending strength and the pullout strength models, were successfully meshed and analyzed. For the bending strength models, the total number of elements and nodes varied from 290,000 to 400,000 and from 436,000 to 580,000, respectively. Their solution time varied from 10 to 30 hours. The maximal tensile stress occurred at either the proximal root radius or the distal root radius of the lag screws (Figure 1C). For the pullout strength models, the total number of elements and nodes ranged from 107,000 to

213,000 and from 230,000 to 382,000, respectively. Their computational time varied from 5 to 20 hours. No deformation occurred in the lag screw of the pullout strength model, and all of the deformation occurred at the bone (Figure 1D). In the convergent studies, the maximal tensile stress obtained from the bending strength model was sensitive to the mesh density compared to the total reaction force obtained from the pullout strength model. Fortunately, both types of finite element models converged properly.

Taguchi Robust Design Methods

The results of the L_{25} orthogonal array (from L-01 to L-25) and five random designs (from V-01 to V-05) for both the maximal tensile stress and the total reaction force are listed in Table 1. To obtain the best combination of the lag screw designs, the maximal tensile stress was transformed into the-smaller-the-better signal-to-noise ratio and the total reaction force was transformed into the-larger-the-better signal-to-noise ratio. Then, the S/N ratio plots of both the maximal tensile stress and the total reaction force at each level for each design factor were obtained (Figure 4A and 4B). The S/N ratio plots of the maximal tensile stress suggested optimum factor level settings of $IP_1 ID_5 RR_{p2} P_3 HA_{p1} TW_2$, which correspond to a fully conical design, an inner diameter of 5 mm, a proximal root radius of 0.55 mm, a pitch of 3.3 mm, a proximal half angle of 5 degrees, and a thread width of 0.15 mm. For the total reaction force, the S/N ratio plots suggested optimum factor level settings of $IP_4 ID_1 RR_{p1} P_2 HA_{p3} TW_1$, which correspond to an initial position of conical angle of 21 mm, an inner diameter of 3.3 mm, a proximal root radius of 0.4 mm, a pitch of 2.95 mm, a proximal half angle of 12.5 degrees, and a thread width of 0.1 mm. The ANOVA tables were developed using the S/N ratios as shown in Table 2. The initial position of the conical angle (63.47%) and the inner diameter (30.29%) were

Figure 4. S/N ratio plots at each level for each design variable: (A) the maximal tensile stress, (B) the total reaction force

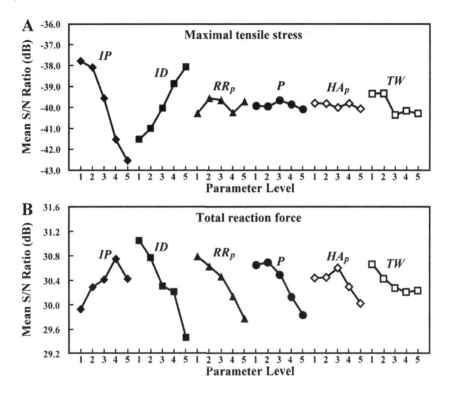

Table 2. ANOVA tables for the bending strength models and the pullout strength models

Parameters	The bending strength models			
	Degree of freedom	Sum of squares	Mean square	Contribution (%)
Initial position of conical angle	4	87.477	21.869	63.47
Inner diameter	4	41.745	10.436	30.29
Proximal root radius	4	2.382	0.595	1.73
Pitch	4	0.507	0.127	0.37
Proximal half angle	4	0.349	0.087	0.25
Thread width	4	5.376	1.344	3.90
Total	24	137.835	—	100
Parameters	The pullout strength models			
	Degree of freedom	Sum of squares	Mean square	Contribution (%)
Initial position of conical angle	4	1.744	0.436	10.41
Inner diameter	4	7.370	1.843	43.99
Proximal root radius	4	3.269	0.817	19.51
Pitch	4	2.716	0.679	16.21
Proximal half angle	4	0.949	0.237	5.66
Thread width	4	0.706	0.177	4.22
Total	24	16.754	—	100

Table 3. The percentage errors and the correlation coefficient for the bending strength models and the pullout strength models

	The maximal tensile stress (The bending strength models)								
	Learning group					Verification group			
	Mean error	Max. error	Min. error	R	Learning cycles	Mean error	Max. error	Min. error	R
ANN-B1	4.68	9.17	0.10	0.98	5,000	5.23	12.86	2.70	1.00
ANN-B2	4.22	10.20	0.53	0.99	6,000	5.12	11.47	2.16	1.00
ANN-B3	3.10	7.67	0.21	0.99	6,000	3.44	9.76	0.29	1.00
ANN-B4	2.19	6.64	0.12	1.00	7,000	3.22	6.96	0.86	1.00
ANN-B5	1.79	3.17	0.32	1.00	8,000	3.60	8.67	0.61	1.00
ANN-B6	0.26	1.43	0.00	1.00	15,000	3.78	6.76	1.01	1.00
ANN-B7	0.98	2.51	0.31	1.00	20,000	3.55	6.78	0.06	1.00
MLR-B1	6.80	26.41	0.18	0.95	—	4.91	11.81	0.25	1.00
MLR-B2	5.09	14.69	0.58	0.97	—	6.55	12.51	1.98	1.00
MLR-B3	4.60	9.76	0.20	0.98	—	7.45	11.00	0.60	1.00
MLR-B4	3.96	12.85	0.26	0.99	—	8.99	14.10	1.60	0.98
	The total reaction force (The pullout strength models)								
	Learning group					Verification group			
	Mean error	Max. error	Min. error	R	Learning cycles	Mean error	Max. error	Min. error	R
ANN-P1	2.29	7.88	0.25	0.95	5,000	2.37	5.45	0.23	1.00
ANN-P2	1.54	5.49	0.05	0.98	6,000	1.77	4.21	0.04	1.00
ANN-P3	1.06	4.46	0.01	0.99	6,000	1.87	4.24	0.68	1.00
ANN-P4	1.03	3.71	0.01	0.99	7,000	1.39	2.87	0.33	1.00
ANN-P5	0.26	0.61	0.03	1.00	8,000	0.97	2.32	0.05	1.00
ANN-P6	0.30	0.73	0.01	1.00	15,000	0.97	2.79	0.09	1.00
ANN-P7	0.29	0.76	0.02	1.00	20,000	0.98	2.53	0.07	1.00
MLR-P1	2.33	7.97	0.23	0.94	—	2.87	4.21	1.32	0.99
MLR-P2	1.42	5.14	0.12	0.98	—	2.49	4.48	1.47	0.96
MLR-P3	1.26	4.14	0.10	0.98	—	2.36	4.05	0.89	0.96
MLR-P4	1.24	3.80	0.10	0.98	—	2.26	4.18	0.69	0.96

significant factors affecting the bending strength of the lag screws. The inner diameter (43.99%), the proximal root radius (19.51%), and the pitch (16.21%) had a higher contribution to the pullout strength of the lag screws.

Artificial Neural Networks

The ANN models of both the bending strength and the pullout strength were successfully developed.

Increasing the number of the neurons in the hidden layer significantly decreased the error between the ANN models and the finite element models, but a larger number of the learning cycles were required (Table 3). The mean error of the learning group was larger than that of the verification group. However, the correlation coefficient between the ANN models and the finite element models for both the learning group and the verification group was quite similar. In addition, the bending strength models had larger mean error compared to the pullout strength models. In the case of the bending strength, ANN-B6 and ANN-B7 revealed similar mean error, maximum error, minimum error, and correlation coefficient values. Thus, ANN-B6 was selected as the best ANN model for predicting the maximal tensile stress of the lag screws. ANN-B6 had a mean error of 0.26%, a maximum error of 1.43%, and a correlation coefficient of 1.0 for the learning group and a mean error of 3.78%, a maximum error of 6.76%, and a correlation coefficient of 1.0 for the verification group. In the case of the pullout strength, ANN-P5, ANN-P6, and ANN-P7 showed similar mean error, maximum error, minimum error, and correlation coefficient values. Therefore, ANN-P5 was selected as the best ANN model for predicting the total reaction force of the lag screws. ANN-P5 had a mean error of 0.26%, a maximum error of 0.61%, and a correlation coefficient of 1.0 for the learning group and a mean error of 0.97%, a maximum error of 2.32%, and a correlation coefficient of 1.0 for the verification group.

Multiple Linear Regressions

The MLR model of the pullout strength could be successfully created, but that of the bending strength could not be accurately developed. Using higher-order equations reduced the error between the MLR models and the finite element models (Table 3). The mean error of the learning group was also larger than that of the verification group, but the correlation coefficient between the MLR models and the finite element models for both the learning group and the verification group had no significant difference. In addition, the bending strength models had larger mean error and the maximum error compared with the pullout strength models. In the case of the bending strength, the smallest mean error of 3.96% and the highest correlation coefficient of 0.99 for the learning group were obtained with MLR-B4, which was superior to the others (MLR-B1, MLR-B2, and

MLR-B3). Unfortunately, MLR-B4 revealed a higher maximum error (12.85% for the learning group and 14.10% for the verification group) compared to the ANN models. In the case of the pullout strength, the smallest mean error and the highest correlation coefficient for the learning group were obtained by MLR-P4, which was superior to the others (MLR-P1, MLR-P2, and MLR-P3). MLR-P4 showed an acceptable error and could be used to predict the results of the finite element models compared to MLR-B4. MLR-P4 had a mean error of 1.24%, a maximum error of 3.8%, and a correlation coefficient of 0.98 for the learning group and a mean error of 2.26%, a maximum error of 4.18%, and a correlation coefficient of 0.96 for the verification group.

Optimal Designs of Orthopedic Screws

The Pareto optimal designs of the lag screws under different weights were obtained using the optimization algorithm. Increasing w increased the bending strength (decreased the maximal tensile stress) and decreased the pullout strength (decreased the total reaction force). In addition, increasing w increased the values for ID, RR_p, and P. However, IP, HA_p, and TW were kept constant (Figure 5A). To determine the optimal designs from the Pareto front, the knee region of the Pareto front was defined as the difference between the normalized bending strength and the normalized pullout strength. A difference of 3% was applied to define the knee region (Figure 5B). In the knee region, w was within the range of 0.42 to 0.68. This range represents the corresponding range of the design variables as follows: 0 mm for IP, 3.63-4.01 mm for ID, 0.40-0.42 mm for RR_p, 2.6 mm for P, 20 degrees for HA_p, and 0.1 mm for TW. The optimal design of the lag screws could be selected within this corresponding range of design variables. Thus, the optimal design of the lag screw was 0 mm for IP, 3.90

Figure 5. The outcomes of a multiobjective optimization: (A) change in normalized objective functions and design variables corresponding to the given weight, (B) the optimal solutions of the lag screws

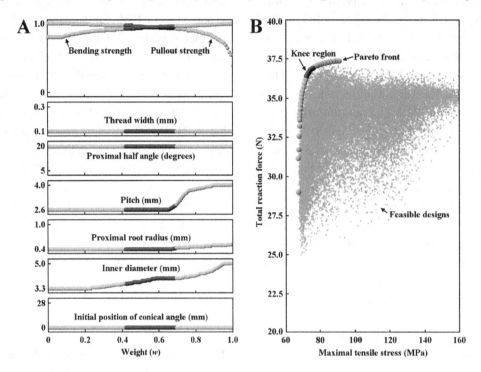

mm for ID, 0.4 mm for RR_p, 2.6 mm for P, 20 degrees for HA_p, and 0.1 mm for TW.

DISCUSSION AND RECOMMENDATIONS

The maximal tensile stress of the lag screws could not be predicted using the MLR method and was difficult to predict using the ANN method compared to the total reaction force. The reason for this difficulty might be that the maximal tensile stress was more sensitive to the local geometry of the lag screws, such as a proximal root radius or a distal root radius, than the total reaction force. Based on the results of the L_{25} orthogonal array, changing the designs of the lag screws could significantly change the maximal tensile stress, but it did not make a significant change in the total reaction force. Thus, the MLR method might

fail and the ANN method might need many neurons in the hidden layer where the relationship between the input variables and the output performance is more complicated. The local geometry of the lag screws could also affect the results of a convergent study. Actually, past research has found that a convergent solution is easy to achieve with the use of the reaction force or the strain energy as the criterion. However, using the stress as the criterion made it difficult to achieve a convergent result (C K Chao, Hsu, Wang, & Lin, 2007; Keyak & Skinner, 1992; Marks & Gardner, 1993). Therefore, the results of the numerical simulations should be carefully evaluated whenever the stress is being used as a convergent criterion. In this research, the variation between the results of the finite element models with different mesh densities was less than 5% for both the maximal tensile stress and the total reaction force.

In constructing the objective functions using the ANN method, both the maximal tensile stress and the total reaction force of the lag screws could be accurately predicted. The best ANN model was the one that produced most accurate results with the fewest learning cycles. The ANN model with six neurons in the hidden layer (ANN-B6) sufficiently predicted the results of the bending strength models. In addition, the ANN model with five neurons in the hidden layer (ANN-P5) sufficiently predicted the results of the pullout strength models. Both ANN-B6 and ANN-P5 had a lower mean error, a smaller maximum error, and a higher correlation coefficient. Although increasing the number of the neurons in the hidden layer could improve the applicability of the ANN models, the unknown coefficients significantly increased from nine for one neuron to fifty-seven for seven neurons. This increase indicates that the learning cycles also significantly increased. In this study, a learning cycle of 5,000 was necessary for the ANN model with one neuron and that of 20,000 was required for the ANN model with seven neurons. Past studies have used the mean error, the maximum error, and the correlation coefficient to evaluate the feasibility of ANN models (Dickey, Pierrynowski, Bednar, & Yang, 2002; Kuzmanovski & Aleksovska, 2003; Schöllhorn, 2004). In this study, these indexes were also selected to evaluate the models. However, the correlation coefficient might be an unsuitable index in this study. The reason is that the ANN model with higher maximum error still produces an excellent correlation coefficient, such as ANN-B1 and ANN-B2. Therefore, only the mean error and the maximum error were used to evaluate the ANN models.

In constructing the objective functions using the MLR method, the maximal tensile stress of the lag screws could not be accurately predicted even though the MLR model with a fourth-order equation was applied. In addition, the maximum error of each MLR model for the bending strength was quite high. This result implies that the optimal lag screw design could not be obtained according to a rough surrogate model. Fortunately, the total

reaction force could be successfully developed using the MLR model with a fourth-order equation. Although the mean error and the maximum error of MLR-P4 were inferior to those of ANN-P5, the former method could also be used in the design optimization process. In this study, the ANN methods were absolutely superior to the MLR methods, possibly because the MLR methods frequently used a polynomial equation to develop the objective function. This type of equation might actually limit its ability to construct the predicted equation as compared to the ANN methods with a sigmoid function.

The Taguchi robust design method used in this study could calculate the contributions of the design variables and provide the best combinations for optimal performance. In addition, an additive model could predict the outcomes of the performances. The initial position of the conical angle and the inner diameter were important factors for the bending strength models. The inner diameter, the proximal root radius, and the pitch were also significant factors for the pullout strength models. Thus, improving these design variables could greatly decrease the maximal tensile stress or increase the total reaction force. An additive model had been used to predict the outcomes of some problems (Ajaal & Smith, 2009; Hwang et al., 2009). Although an additive model could be used to predict either the maximal tensile stress or the total reaction force in this study, it would not be suitable for use as a predictor. There are two reasons that could explain this. First, the additive model used the combinations of the design factors with discrete levels. Thus, the design factors with continuous levels were not allowed for the additive model, which implied that the optimal design provided by the additive model might be incorrect. Second, the additive model consisted of linear terms, which meant that it could not present the results due to the stronger interactions arising from nonlinear problems. These interactions would greatly affect the accuracy and feasibility of this model.

In clinical applications, fatigue failure and screw loosening of the lag screws used in the double screw nail were found. The maximal tensile stress and the total reaction force could represent fatigue failure and screw loosening problems, respectively. The conclusions of past studies on the maximal tensile stress and the total reaction force of the orthopedic screws severely conflict with each other (C. K. Chao, Lin, Putra, & Hsu, 2010; C C Hsu et al., 2006). Improving the maximal tensile stress would threaten the total reaction force and vice versa. Additionally, it is impossible to find a single optimal screw design with respect to all aspects of performance and difficult to select one best solution from a huge number of Pareto fronts. For the knee region, the optimal lag screw designs obtained in this study could provide better bending strength and pullout strength simultaneously.

FUTURE RESEARCH DIRECTIONS

Design optimization can be applied to different types of products and different fields. For the development of medical devices in the bioengineering field, design optimization is a relatively new approach, and there are few studies that apply this approach for designing the devices. Although commercial software provides powerful techniques to solve optimization problems, many design optimization problems cannot be conducted because of a limited capacity of hardware. To compromise for this limited capacity, a real design optimization problem, which may be a three-dimensional nonlinear problem, is usually simplified to a three-dimensional linear problem, a two-dimensional nonlinear problem, or a two-dimensional linear problem. Actually, the results obtained from these simplified problems might be incorrect. To eliminate the limited capacity of hardware and the incorrectness of the simplified problems, a surrogate method is necessary. Artificial neural networks or multiple linear regressions are frequently applied as surrogate methods. However, how to accurately and easily develop a surrogate model is an important and challenging research issue. In addition, discovering an innovative surrogate method might be another research issue.

CONCLUSION

The ANN method can accurately construct objective functions for the lag screws used in the double screw nail for both the bending strength and the pullout strength. The MLR method can successfully develop the objective function of the lag screws for the pullout strength, but it failed to construct the objective function for the bending strength. The optimal design for the lag screws could be obtained using the ANN method and genetic algorithms. The ANN-based GAs could effectively decrease the time and effort required for developing the new designs of the orthopedic screws and might directly help orthopedic surgeons select a suitable implant for their patients.

ACKNOWLEDGMENT

I would like to thank Prof. Ching-Kong Chao (Department of Mechanical Engineering, National Taiwan University of Science and Technology) and Prof. Jinn Lin (Department of Orthopedic Surgery, National Taiwan University Hospital) for their kind support and suggestions during preliminary investigations. In addition, I would like to thank Lin-Zaw Win for his assistance and contributions.

REFERENCES

Ajaal, T. T., & Smith, R. W. (2009). Employing the Taguchi method in optimizing the scaffold production process for artificial bone grafts. *Journal of Materials Processing Technology, 209*, 1521–1532. doi:10.1016/j.jmatprotec.2008.04.001

Banan, H., Al-Sabti, A., Jimulia, T., & Hart, A. J. (2002). The treatment of unstable, extracapsular hip fractures with the AO/ASIF proximal femoral nail (PFN)—our first 60 cases. *Injury-International Journal of the Care of the Injured, 33*, 401–405.

Bellabarba, C., Herscovici, D., Ricci, W. M., & Hudanich, R. (2003). Percutaneous treatment of peritrochanteric fractures using the gamma nail. *Journal of Orthopaedic Trauma, 17*(8), S38–S50. doi:10.1097/00005131-200309001-00009

Brown, A. M. (2001). A step-by-step guide to non-linear regression analysis of experimental data using a Microsoft Excel spreadsheet. *Computer Methods and Programs in Biomedicine, 65*, 191–200. doi:10.1016/S0169-2607(00)00124-3

Bucholz, R. W., Heckman, J. D., & Court-Brown, C. (2006). *Fractures in adult*. Philadelphia, PA: Lippincott Williams & Wilkins.

Chao, C. K., Hsu, C. C., Wang, J. L., & Lin, J. (2007). Increasing bending strength of tibial locking screws: Mechanical tests and finite element analyses. *Clinical Biomechanics (Bristol, Avon), 22*, 59–66. doi:10.1016/j.clinbiomech.2006.07.007

Chao, C. K., Lin, J., Putra, S. T., & Hsu, C. C. (2010). A neurogenetic approach to a multiobjective design optimization of spinal pedicle screws. *Journal of Biomechanical Engineering-Transactions of the ASME, 132*(9), 091006–0910066. doi:10.1115/1.4001887

Dickey, J. P., Pierrynowski, M. R., Bednar, D. A., & Yang, S. X. (2002). Relationship between pain and vertebral motion in chronic low-back pain subjects. *Clinical Biomechanics (Bristol, Avon), 17*, 345–352. doi:10.1016/S0268-0033(02)00032-3

Fowlkes, W. Y., & Creveling, C. M. (1995). *Engineering methods for robust production design using Taguchi method in technology and product development*. Reading, MA: Addison Wesley.

Gatti, C. J., Doro, L. C., Langenderfer, J. E., Mell, A. G., Maratt, J. D., & Carpenter, J. E. (2008). Evaluation of three methods for determining EMG-muscle force parameter estimates for the shoulder muscles. *Clinical Biomechanics (Bristol, Avon), 23*, 166–174. doi:10.1016/j.clinbiomech.2007.08.026

Gismondi, R. C., Almeida, R. M. V. R., & Infantosi, A. F. C. (2002). Artificial neural networks for infant mortality modelling. *Computer Methods and Programs in Biomedicine, 69*, 237–247. doi:10.1016/S0169-2607(02)00006-8

Hartford, J. M., Patel, A., & Powell, J. (2005). Intertrochanteric osteotomy using a dynamic hip screw for femoral neck nonunion. *Journal of Orthopaedic Trauma, 19*(5), 329–333.

Hernández, J. A. (2009). Optimum operating conditions for heat and mass transfer in foodstuffs drying by means of neural network inverse. *Food Control, 20*, 435–438. doi:10.1016/j.foodcont.2008.07.005

Hesse, B., & Gächter, A. (2004). Complications following the treatment of trochanteric fractures with the gamma nail. *Archives of Orthopaedic and Trauma Surgery, 124*, 692–698. doi:10.1007/s00402-004-0744-8

Hsu, C. C., Chao, C. K., Wang, J. L., Hou, S. M., Tsai, Y. T., & Lin, J. (2005). Increase of pullout strength of spinal pedicle screws with conical core: Biomechanical tests and finite element analyses. *Journal of Orthopaedic Research, 23*(4), 788–794. doi:10.1016/j.orthres.2004.11.002

Hsu, C. C., Chao, C. K., Wang, J. L., & Lin, J. (2006). Multiobjective optimization of tibial locking screws design using a genetic algorithm: Evaluation of mechanical performance. *Journal of Orthopaedic Research, 24*, 908–916. doi:10.1002/jor.20088

Hsu, C. C., Lin, J., Amaritsakul, Y., Antonius, T., & Chao, C. K. (2009). Finite element analysis for the treatment of proximal femoral fracture. *CMC-Computers. Materials & Continua, 11*(1), 1–13.

Hwang, R. L., Lin, T. P., Liang, H. H., Yang, K. H., & Yeh, T. C. (2009). Additive model for thermal comfort generated by matrix experiment using orthogonal array. *Building and Environment, 44*, 1730–1739. doi:10.1016/j.buildenv.2008.11.009

Keyak, J. H., & Skinner, H. B. (1992). Three-dimensional finite element modeling of bone: Effects of element size. *Journal of Biomechanical Engineering-Transactions of the ASME, 14*, 483–489.

Kouvidis, G. K., Sommers, M. B., Giannoudis, P. V., Katonis, P. G., & Bottlang, M. (2009). Comparison of migration behavior between single and dual lag screw implants for intertrochanteric fracture fixation. *Journal of Orthopaedic Surgery and Research, 4*(16), 1–9.

Kubiak, E. N., Bong, M., Park, S. S., Kummer, F., Egol, K., & Koval, K. J. (2004). Intramedullary fixation of unstable intertrochanteric hip fractures. *Journal of Orthopaedic Trauma, 18*(1), 12–17. doi:10.1097/00005131-200401000-00003

Kuzmanovski, I., & Aleksovska, S. (2003). Optimization of artificial neural networks for prediction of the unit cell parameters in orthorhombic perovskites. Comparison with multiple linear regression. *Chemometrics and Intelligent Laboratory Systems, 67*, 167–174. doi:10.1016/S0169-7439(03)00092-3

Lee, D. C., & Lee, J. I. (2004). Structural optimization design for large mirror. *Optics and Lasers in Engineering, 42*, 109–117. doi:10.1016/S0143-8166(03)00079-4

Lin, J. (2006). Encouraging results of treating femoral trochanteric fractures with specially designed double screw nails. *The Journal of Trauma Injury Infection and Critical Care, 63*(4), 866–874. doi:10.1097/TA.0b013e3180342087

Lorich, D. G., Geller, D. S., & Nielson, J. H. (2004). Osteoporotic pertrochanteric hip fractures. *The Journal of Bone and Joint Surgery. American Volume, 86*, 398–410.

Marks, L. W., & Gardner, T. N. (1993). The use of strain energy as a convergence criterion in the finite element modeling of bone and the effect of model geometry on stress convergence. *Journal of Biomechanical Engineering-Transactions of the ASME, 15*, 474–476.

Michalewicz, Z. (1992). *Genetic algorithms + Data structures = Evolution programs*. Berlin, Germany: Springer.

Mitchell, M. (1996). *An introduction to genetic algorithms*. Cambridge, MA: Bradford.

Pervez, H., & Parker, M. J. (2001). Results of the long gamma nail for complex proximal femoral fractures. *Injury-International Journal of the Care of the Injured, 32*, 704–707.

Schipper, I. B., Steyerberg, E. W., & Castelein, R. M. (2004). Treatment of unstable trochanteric fractures: Randomized comparison of the gamma nail and the proximal femoral nail. *The Journal of Bone and Joint Surgery. British Volume, 86*, 86–94.

Schmid, F., Hirschen, K., Meynen, S., & Schäfer, M. (2005). An enhanced approach for shape optimization using an adaptive algorithm. *Finite Elements in Analysis and Design, 41*, 521–543. doi:10.1016/j.finel.2004.07.005

Schneider, P., Schneider, A., & Schwarz, P. (2002). A modular approach for simulation-based optimization of MEMS. *Microelectronics Journal, 33*, 29–38. doi:10.1016/S0026-2692(01)00101-X

Schöllhorn, W. I. (2004). Applications of artificial neural nets in clinical biomechanics. *Clinical Biomechanics (Bristol, Avon), 19*, 876–898. doi:10.1016/j.clinbiomech.2004.04.005

Shokrieh, M. M., & Rezaei, D. (2003). Analysis and optimization of a composite leaf spring. *Composite Structures, 60*, 317–325. doi:10.1016/S0263-8223(02)00349-5

Uysal, H., Gul, R., & Uzman, U. (2007). Optimum shape design of shell structures. *Engineering Structures, 29*, 80–87. doi:10.1016/j.engstruct.2006.04.007

Viceconti, M., Casali, M., Massari, B., Cristofolini, L., Bassini, S., & Toni, A. (1996). The 'Standardized femur program' proposal for a reference geometry to be used for the creation of finite element models of the femur. *Journal of Biomechanics*, (9): 1241. doi:10.1016/0021-9290(95)00164-6

Wang, C. J., Brown, C. J., Yettram, A. L., & Procter, P. (2000). Intramedullary femoral nails: One or two lag screws? A preliminary study. *Medical Engineering & Physics, 22*, 613–624. doi:10.1016/S1350-4533(00)00081-3

Willoughby, R. (2005). Dynamic hip screw in the management of reverse obliquity intertrochanteric neck of femur fractures. *Injury-International Journal of the Care of the Injured, 36*, 105–109.

ADDITIONAL READING

Andrisevic, N., Ejaz, K., Rios-Gutierrez, F., & Alba-Flores, R. (2005). Detection of heart murmurs using wavelet analysis and artificial neural networks. *Journal of Biomechanical Engineering-Transactions of the ASME, 127*(6), 899–904. doi:10.1115/1.2049327

Cigizoglu, H. K., & Alp, M. (2006). Generalized regression neural network in modelling river sediment yield. *Advances in Engineering Software, 37*(2), 63–68. doi:10.1016/j.advengsoft.2005.05.002

Davis, D. P., Peay, J., Good, B., Sise, M. J., Kennedy, F., & Eastman, A. B. (2008). Air medical response to traumatic brain injury: A computer learning algorithm analysis. *The Journal of Trauma Injury Infection and Critical Care, 64*(4), 889–897. doi:10.1097/TA.0b013e318148569a

Fan, S. S., Liang, Y. c., & Zahara, E. (2004). Hybrid simplex search and particle swarm optimization for the global optimization of multimodal functions. *Engineering Optimization, 36*(4), 401–418. doi:10.1080/03052150410001685521

Ghaboussi, J., Kwon, T. H., Pecknold, D. A., & Hashash, Y. M. A. (2009). Accurate intraocular pressure prediction from applanation response data using genetic algorithm and neural networks. *Journal of Biomechanics, 42*(14), 2301–2306. doi:10.1016/j.jbiomech.2009.06.020

Gharagheizi, F. (2008). QSPR studies for solubility parameter by means of genetic algorithm-based multivariate linear regression and generalized regression neural network. *Molecular Informatics, 27*(2), 165–170.

He, J., Valeo, C., Chu, A., & Neumann, N. F. (2011). Prediction of event-based stormwater runoff quantity and quality by ANNs developed using PMI-based input selection. *Journal of Hydrology (Amsterdam)*, *400*, 10–23. doi:10.1016/j.jhydrol.2011.01.024

He, S., Prempain, E., & Wu, Q. H. (2004). An improved particle swarm optimizer for mechanical design optimization problems. *Engineering Optimization*, *36*(5), 585–605. doi:10.1080/0305 2150410001704854

Hedia, H. S., & Mahmoud, N. A. (2004). Design optimization of functionally graded dental implant. *Bio-Medical Materials and Engineering*, *14*(2), 133–143.

Kwon, Y. K., & Moon, B. R. (2007). A hybrid neurogenetic approach for stock forecasting. *IEEE Transactions on Neural Networks*, *18*(3), 851–864. doi:10.1109/TNN.2007.891629

Lei, J., & Li, Y. (2009). An approaching genetic algorithm for automatic beam angle selection in IMRT planning. *Computer Methods and Programs in Biomedicine*, *93*(3), 257–265. doi:10.1016/j.cmpb.2008.10.005

Lin, C. S., Chiu, J. S., Hsieh, M. H., Mok, M. S., Li, Y. C., & Chiu, H. W. (2008). Predicting hypotensive episodes during spinal anesthesia with the application of artificial neural networks. *Computer Methods and Programs in Biomedicine*, *92*(2), 193–197. doi:10.1016/j.cmpb.2008.06.013

Mathias, J. D., Balandraud, X., & Grediac, M. (2006). Applying a genetic algorithm to the optimization of composite patches. *Computers & Structures*, *84*, 823–834. doi:10.1016/j.compstruc.2005.12.004

Muniz, A. M. S., Liu, H., Lyons, K. E., Pahwa, R., Liu, W., & Nobre, F. F. (2010). Comparison among probabilistic neural network, support vector machine and logistic regression for evaluating the effect of subthalamic stimulation in Parkinson disease on ground reaction force during gait. *Journal of Biomechanics*, *43*(4), 720–726. doi:10.1016/j.jbiomech.2009.10.018

Njubi, D. M., Wakhungu, J. W., & Badamana, M. S. (2010). Use of test-day records to predict first lactation 305-day milk yield using artificial neural network in Kenyan Holstein–Friesian dairy cows. *Tropical Animal Health and Production*, *42*, 639–644. doi:10.1007/s11250-009-9468-7

Polak, A. G. (2011). Analysis of multiple linear regression algorithms used for respiratory mechanics monitoring during artificial ventilation. *Computer Methods and Programs in Biomedicine*, *101*(2), 126–134. doi:10.1016/j.cmpb.2010.08.001

Scalabrin, G., Piazza, L., & Condosta, M. (2003). Convective cooling of supercritical carbon dioxide inside tubes: Heat transfer analysis through neural networks. *International Journal of Heat and Mass Transfer*, *46*, 4413–4425. doi:10.1016/S0017-9310(03)00256-4

Seyhan, A. T., Tayfur, G., Karakurt, M., & Tanoğlu, M. (2005). Artificial neural network (ANN) prediction of compressive strength of VARTM processed polymer composites. *Computational Materials Science*, *34*, 99–105. doi:10.1016/j.commatsci.2004.11.001

Tayfur, G., & Singh, V. P. (2006). ANN and fuzzy logic models for simulating event-based rainfall-runoff. *Journal of Hydraulic Engineering*, *132*(12), 1321–1330. doi:10.1061/(ASCE)0733-9429(2006)132:12(1321)

Tayfur, G., & Singh, V. P. (2011). Predicting mean and bankfull discharge from channel cross-sectional area by expert and regression methods. *Water Resources Management*, *25*, 1253–1267. doi:10.1007/s11269-010-9741-6

Tiryaki, B. (2008). Application of artificial neural networks for predicting the cuttability of rocks by drag tools. *Tunnelling and Underground Space Technology*, *23*, 273–280. doi:10.1016/j.tust.2007.04.008

Xu, L., Reinikainen, T., Ren, W., Wang, B. P., Han, Z., & Agonafer, D. (2004). A simulation-based multi-objective design optimization of electronic packages under thermal cycling and bending. *Microelectronics and Reliability*, *44*, 1977–1983. doi:10.1016/j.microrel.2004.04.024

Yamamura, S., Kawada, K., Takehira, R., Nishizawa, K., Katayama, S., & Hirano, M. (2004). Artificial neural network modeling to predict the plasma concentration of aminoglycosides in burn patients. *Biomedicine and Pharmacotherapy*, *58*, 239–244. doi:10.1016/j.biopha.2003.12.012

Yin, Y. G., & Ding, Y. (2009). A close to real-time prediction method of total coliform bacteria in foods based on image identification technology and artificial neural network. *Food Research International*, *42*, 191–199. doi:10.1016/j.foodres.2008.10.006

Zhang, G. P. (2003). Time series forecasting using a hybrid ARIMA and neural network model. *Neurocomputing*, *50*, 159–175. doi:10.1016/S0925-2312(01)00702-0

KEY TERMS AND DEFINITIONS

Artificial Neural Networks: A mathematical model for a learning process that is based on the concept of the biological nerve system.

Genetic Algorithm: An optimization technique or searching tool that is inspired by the evolution process in nature featuring inheritance, selection, mutation, and crossover.

Multilayer Perceptron: A fully connected network between layers in ANNs' structure that consists of one or several nodes inside each layer.

Multiple Linear Regressions: A statistical method that represents a relationship between several independent variables and one dependent variable.

Orthopedic Screw: A screw used inside the body to heal the fractures of bone.

Surrogate Model: An approximation model that can produce the result or the behavior of the inputs for a specific objective.

Taguchi Robust Design Method: This is one statistical method for the optimal design of the product or process using the benefit of "Orthogonal arrays" and "ANOVA analysis."

Chapter 10
Dashboard to Support the Decision-Making within a Chronic Disease:
A Framework for Automatic Generation of Alerts and KPIs

Leonor Teixeira
University of Aveiro / GOVCOPP / IEETA, Portugal

Vasco Saavedra
University of Aveiro, Portugal

João Pedro Simões
Accenture, Portugal

ABSTRACT

This chapter describes a monitoring system based on alerts and Key Performance Indicators (KPIs), applied in clinical context, within a chronic disease (haemophilia). This kind of disease follows the patient through his/her life, and its treatment requires an almost permanent exchange of data/information with healthcare professional (HCPs), with the information and communications technologies (ICTs) a key contribution in this process. However, most applications based on those ICTs do not allow the analysis of heterogeneous data in real-time, requiring the availability of clinicians to check the data and analyze the information to support the clinical decision process. Since time is a scarce resource in the context of healthcare providers, and information a crucial resource in the decision support process, real-time monitoring systems can help finding the right balance between those two resources, presenting the key information in an appropriate format, through alerts and KPIs. The system described in this chapter, named hemo@care_dashboard, aims to support clinical decision-making of healthcare professionals of a specific chronic disease, providing real-time information in a push-logic through alerts and KPIs, displayed on a dashboard.

DOI: 10.4018/978-1-4666-1803-9.ch010

INTRODUCTION

Currently, we have witnessed an explosion of different Information and Communication Technologies (ICTs) with the aim to help the management of clinical information and support the decision-making process. These ICTs have appeared sporadically in time and independently structured, resulting in the existence of different applications, each with its own purpose, and without any effective mechanism for their integration in the context of an institution. This fact, not only contributes to data redundancy and time spent on analysis and maintenance of data, but can also be a source of errors due to the possibility of the inconsistency of information. Usually the amount of the data contained on Health Information Systems (HISs) is very large, and consequently the process of retrieving the information necessary to answer a particular clinical question may be both difficult and time consuming. Moreover, it is no coincidence that on the top of the needs of the research in HISs are issues relating to interoperability. The need for system integration solutions in healthcare reported in the literature, not only confirms the existence of a wide variety of heterogeneous systems, but also highlights the negative impact associated with the severity of data inconsistency when used to support decision-making. Least explored in the literature are the types of applications that try to compensate the lack of availability that usually exists in healthcare providers to select and analyze the amount of scattered data by the different HISs, in order to support the clinical decision process. In the context of chronic diseases, as in haemophilia, this situation requires more attention due to the constant flow of data entry, sometimes requiring immediate analysis and interpretation by clinicians in order to take clinical action. In fact, the main mission of the clinicians is to provide healthcare and therefore it is not expected that they spend much of their available time analyzing the information needed for decision-making.

Furthermore, managing this continuously growing of clinical information within the finite amount of time available to clinicians can be difficult.

Given those two resources of extreme importance within the provision of health services (information and time), we believe that monitoring systems can help healthcare providers finding the balance between the use of those two resources, providing the relevant information in real-time, through alerts and Key Performance Indicators (KPIs), displayed in a dashboard, on a push-logic supply. This type of applications, based on dashboards, although widely used in healthcare, more specifically associated with the capture of vital signs and symptoms of chronic patients through remote monitoring devices (e.g., (Blount, *et al.*, 2007; Castro, *et al.*, 2010; Kroch, *et al.*, 2006; Rosow, Adam, Coulombe, Race, & Anderson, 2003), is still an underexplored approach in real-time monitoring of clinical data stored in different HISs.

This chapter aims to present a data monitoring system based on alerts and KPIs, applied in the chronic diseases, more specifically in haemophilia care. This application uses heterogeneous data from an integrated clinical information management system, in the haemophilia care, developed in collaboration with the *Haematology Service of Coimbra Hospital Centre* (SH_CHC) to provide a quick reading of the relevant information for decision-making through a set of alerts and KPIs displayed on a dashboard (*hemo@care_dashboard*). With this solution, it is possible to present in real-time a wide range of data in an easy format visualization to a group of professionals, contributing to an increase of the healthcare service quality.

BACKGROUND: THE IMPORTANCE OF INFORMATION IN REAL-TIME IN A CHRONIC DISEASE CARE

Since the appearance of the first HISs we witness to a constant change in the needs and requirements in the health information area, which lead to the existence of different kinds of applications. These changes are not only caused by the technology acceleration, but are also due to socioeconomic changes associated with the provision of health-care (Ball, Weaver, & Kiel, 2004). Haux (2006) refers to the existence of several factors that led to those changes, which in turn contribute to the creation of new HISs approaches to support the clinical information management process. The need for globalization was one of those factors, initially having HISs conceived to serve the local needs (at a departmental and institutional level), but nowadays, nobody thinks of the HIS development process without considering a global scope. Another important factor is the paradigm shift in the clinical information process, in which even the patient is taking an increasingly prominent role as a direct consumer of that information, also providing a great contribution with valuable feedback, that could possibly result in new data/ information.

In the scope of the clinical practice of chronic diseases, the needs for the use of ICTs in the support of the information management process is strengthened by the steady flow of data information involved in the patients monitoring process (Bodenheimer, Lorig, Holman, & Grumbach, 2002). Following this increased flow, it is also involved a greater amount of data and information processing, essential for the decision making process, in order to support the clinical responses, usually with particularities to each case. This is exactly the reality presented in most of the clinical practice of chronic diseases, like the one which led to this work – the haemophilia.

The haemophilia, in addition of being a chronic disease, is also a rare disease, and as such, quite expensive for the National Health Service (NHS) due to the cost associated with the drugs used in treatments (Coagulation Factor Concentrate - CFC). As such, an effective management of this disease involves not only the information management process, but also the coordination and management of the others associated resources. People who suffer from this type of disease are associated with a treatment regimen throughout his/her life, by intravenous administration of the CFC. For greater convenience to patients, this treatment can be done in his/her own residence, being subject to certain responsibilities. Within these responsibilities, the patients on home-treatment are required to registry a set of data, namely, the episodes that led to treatments, the administered CFC measured in a number of international units (IU), as well as the treatment evaluation and efficiency. All these data should be returned to the hospital responsible by the patient in order to be processed and analyzed by clinicians. In reality we are faced with a constant flow of data inputs, which need to be analyzed in order to generate the information required to support the decisions for future treatments.

In this scope, ICTs have made a great contribution, with several studies that show strong advantages for their use in the clinical information management and data sharing/ communication. For example, in the specific case of haemophilia, the pathology involved in this study, we highlight the works of Collins *et al.* (2003), Baker, Laurenson, Winter and Pritchard (2004), and Walker, *et al.* (2004) with empirical contributions, as well as Mondorf, *et al.* (2009) and Pattacini, Rivolta, perna, Riccardi and Tagliaferri (2009) with more practical contributions, demonstrating the advantages of using ICTs in the management process of haemophilia.

However, these type of applications, with all its merits in the storage, management and distribution of the data/information, in most cases do not allow the analysis of heterogeneous data in real-time, requiring by clinicians the availability to check the data and analyze the information to support the clinical decision process. Since time is a scarce resource in the context of healthcare providers, and information a crucial resource in the decision support process, real-time monitoring systems can help finding the right balance between those two resources, presenting the important information in an appropriate format, through alerts and KPIs. The system described in this chapter, named *hemo@care_dashboard*, aims to support clinical decision-making of healthcare professionals of a specific chronic disease, providing real-time information in push-logic through alerts and KPIs, displayed on a dashboard.

HEMO@CARE DASHBOARD: A REAL-TIME MONITORING SYSTEM BASED ON ALERTS AND KPIS

The *hemo@care_dashboard* appears as an extension of a specific Web-based application that aims to manage clinical information in haemophilia care, named *hemo@care*.

Brief Description of hemo@care and its Relationship with the hemo@care_dashboard

The *hemo@care* is a Web-based application to manage the clinical information in haemophilia care, developed to be used by haematologists, nursing staff, and patients suffering from haemophilia. It incorporates an extensive dataset, including medical information (medical history, physical examination results, laboratory data, detailed information on the primary diagnosis, symptoms and manifestations, treatments, potential complications, etc.) and non-medical information (demographic information, sociopsychological background, etc). In a nutshell, it provides healthcare professionals (HCP) the tools to manage all the essential information regarding patients' data and treatments. This application was developed in collaboration with the *Haematology Service of Coimbra Hospital Centre*, and consists of a wide range of information, providing different functionality based on a comprehensive and complex data model, aggregating three different modules: Patient Clinical Data Management

(PCDM), Treatment Data Management (TDM) and CFC Stock Data Management (CFCSDM).

- **Patient Clinical Data Management (PCDM) Module**: This module manages the patient's clinical data. Although parts of this data are available from other Information Systems (IS), it is very difficult to obtain aggregated reports to support clinical treatment analysis. Moreover, there is a large number of data related to the specifications of the haemophilia pathology that are not supported by other ISs, and are stored in paper files or in isolated ISs. This module (PCDM) aims to provide physicians with the tools to manage the patient's clinical data, also providing the means to transform the flat information records stored in other ISs in relevant information which can be aggregated in several different views.

- **Treatment Data Management (TDM) Module**: This module is responsible for the management of the patient treatment information lifecycle, which data is generated in the scope of CFC treatments. There are three actors that interact with this module: the nurse, the patient and the physician. The nurse and the patient are responsible by inserting treatments result data, respectively, in a hospital and homemade regime, including the bleeding episode associated and the CFC administrated in the scope of that treatment. The physician controls the treatment evaluation process, consulting the related information and is responsible for the insertion of the specific treatment protocol.

- **CFC Stocks Data Management (CFCSDM) Module**: In a nutshell, this module provides the tools for managing the stocks of the products used in the haemophilia treatment, specifically the CFC. This module is integrated with the TDM,

Figure 1. The hemo@care_dashboard, suported by the DB of hemo@care

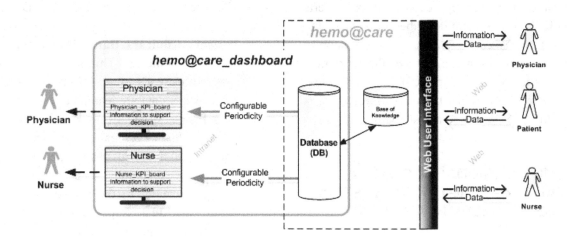

providing an automatic management of CFC products. The nurse and the patient represent the main actors that interact with this module.

The *hemo@care* isn't just a system for managing the clinical information. It includes a decision support system (DSS) based on an alert system activated by a pre-established base of knowledge. This functionality is dependent on the intrinsic behaviour of the application, which makes the system somewhat inflexible, particularly when it necessary to define new functionalities of alerts and KPIs. On the other hand, with a repository of information such extensive as the one that supports the *hemo@care* which integrates multiple channels of data entry by patients, nurses and the clinicians, motivated the need to create a complementary application in order to provide the immediate reading of data, analysis and real-time information display. Also the fact that the data of the CFCSDM are strongly dependent on the state and evolution of the data of the module TDM has contributed to the demand for monitoring those modules, in order to support the associated administrative decisions, for example, orders for new drugs. It was in this context that arise the *hemo@ care_dashboard*, a framework for presenting a

set of charts and alarms by configuration, which analyze and provides real-time information in a push-logic through alerts and KPIs, displayed on a dashboard, Figure 1.

This dashboard, although based on the database of the *hemo@care* application, was developed in order to be flexible, reusable, configurable, providing an easy way to create new alerts or KPIs, and having a great potential to monitoring real-time data on dynamic environment (constant flow of data entry), as those who normally support the clinical practice of chronic disease. The dashboard is a panel that displays information in a push-logic, on a synthesized form and preferably using charts (Marcus, 2006). According to Park, Smaltz, McFadden and Souba (2009), such a panel should appear in context and guided by knowledge, i.e. display information relevant to the decision-maker and directed to target. With a dashboard, the appropriate information is made available at the right time and place. Based on this approach, and considering that the relevant decision-makers in the context in which the *hemo@care_dashboard* was developed are the 'Physician' (with clinical decisions) and the 'nurse' (with decisions within clinical and administrative assistance), two panels were defined: *physician_ KPI_board*, to support clinical decisions for doctors and *nurse_ KPI_* *board* to support the decisions for nurses (see Figure 1). These panels were defined in order to display important information in the form of alerts and KPIs, updated with a defined frequency, event-driven, and not allowing any input interaction by the stakeholders, with the exception of the actions for recognition alerts. The aim of this solution is just to inform the state of the data in the *hemo@care* application, and any feedback through the data entry will have to be made directly in the *hemo@care*. The *hemo@care_dashboard* is viewed through a Web browser, available on the intranet of the Hospital.

hemo@care_dashboard: Content and Format

As mentioned, the *hemo@care_dashboard* presents the information in a set of alerts and KPIs. A KPI is a metric that represents a performance indicator, which can be used in order to support the decision. The KPI presentation should be, wherever possible, in a graphical format, due to its effortlessness in transmitting information. Some KPIs presented in the *hemo@care_dashboard* allow drill-down, enabling the visualization of other levels of information in a more detailed format. Table 1 presents some examples of the KPIs available on the *hemo@care_dashboard*, the type of decision that supports (clinical or administrative), the target actor (Doctor or Nurse), and a brief description of the type of the decision that supports, as well as the drill-down information, if available.

The alerts intend to notify decision-makers of exceptional situations that require attention, often pursued with a particular action. They usually appear as information, in the form of a message, with an image displaying the level of priority. The time display of the warning on the dashboard is defined according to the priority level. The top priority events require an action from the actor to disappear from the panel. Table 2 illustrates some examples of the alerts available on *hemo@*

care_dashboard, its target actor (Doctor or Nurse), the condition to appear on the panel, and the priority that should be checked and resolved.

Using the examples of KPIs and alerts defined in Table 1 and Table 2, the interfaces presented in the Figure 2 and Figure 3 represent examples of panels to the 'Doctor' and 'Nurse', respectively, appearing in the restrict place, 24 hours a day, with periodic updates at pre-determined times.

hemo@care_dashboard: Technology Overview

One of the ideas in the design of this application is to develop a technologic solution as much open and flexible as possible, in order to simplify the integration of news Alerts and KPIs, as well as to facilitate its adaptation to other domains. The *hemo@care_dashboard* was implemented using a set of open source solutions, Table 3.

Development Framework of the hemo@care_dashboard

The framework used in the development of the *hemo@care_dashboard* was the *Ext-GWT* (Slender, 2009), which is based on *GWT*. The Google Web Toolkit (GWT) is a development toolkit for building and optimizing complex browser-based applications.

GWT allows the deployment of high performance RIAs (*Rich Internet Applications*), with the same level of interactivity and performance as the desktop applications, and with the guarantee of identical running in different browsers (Cooper & Collins, 2008). The development using the GWT framework is made using the JAVA programming language, the GWT performing the conversion to Web language (HTML, JavaScript, CSS, etc.). Thus, the programmer is abstracted of the specific Web *quirks*, not being required solid knowledge of HTML, JavaScript and CSS. Moreover, given that the inconsistencies between browsers can be caused by several factors (different browsers,

Table 1. Examples of KPIs presented in hemo@care_dashboard

KPI (Target actor)	How it helps the decision process	Drill-down
• *Average Effectiveness of Treatments (Doctor)*	Provides a general overview of the average effectiveness of the treatment used by patients in a pre-defined timeline.	Display the effectiveness of treatments per patient, in the same pre-defined timeline.
• *Record of Treatment (Doctor and Nurse)*	Provides a distribution of the number of treatments per day introduced in order to detect and analyze the peaks of records, on a comparative time base.	Displays the patients who have registered treatments on a selected day.
• *Evolution of Hospital Stock of the drugs - CFC (Doctor and Nurse)*	Displays the evolution of stock levels by type of drug (CFC) in order to take timely decisions on the need for new orders.	*NA*
• *Evolution of Consumption of Drugs (Doctor and Nurse)*	Displays the level of CFC product consumption, per patient, a pre-defined timeline in order to detect abnormal situations.	Displays the distribution of consumption of a patient in the same pre-defined timeline.
• *Requested and Unanswered Aid (Doctor and Nurse)*	Displays the number of messages sent by patients and not answered by the clinician.	*NA*
• *Response Rate (Doctor)*	Displays the percentage of clinical response to messages from patients.	*NA*

Table 2. Examples of the alerts presented in hemo@care_dashboard

Alert (Actor)	Raise Condition	Priority
• *Out of Stock (Nurse)*	When a product goes out of stock.	High
• *Safety Stock (Nurse)*	When stock levels reach the safety stock defined.	Average
• *Unusable Batch (Nurse)*	When a lot is unusable for some reason (validity expiry date, poor storage, broken batch).	Low
• *Best before date Approaching (Nurse)*	When the validity of a batch is about to expire.	Average
• *Home Treatment Inserted (Doctor)*	When a patient inserts a treatment at home.	Low
• *New Mail Message (Doctor)*	When aid is requested by a patient using an email message.	High
• *Consecutive Treatments (Doctor)*	When two consecutive treatments are recorded for the same episode.	High
• *Maximum Dose reached (Doctor)*	When a single dose administration exceed 6000 IU.	High
• *Treatment without protocol (Doctor)*	When a prophylactic treatment protocol is prescribed, without the existence of the corresponding treatment record.	High

different versions of the same browser, browser specific extensions, etc.) and increase by about 25% the cost of development, this all may be easily eliminated with the use of GWT, because it generates optimized versions for the client browser specificities.

Ext-GWT, known as GXT, is a framework based on GWT developed by *ExtJS*, the company responsible for the development of a JavaScript library with the same name. As extension to GWT,

GXT adds a set o interactive *widgets*, a complete data model, cache and a simplified version of the Model-View-Controller (MVC) paradigm.

Data Binding Framework XML/JAVA

The framework Castor was used to perform the mapping between XML and Java objects. It is an open source technology that allows conversion between Java objects, XML documents and relational

Figure 2. Interface of hemo@care_dashboard to the role 'Doctor' (interface in Portuguese)

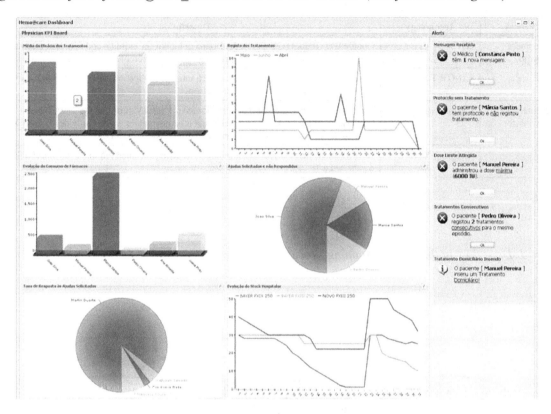

Figure 3. Interface of hemo@care_dashboard to the role 'Nurse' (interface in Portuguese)

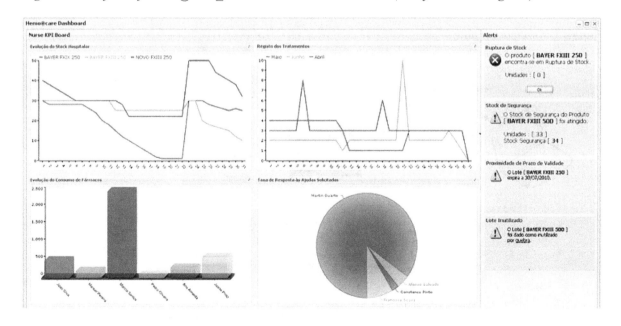

Table 3. Main technologies used in the development of the hemo@care_dashboard

Category	Technology	Description
Development Framework	**GWT**	Google Web Toolkit (GWT) is a development toolkit for building and optimizing complex browser-based applications. (http://code.google.com/webtoolkit/)
	Ext-GWT	Ext GWT is a Java library for building rich internet applications with Google Web Toolkit (GWT). (http://www.sencha.com/products/gwt/)
Data binding framework for Java	**Castor**	Castor is an Open Source data binding framework for Java[tm]. It's the shortest path between Java objects, XML documents and relational tables. Castor provides Java-to-XML binding, Java-to-SQL persistence, and more. (http://www.castor.org/)
	XSD ←→XML	An XML Schema describes the structure of an XML document. (http://www.w3schools.com/schema/)

Figure 4. Data flow in the Castor mapping process.

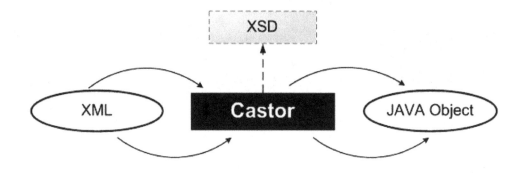

Figure 5. Application flow

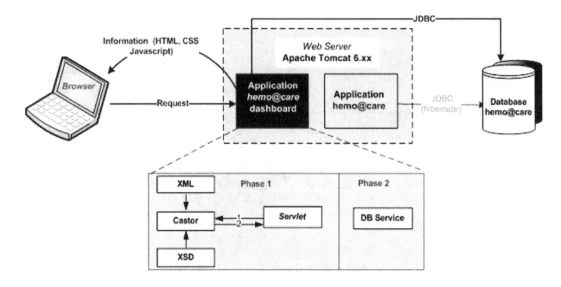

databases (RDB). For the automatic creation of Java objects is needed to define an XSD Schema, which will be used by Castor to generate the set of JAVA objects. This XSD defines the structure, as well as the elements and attributes allowed in the XML file. In the process of mapping XML to JAVA, Castor uses the XSD to validate the XML file. Once validated the generated Java object will be populated with the data in XML file, Figure 4.

hemo@care_dashboard: Process of Defining KPIs and Alerts

As mentioned, the main advantage of this application is the ease with which new KPIs and alerts can be created, just by configuring an XML file. Once configured in the file, the new KPI or alert is automatically presented in the Web-based application. This framework allows the creation and the visualization of information quickly, easily and graphically. As can be seen in the representation of Figure 5, the *hemo@care_dashboard* application runs on an Apache Tomcat Web server and is activated by a request made by the browser.

The flow of the *hemo@care_dashboard* application is divided into two steps: firstly the application is processed by a *servlet*, which reads a file with the XML configuration. The data presented in the file are interpreted by the Castor framework (and validated by the XSD Schema) and a set of Java objects are automatically generated using the existing information in the XML file. These objects transport the configuration information and are returned to the browser that made the request. The browser interprets these instructions and prepares the system interface for the presentation of a set of charts and alerts. In the second phase, each component of the dashboard (chart or warning) is responsible for performing a service request to a database that performs the query specified in the query attribute directly to the *hemo@care* database (via JDBC).

Since the system configuration allows collecting any kind of data, this service is based on meta information to perform data processing. According to Parsian (2006), the metadata describes the data properties, but not the data "*per si*", allowing to dynamically obtain the number of columns, data type, and the number of rows returned. By analyzing this meta-information, it is possible to perform data processing and build a standardized structure that is returned to the system, being automatically generated the corresponding chart or alert.

In fact, the *hemo@ care_dashboard* application works through direct queries to the *hemo@ care* database, thereby enabling the extraction off any kind of simple or aggregate information. The data collection is done using the universal *structured query language* (SQL). Configuration is done through an XML document, which defines the type of presentation (Chart or Warning), the SQL statement to obtain the data, and may also define other attributes such as positioning, co-

Table 4. Statisticsconfigurexml configuration file

'Average Effectiveness of Treatments' XML configuration	

Information type	`<chart xsi:type="BarChart" title="Média da Eficácia dos Tratamentos" style="font-size: 14px; font-family: Verdana;" background="#ffffff0" tooltip="#val#" color="#ff00ff" animateOnShow="false">`
	`<XAxis labelDegree="45" labelSize="10" labelColour="#000000" gridColor="-1" zDepth3D="5"/>`
	`<YAxis min="0" max="9" gridColor="-1"/>`
	`<barChartQueryConfig label="1" value="0"/>`

SQL statement	`<query>`
	select avg(tratamento.eficacia), paciente.nome
	from paciente, tratamento
	where paciente.pacienteid=tratamento.pacienteid
	group by paciente.nome
	`</query>`

Drill-down	`<drilldown>`
	`<subchart xsi:type="BarChart" title="#val#">`
	`<query>`
	select eficacia, to_char(datatratamento, 'YYYY/MM/DD')
	from tratamento where tratamento.paciente_nome=?
	order by to_char(datatratamento, 'YYYY/MM/DD')
	`</query>`
	`<barChartQueryConfig label="1" value="0"/>`
	`</subchart>`
	`</drilldown>`

	`</chart>`

lours, among others. Table 4 presents the snippet exemplifying the XML configuration to present the '*Average Effectiveness of Treatments*', in a bar chart widget, enabling to display, by drill-down, the effectiveness of treatments per patient, in the same pre-defined timeline.

This way it is possible to present to potential decision-makers (for example physician) the information in an easy interpretation format. The basic idea is to use images (charts) generated by the Framework as a mean to achieve greater understanding and gathering of the information that is present in the data and their relationships. It is a simple and powerful concept that has created tremendous impact on various areas of engineering, science and medicine.

CONCLUSION

This chapter described a graphical application based on alerts and KPIs, with the aim to present a set of metrics in real-time for helping the decision support in the context of a specific chronic disease. People with chronic diseases, due to having to live daily with the disease, have a greater need of interaction/communication with their healthcare providers. This kind of interaction can be easily promoted through technology platforms that ensure the constant flow of exchanges of data and information. However, most of these applications, in most cases do not allow the analysis of heterogeneous data in real-time, requiring on the part of clinicians the time and the availability to check the data and analyze the information. The importance of the information resources in the clinical context led to seek a solution of monitoring data in real-time, named *hemo@care_dashboard*. This technological solution complements the role of other application developed to manage the

clinical information in the area of haemophilia (*hemo@care*), that by the quantity of the data involved does not allow its analysis and presentation in real-time. The need for the definition of new KPIs and alerts in the context of chronic diseases contributed to the development of a potential solution that would facilitate the definition of new features, without involving too much effort for its implementation. The *hemo@care_dashboard* appears as a solution to this supposed problem, and can easily respond to the need to quickly create new KPIs and alerts through a simple setup process, allowing the analysis of a large set of heterogeneous data spread over several applications, with the presentation of the information in an suitable format, at an appropriate time for right decision-makers.

REFERENCES

Baker, R., Laurenson, L., Winter, M., & Pritchard, A. (2004). The impact of information technology on haemophilia care. *Haemophilia*, *10*(4), 41–46. doi:10.1111/j.1365-2516.2004.00995.x

Ball, M. J., Weaver, C. A., & Kiel, J. M. (2004). *Healthcare information management systems: Cases, strategies, and solutions* (3rd ed.). New York, NY: Springer.

Blount, M., Batra, V. M., Capella, A. N., Ebling, M. R., Jerome, W. F., & Martin, S. M. (2007). Remote health-care monitoring using personal care connect. *IBM Systems Journal*, *46*(1), 95–113. doi:10.1147/sj.461.0095

Bodenheimer, T., Lorig, K., Holman, H., & Grumbach, K. (2002). Patient self-management of chronic disease in primary care. *Journal of the American Medical Association*, *288*(19), 2469–2475. doi:10.1001/jama.288.19.2469

Castro, R., Kneupner, K., Vega, J., De Arcas, G., López, J. M., & Purahoo, K. (2010). Real-time remote diagnostic monitoring test-bed in JET. *Fusion Engineering and Design*, *85*(3-4), 598–602. doi:10.1016/j.fusengdes.2010.03.050

Collins, P., Bolton-Maggs, P., Stephenson, D., Jenkins, B., Loran, C., & Winter, M. (2003). Pilot study of an Internet-based electronic patient treatment record and communication systems for haemophilia, Advoy.com. *Haemophilia*, *9*(3), 285–291. doi:10.1046/j.1365-2516.2003.00747.x

Cooper, R., & Collins, C. (2008). *GWT in practice*. Manning Publications Co.

Haux, R. (2006). Health information systems - Past, present, future. *International Journal of Medical Informatics*, *75*(3-4), 268–281. doi:10.1016/j.ijmedinf.2005.08.002

Kroch, E., Vaughn, T., Koepke, M., Roman, S., Foster, D., & Sinha, S. (2006). Hospital boards and quality dashboards. *Journal of Patient Safety*, *2*(1), 10–19.

Marcus, A. (2006). Dashboards in your future. *Interaction*, *13*(1), 48–60. doi:10.1145/1109069.1109103

Mondorf, W., Siegmund, B., Mahnel, R., Richter, H., Westfeld, M., & Galler, A. (2009). Haemoassist 'TM' - A hand-held electronic patient diary for haemophilia home care. *Haemophilia*, *15*(2), 464–472. doi:10.1111/j.1365-2516.2008.01941.x

Park, K. W., Smaltz, D., McFadden, D., & Souba, W. (2009). The operating room dashboard. *Journal of Surgical Research*, *164*(2), 294-300. doi: 10.1016/j.jss.2009.09.011

Parsian, M. (2006). *JDBC metadata, MySQL, & Oracle recipes: A problem-solution approach*. Apress Academic.

Pattacini, C., Rivolta, G. F., Perna, C. D., Riccardi, F., & Tagliaferri, A. (2009). A web-based clinical record 'xl'Emofilia^{®}' for outpatients with haemophilia and allied disorders in the Region of Emilia-Romagna: Features and pilot use. *Haemophilia*, *15*(1), 150–158. doi:10.1111/j.1365-2516.2008.01921.x

Rosow, E., Adam, J., Coulombe, K., Race, K., & Anderson, R. (2003). Virtual instrumentation and real-time executive dashboards: Solutions for health care systems. *Nursing Administration Quarterly*, *27*(1), 58–76.

Slender, G. (2009). *Overview of Ext GWT and GWT*. Springer. doi:10.1007/978-1-4302-1941-5

Walker, I., Sigouin, C., Sek, J., Almonte, T., Carruthers, J., & Chan, A. (2004). Comparing hand-held computers and paper diaries for haemophilia home therapy: A randomized trial. *Haemophilia*, *10*(6), 698–704. doi:10.1111/j.1365-2516.2004.01046.x

KEY TERMS AND DEFINITIONS

Alerts: A warning to notify decision-makers of exceptional situations that require attention.

Dashboard: A panel that displays information in a push-logic, on a synthesized form.

Haemophilia: A kind of chronic and rare disease.

Hemo@care: A web-based Information System to management the clinical information in haemophilia care.

Home Therapy: A process where hemophilic patients perform treatment with coagulation-factor concentrates (CFC) in their homes.

KPI: A metric that represents a performance indicator, which can be used to support the decision.

Web-Based Application: A technological application that is accessed with a Web browser over a network such as the Internet or an Intranet.

Chapter 11
Identification of Motor Functions Based on an EEG Analysis

Aleš Belič
University of Ljubljana, Slovenia

Vito Logar
University of Ljubljana, Slovenia

ABSTRACT

A combination of several techniques is necessary for a reliable identification of activities based on EEG signals. A separation of the overlapping patterns in the EEG signals is often performed first. These separated patterns are then analysed by some artificial intelligence methods in order to identify the activity. As pattern separation and activity identification are often linked, the two processes must be tuned to a specific problem, thus losing some generality of the procedure. The complexity of the patterns in EEG signals is often too great for completely automated pattern recognition. In this case, phase demodulation was introduced as a procedure for the extraction of the phase properties of the EEG signals. These phase shifts are known to correlate with the brain activity; therefore, phase-demodulated EEG signals were used to predict the motor activity. Three studies with off-line identification of the motor activities have been performed so far. In the first study, a continuous gripping force was predicted. In the second study, index- and middle-finger activation was predicted, and in the final study, wrist movements were analysed. The presented procedure can be used for designing a continuous brain-computer interface.

DOI: 10.4018/978-1-4666-1803-9.ch011

INTRODUCTION

While several fictional films show the extensive use of brain-computer interfaces (BCIs), reality lags a long way behind. The reason is the complexity of the brain functions and their adaptive character, which keeps changing the patterns of brain activity. Several methods for measuring brain activity are nowadays used in medicine, such as functional magnetic resonance imaging (fMRI), magnetoencephalography (MEG), electroencephalography (EEG) with surface and, in special cases, with implanted electrodes. fMRI measures changes in the blood flow, while MEG and EEG measure the electric activity of the brain. All of these methods produce data that characterise certain aspects of brain activity and can be used as the basis for BCI development. However, fMRI and MEG are extremely expensive, while implanted electrodes present certain health risks. Therefore, a BCI with surface-mounted EEG electrodes seems to be the most feasible technology of the moment. Several BCI systems have been developed on the basis of EEG so far (Birbaumer et al., 1999; Wolpaw & McFarland, 2004; Taylor et al., 2002; Wessberg et al., 2000); however, their common feature is a discrete-event type of functioning. As soon as the BCI detects a certain pattern in the EEG signals, it triggers a series of pre-programmed events. The discrete-event functioning of BCIs somewhat limits their use and reduces the computer functionality. The alternative is to develop a BCI with the possibility for the continuous control of machines. Our group introduced a phase-demodulation (PD) approach that was successfully applied for the off-line identification of several motor activities in humans (Logar et al., 2008a; Logar et al., 2008b; Logar & Belič, 2011). The main problem for continuous BCI systems is represented by a reliable identification of the patterns associated with the force- and position-control functions in the brain.

In this chapter, we would like to show several aspects of EEG signals analyses, especially the necessity of combining several methods, as well as expert knowledge, in order to identify the specific patterns of the EEG signals that are associated with the position and force control of the hands.

BACKGROUND

The history of the discovery of the EEG started with Richard Caton, a Liverpool physician and medical school professor, who discovered electrical brain signals by probing the surface of the exposed brains of animals. He published his first results in 1875. Two years later, Caton reported that when he interrupted light falling on an animal's eye, he detected negative variations in the electrical activity of the brain. He also discovered that electrical activity in the brain occurred on the opposite side from the eye. Adolph Beck of Poland repeated and published his work about 15 years after Caton, in 1890. However, he went beyond Caton when he found that though a sensory stimulus, such as a sound clap, induced a response at a single point, there was also a brain-wide interruption of the slow, even pattern of the brain waves. It was not until 1949 that the reticular activating system of the brain was discovered, which had an important role in controlling the states of the brain. Hans Berger, an Austrian psychiatrist was the first to record electroencephalographs from humans. In 1897, Berger became aware of Richard Caton's work. His experiments with animals were inconclusive by 1910, but after the First World War he decided to look for the EEG in the human brain. In the early years of the 1920s Berger obtained his first results in subjects who had skulls with gaps under the skin where a piece of bone was missing. He made recordings on moving photographic paper with a wavy spot of light. This was how Berger found the regular waves at about 10 cycles per second that he named the Alpha waves. Later

Berger found that Alpha waves diminish during sleep, general anaesthesia, and cocaine stimulation. While Alzheimer's disease and multiple sclerosis altered EEG, he was rather disappointed that many illnesses including schizophrenia and aphasia showed only little or no obvious effect on the recorded EEG. He reported that the Alpha wave frequency was decreased in patients with high intra-cranial pressure resulting from injuries and found, significantly, that epileptic patients had large amplitude waves. Nowadays, EEG is a conventional technique for measuring the brain's activity and for diagnosing various nervous complaints (Yamada & Meng, 2010).

The exact genesis of EEG is still unknown; however, it is known that the brain waves originate in the cortex, because poor conductivity of the brain tissue prevents the detection of the potential and current changes to the deeper brain structures on the surface. Another problem is the voltage drop caused by the good conducting properties of the liquor, which is located between the cortex and the top of the skull. Good conducting properties of the liquor represent an almost short circuit for the currents that are generated in the brain. That is the reason why in some positions on the scalp hardly any changes of potential can be measured. One has to be aware that the EEG recordings also consist of the potentials that do not originate in the brain and are called artefacts. For example, eye-blinking or swallowing produce large signals in the EEG. For the diagnosis it is important to recognize such artefacts as they could lead to a false diagnosis. EEG has a very high temporal resolution (in the millisecond range) and can be set up with various numbers (16-128) and positioning systems of the electrodes that affect its spatial resolution; however, the spatial resolution remains relatively low due to conductivity issues associated with the underlying tissues (Nunez & Srinivasan, 2006).

The brain can be considered as a huge system of highly interconnected oscillators - groups of neurons whose membranes repeatedly polarise and depolarise, thus causing electrical currents to flow and conduct the information through the network. Groups of neurons can synchronise themselves, forming well-known brain rhythms (alpha, beta, etc.) whose properties are defined by their physico-chemical characteristics as well as by the structure of the network. The brain rhythms may be interpreted as natural (resonance, idle) rhythms of neuronal groups. External or internal stimuli cause temporal desynchronisations of the oscillators, resulting in changed patterns of the oscillations. The brain most probably operates in the mode of distributed processing; therefore, specific regions must join their efforts when solving complex tasks. The theory of binding tries to explain how different aspects of perception and action functionally integrate into the brain to form a unitary experience and action (Basar et al., 2001; Fingelkurts et al., 2005; Ivanitsky et al., 2001; von der Malsburg, 1985; von der Malsburg & Schneider, 1986; Manganoti et al., 1998; Pfurtscheller & Andrew, 1999; Schnitzler & Gross, 2005; Singer & Gray, 1995). Electrical potentials that can be measured on the scalp are the result of a cumulative electrical activity of the underlying neural networks and are detected with EEG. These EEG signals are one of the most complex signals known to man. The numerous parallel processes of the brain are perpetually reflected in the EEG signals. As all the processes cannot be completely voluntarily controlled it is never possible to measure the EEG signals of a living organism that would result from a single process. The EEG signals are also statistically non-stationary, which further complicates the problem of brain-activity identification on the basis of EEG analysis. Considering all of the above, it is clear that EEG signals are information-rich; however, the information of several sources is mixed. With the era of digitally recorded EEG, several numerical methods were applied to EEG analysis with variable rates of success. The main problems represent non-stationary properties of the signals and time-variable mixing of the information which cannot be overcome with the automatic use of signal processing methods. The brain works in feedback and feed-forward modes, which are mixed according to the history of the performed activity. Also, several activities are performed in parallel; however, their relative intensity varies with time. Currently, there is no method for the identification of the activity that could ideally filter out all the mentioned variability of the EEG signal in order to find the specific patterns associated with the observed activity. In order to separate typical patterns in EEG signals that could be associated with specific processes, a combination of several techniques is necessary. Principal component analysis (PCA) (Jackson, 1991) or, in some cases the more suitable, independent component analysis (ICA) (Hyvärinen, et al., 2001) is usually the first step in the decomposition process that should separate the superimposed patterns of the parallel processes (sources). Next, the identification of the complex patterns of EEG signals is performed with an artificial intelligence (AI) method.

IDENTIFICATION OF HAND MOVEMENTS

The identification of the motor activity from EEG signals is a complex process that is composed of several not entirely independent tasks. As the number of measured signals in the EEG was large and at least the signals of the nearby electrodes were correlated, the reduction in the number of signals was made as the first step, using PCA and ICA. The signal number reduction produces uncorrelated components that can be considered as the estimates of the source signals of the studied activity, while most of the total signal set information is retained. In the following steps the correlation between the EEG signal components and the measured activity was established. Our group introduced a phase demodulation (PD) approach

that was successfully applied in the identification of several motor activities in humans (Logar et al., 2008a; Logar et al., 2008b; Logar & Belič, 2011).

Experimental Designs

The data from three studies was used for the offline identification of motor activity. In all three studies a 32-channel EEG with a 10-20 international positioning system was used. The first study consisted of three tasks: a visuo-motor task (VM), where feedback control of the squeezing force by visual feedback was measured; a motor task (M), where open-loop squeezing was performed by test subjects in a similar manner as in the visuo-motor task; and a visual and motor task (V&M), where the open-loop motor activity was performed in combination with a distractive visual signal. Each task was divided into 20 blocks, of which the first part was active and lasted 25s and the second part was a pause that lasted 25s. Five healthy volunteers were enrolled in the study.

The second study involved the identification of yes/no answers performed by the index finger and the middle finger, respectively. In this study we used the data from three healthy, male subjects. The modified Sternberg paradigm consisted of four tasks and involved a presentation of verbal-visual and goal stimuli to the subject before and after a short retention period, respectively. The activity tasks performed were as follows: memorize-reorder (M-R), reorder (R), memorize (M) and wait (W). All four tasks required an observation of different character sets, their manipulation and a response according to the task's instruction. Randomly, after every few activity tasks, the subjects were allowed 10 seconds of relaxation. The sequence of tasks was randomly chosen by a computer. The number of repetitions of each task was approximately the same. Every task consisted of an instruction about which task had to be performed, a presentation of the character set, a start signal, a retention period, a probe question, a response and a pause. The total time of each task was 10 seconds. All the characters and their positions in the presentation set were random and chosen by a computer.

The third study was again a visuo-motor task, where wrist-movement regulation was studied with respect to the reference that was visually represented. The task required the subjects to observe a randomly generated continuous signal, representing the amplitude of the desired joystick movement on the screen and following its time-course by applying the wrist shift to the joystick as precisely as possible. Only the two dots that indicated the desired and the actual wrist-shift (joystick) were displayed to the subject during the performance of the task. The wrist shifts that needed to be applied were limited to 70% of the joystick's maximum shift to prevent any possible hardware non-linearities, while the upper frequency limit of the target signal was 0.15Hz. Each task was divided into 10 blocks, of which the first part was active and lasted 30 seconds and the second part was a pause that lasted 30 seconds. Four subjects were enrolled in the study.

Dimension-Reduction Issues for EEG Signals

When several signals that characterise different aspects of the system are measured, it is quite often that the signals are correlated. In such cases it is possible to reduce the number of signals without information loss, using PCA, ICA, or similar methods. However, non-linear relations between the EEG signals and their non-stationary character complicate the issue. The conductivity of the liquor and the adaptation of the brain activity cause complicated mixing of the source electrical signals on the scalp; therefore, it is difficult to identify the original source signals. The sources are not really located in a point of space but rather composed of relatively large areas in the brain that sometimes cooperate with each other. Also, the source localisation problem cannot be numerically,

uniquely solved; therefore, none of the techniques can provide ideal results. In our studies we tested PCA and ICA (fast ICA algorithm) for the reduction of the number of EEG signals. The PCA and ICA results for the first study motor task EEG signal analyses are shown here: first, a single 25s activity interval was analysed; next, all the 25s activity intervals were averaged and analysed; and finally, the whole duration of the signals was analysed. Figures 1 and 2 show the analysis results. The results are presented as interpolated eigenvector maps projected on to the head, using general electrode positions. Each electrode signal contributes to the component and its contribution is described by the weight, which is the eigenvector component corresponding to the specific EEG signal. The five most significant components are shown, representing approximately 95% of the total signals variability.

As can be seen in Figure 1, the first four principal components are quite similar, regardless of the analysed EEG signal interval, while the fifth components are more variable; however, there is still some resemblance among them. In Figure 2 the independent component compositions differ significantly with respect to the analysed intervals; only some vague similarity can be found in some of the components. Every run of the ICA also produced different component compositions due to its optimisation procedure. There is also an issue in the physiological interpretability of the results. The PCA results indicate that the origins of the components 1, 2, and 4 are somewhere in the central area (motor cortex), with radial (1 and 4) and tangential (2) orientations of the source dipoles, while the components 3 and 5 have a less obvious source. The ICA results cannot be interpreted in the sense of simple sources, suggesting that the independent components are still composed of signals that are emitted from several sources. While ICA is successfully being used for the muscular artefact elimination from the EEG signals, it was less efficient in our case. ICA uses the optimisation method for the generation of the

Figure 1. Interpolated normalised values of the five most significant principal components compositions (eigenvectors) from the EEG signals of the motor task when analysing one activity period (upper row), the averaged signal of all the activity periods (middle row), and the whole signal (lower row). Colour code: White – 1, Black - -1.

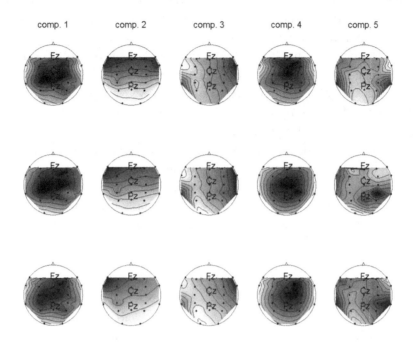

Figure 2. Interpolated, normalised values of the five most significant independent component compositions (eigenvectors) from the EEG signals of the motor task when analysing one activity period (upper row), averaged signal of all the activity periods (middle row), and the whole signal (lower row). Colour code: White – 1, Black - -1.

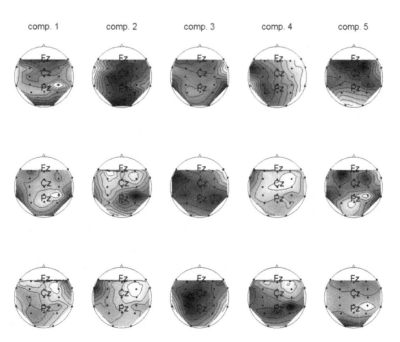

components that have unique distributions of values, and only one of them is Gaussian, while PCA assumes Gaussian distributions for all the components and separates the components on the basis of the covariance matrix of the original signals. In the case of the elimination of muscular artefacts, the muscular artefacts have different origins than the EEG signals and may also have unique distributions that separate them from the EEG sources, which is an ideal case for ICA application. In the case of the separation of EEG sources, the results would suggest that the source signals' values might have similar distributions, which suggests that PCA is a more suitable method. However, as the distributions are most likely not Gaussian, the PCA results are not optimal. Finally, the five most significant principal components were used as representative signals for the motor activity.

Modeling the EEG-Hand-Motion Relation Using Phase Demodulation

The next step is a model design of the EEG and the hand-motion relation. This requires a model that would have EEG signal components as the inputs and would calculate the parameters of the moving hand. There are several possible techniques that can be used for modelling. As it is not completely clear how the EEG signals relate to the brain activity, there are also no specific guidelines for designing a model. This would suggest a black-box model identification. As the EEG signals do not resemble the hand-motion trajectories, we can assume a highly non-linear relation. Several AI methods are available for solving this class of problems. In our case, we tested artificial neural networks (ANNs) and fuzzy models. While both types can model an arbitrary non-linear function, their ability to describe non-linear relations is not equal and some advantages of one over another can be observed. Unfortunately, there is no rule that would serve as a guideline for selecting the model type with respect to the expected relation.

The ANNs are usually capable of a better description of highly non-linear relations; however, the repeated training runs may result in significantly different non-linear hyper-surfaces. The variability depends on the training algorithm, the final goal settings, the quality and the size of the database, and the complexity of the network, and is usually rather large. Fuzzy models do not perform as well as ANNs with highly non-linear relations; however, the training procedure is deterministic, which can be an important advantage.

In the case of modeling the EEG-hand-motion relation none of the two models could model the relation, regardless of whether the raw EEG signals, the principal or independent components, the specific frequency band of the inputs or even combinations with the delayed version of the signals were used. This is a common problem associated with AI methods when the modelled relation is too complex. The AI methods use special optimisation procedures for training and complex relations in combination with an incomplete training dataset produce an objective function with several local minima that can confuse the optimisation procedure. In that case, expert knowledge that can simplify the relation is needed. The procedure involves the separation of the relation into two or more sub-models, where at least some of the sub-models are based on physical or other consistent laws. Therefore, only the completely unknown part of the relation is modelled as a black-box model, which is simpler to identify than the whole relation. We used the phase demodulation of the input components as a sub-model. The EEG signals are generated as synchronous oscillations of the underlying cortex structures from an area of approximately $1cm^2$ around each electrode. The signals are supposed to be the strongest when all the neurons in the area are synchronized; however, their synchronicity also suggests low activity. As soon as the external stimuli are received by the structure, the synchronous oscillations are disrupted. Apart from a decreased signal power, desynchronisations can also be observed in the phase characteristics of the EEG signals (Jensen, 2001). The phase demodulation thus decodes the information that can be related to the activity. The phase modulation is described by the equation:

$$y(t) = A \cdot \sin(2 \cdot \pi \cdot f + x(t)).$$

In the equation the symbols have the following meaning: $y(t)$ – the modulated sine wave, A – the amplitude of the modulated signal, f – frequency of the modulated signal (carrier frequency), and $x(t)$ – modulation signal (useful information). According to the current knowledge of the genesis of EEG signals, the EEG signals resemble the modulated sine wave $y(t)$ where the frequency is defined by the oscillatory properties of the network and represents a resonance frequency of the network. Although the network complexity would more likely suggest the multi-frequency resonance oscillations than a single frequency, this is a simplified model of the EEG generation process. The information on activity is, therefore, hidden in the modulating signal $x(t)$. In order to get to the signal, a demodulation procedure must be used. A Hilbert transform can be used for the demodulation process:

$$\hat{x}(t) = \mathrm{H}\left\{y(t)\right\} = h(t) * y(t) = \frac{1}{\pi} \int_{-\infty}^{\infty} \frac{y(\tau)}{t - \tau} \, d\tau.$$

The problem is the identification of the natural resonance frequency of the network. Since we have no method to identify the frequency, a demodulation result must be used as a measure of how well the selected frequency describes the correct value. When the selected frequency describes the real resonance oscillations $\hat{x}(t)$ has no drift. As the procedure of identifying the resonance frequency is quite time-consuming, a simplification can be used. It can be shown that high-pass filtering can produce reasonable approximations to the $\hat{x}(t)$ calculated with an ideal resonance frequency.

The non-linear relation between the phase-demodulated signals and motor activity can be described with ANNs, fuzzy models or any other general non-linear functions. The ANNs are based on neural structures of the brain and known as general non-linear approximators. Among the numerous ANN structures (Hagan et al., 1996), the feed-forward networks are simple to use and perform well as general non-linear approximators. When using ANNs, the choice of training algorithm is quite important. The Levenberg-Marquadt algorithm (Hagan et al., 1996) is currently considered as one of the most efficient algorithms for ANN training and is a modification of the Newton optimisation method. Fuzzy models (Kosko, 1994) are based on the non-exact nature of human reasoning. Hence, a persons' age is described in terms of young or old instead of numbers. However, as the fuzzy models are used to describe non-linear relations a transformation called fuzzyfication is used to transform the numerical values into the so-called linguistic or fuzzy variables. The transformation is carried out via the membership functions that describe the membership of each number to the linguistic variable. In the case of age, a 5-year-old would belong to the linguistic variable young with 100% and to the variable old with 0%, while the membership rates of ages after 20 depend on the specificity of the modelled relation. There are two general types of fuzzy models, Mamdani and Takagi-Sugeno (TS), named after their authors. The main difference between the two types is in the calculation of the model output. The Mamdani-type model requires a de-fuzzyfication of the fuzzy output functions, while the TS-type uses a linear combination of linear or some low-order polynomial functions as outputs and is thus a bit simpler to use. The main effort for training the TS fuzzy model is put on the model-input space partitioning by the fuzzy membership function. Often Gaussian functions are used as the membership functions. Their number, shape and position define the partitioning of the model-input space.

Figure 3. Signal processing scheme used for the identification of the motor activity from the EEG signals

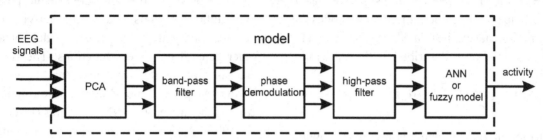

Figure 4. Measured (thick line) and predicted (thin line) gripping force of the first study, visuo-motor task in test subject 1. The training period denotes the data used for the ANN training, while in the validation periods the trained ANN was used for prediction, mse - mean squared error between the prediction and the reference signal.

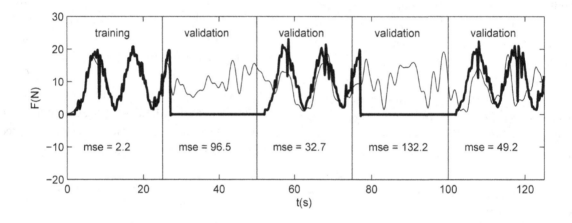

Fuzzy c-means clustering is an algorithm that tries to partition the input space in such a way that data clusters are identified; therefore, a minimum number of membership functions is needed to describe the information.

Solutions and Recommendations

Using the signal-processing scheme, as shown in Figure 3, we were able to identify the motor activities described above.

The off-line system was implemented in MAT-LAB 7.4 (The Mathworks inc., Nattick, USA), using the PCA algorithm in the Neural Networks Toolbox, 3rd-order Butterworth filters for the band-pass and high-pass filter, the phase de-

modulation was performed with the *demod* function, while the feed-forward network with the Levenberg-Marquadt training algorithm (Neural networks toolbox) or Takagi-Sugeno fuzzy model with the c-means clustering algorithm (Fuzzy toolbox) was applied as the non-linear relation estimator.

The results of the proposed scheme with an ANN as the non-linear estimator for the VM task of the first study (force estimation) are shown in Figure 4.

As can be observed in Figure 4, it is possible to train the ANN to mimic the relation; however, the quality of the prediction slowly worsens with time. To achieve the results, all the procedures shown in Figure 3 must be optimized to the problem. The best results were obtained if the PCA was performed on the whole length of the signals. The same component composition was used throughout the training and validation procedures. Only the five most significant components needed to be used. The next important issues were the cut-off frequencies of the band-pass filter. The ideal cut-off frequencies had to be set for each subject individually; however, even the general bandwidth of beta rhythms worked reasonably well for the VM tasks. The rest of the procedures were not as critical and had only a minor effect on the prediction quality. In some cases the model was able to predict the VM tasks for all subjects without additional training, suggesting relatively small inter-subject differences of the identified patterns.

For the second study, an approximately 80% accuracy of the answer predictions was achieved with the system.

In the third study, an additional frequency band had to be introduced (additional 5 inputs to the model) to obtain a similar prediction quality as for the first study. For more details on the results see Logar et al., (2008a); Logar et al., (2008b); and Logar & Belič, (2011).

FUTURE RESEARCH DIRECTIONS

The major issue is to find the transformation that would be able to find some more static features in the EEG signals related to the specific activity. Current methods are mostly developed for statistically static signals and provide results with limited temporal validity for the EEG signals analysis. To establish a long-term correlation for the predicted motion, the parameters of the process of phase-demodulation can be optimised. One possibility is to find the procedure that would demodulate the signals at different frequencies, which should decompose the EEG signal into orthogonal components, similar to a Fourier transform. As we can assume that realistic resonance oscillations are quasi-periodic signals, this would be an attempt to identify the realistic carrier wave. As the processes are most likely of a chaotic nature, this might provide the stabilising effect for the time-evolvement of the patterns in the phase-demodulated EEG signals.

In order to achieve a reliable identification of continuous motion control of the motor system the algorithms must be tested in a real-time environment as well. The ability to consciously modulate the EEG signals is one of the important mechanisms that is used for BCI development and might also be useful in continuous motion control BCI. However, it cannot be tested with an off-line signal analysis. The ability to modulate the EEG patterns could improve the long-term correlation as well as the precision of continuous BCI.

CONCLUSION

Although the results are far from useful for direct implementation in a BCI, they still indicate that a continuous interface could be possible. However, several improvements are still necessary. The separation of sources is an important problem that needs to be further investigated. As was already mentioned, the bandwidth selection of EEG signals is quite important for the quality of the prediction, and is also task related. For open-loop force-prediction experiments higher bandwidths (above beta) provided better results, while the tasks that involved feedback control (visuo-motor tasks) required beta bandwidth signals (data not shown). For a prediction of the activities that involved working-memory tasks the added theta band improved the prediction.

While both the fuzzy model and the ANNs were able to model the relation, each had its advantages and problems. The fuzzy-model identification was a deterministic process and provided consistent results; however, it was never as precise as the best ANN results. In contrast, ANN training had to be repeated even a few thousand times to obtain reasonable results, which was not practical. The choice of the model also had some effect on the selection of the ideal bandwidth, indicating that we could not separate the complex procedure into completely independent tasks.

Demodulation seems to be the most important procedure for the prediction. One reason could be that it resembles the inverse process of EEG generation; however, it also introduces some dynamical properties of the processes that generate the EEG signals, since at least two time-points of the signals are needed for the calculation. As the brain is a highly dynamic structure, the information on its dynamics, as reflected in the phase-demodulated signals, could be important for the relation identification as well.

REFERENCES

Başar, E., Schürmann, M., Demiralp, T., Başar-Eroglu, C., & Ademoglu, A. (2001). Event-related oscillations are "real brain responses" – Wavelet analysis and new strategies. *International Journal of Psychophysiology, 39*, 91–127. doi:10.1016/S0167-8760(00)00135-5

Birbaumer, N., Flor, H., Ghanayim, N., Hinterberger, T., Iverson, I., & Taub, E. (1999). A brain-controlled spelling device for the completely paralyzed. *Nature, 398,* 297–298. doi:10.1038/18581

Fingelkurts, A. A., Fingelkurts, A. A., & Kähkönen, S. (2005). Functional connectivity in the brain – Is it an elusive concept? *Neuroscience and Biobehavioral Reviews, 28,* 827–836. doi:10.1016/j.neubiorev.2004.10.009

Hagan, T. M., Demuth, H. B., & Beale, M. (1996). *Neural network design.* Boston, MA: PWS Publishing Company.

Hyvärinen, A., Karhunen, J., & Oja, E. (2001). *Independent component analysis.* New York, NY: John Wiley & Sons, inc. doi:10.1002/0471221317

Ivanitsky, A. M., Nikolaev, A. R., & Ivanitsky, G. A. (2001). Cortical connectivity during word association search. *International Journal of Psychophysiology, 42,* 35–53. doi:10.1016/S0167-8760(01)00140-4

Jackson, J. E. (1991). *A user guide to principal components.* New York, NY: John Wiley & Sons, inc.

Jensen, O. (2001). Information transfer between rythmically coupled networks: Reading the hippocampal phase code. *Neural Computation, 13,* 2743–2761. doi:10.1162/089976601317098510

Kosko, B. (1994). Fuzzy systems as universal approximators. *IEEE Transactions on Computers, 43*(11), 1329–1333. doi:10.1109/12.324566

Logar, V., & Belič, A. (2011). Brain-computer interface analysis of a dynamic visuo-motor task. *Artificial Intelligence in Medicine, 51*(1), 43–51. doi:10.1016/j.artmed.2010.10.004

Logar, V., Belič, A., Koritnik, B., Brežan, S., Zidar, J., Karba, R., & Matko, D. (2008a). Using ANNs to predict a subject's response based on EEG traces. *Neural Networks, 21*(7), 881–887. doi:10.1016/j.neunet.2008.03.012

Logar, V., Škrjanc, I., Belič, A., Brežan, S., Koritnik, B., & Zidar, J. (2008b). Identification of the phase code in an EEG during gripping-force tasks: A possible alternative approach to the development of the brain-computer interfaces. *Artificial Intelligence in Medicine, 44*(1), 41–49. doi:10.1016/j.artmed.2008.06.003

Manganotti, P., Gerloff, C., Toro, C., Katsuta, H., Sadato, N., & Zhuang, P. (1998). Task-related coherence and task-related spectral power changes during sequential finger movements. *Electroencephalography and Clinical Neurophysiology, 109,* 50–62. doi:10.1016/S0924-980X(97)00074-X

Nunez, P. L., & Srinivasan, R. (2006). *Electric fields of the brain*. New York, NY: Oxford University Press. doi:10.1093/acprof:oso/9780195050387.001.0001

Pfurtscheller, G., & Andrew, C. (1999). Event-related changes of band power and coherence: Methodology and interpretation. *Journal of Clinical Neurophysiology*, *16*, 512–519. doi:10.1097/00004691-199911000-00003

Schnitzler, A., & Gross, J. (2005). Normal and pathological oscillatory communication in the brain. *Nature Reviews. Neuroscience*, *6*, 285–296. doi:10.1038/nrn1650

Singer, W., & Gray, C. M. (1995). Visual feature integration and the temporal correlation hypothesis. *Annual Review of Neuroscience*, *18*, 555–586. doi:10.1146/annurev.ne.18.030195.003011

Taylor, D. M., Tillery, S. I. H., & Schwartz, A. B. (2002). Direct cortical control of 3D neuroprosthetic devices. *Science*, *296*, 1829–1832. doi:10.1126/science.1070291

von der Malsburg, C. (1985). Nervous structures with dynamical links. *Berichte der Bunsengeselschaft Physical Chemistry*, *89*, 703–710.

von der Malsburg, C., & Schneider, W. (1986). A neural coctail-party processor. *Biological Cybernetics*, *54*, 29–40. doi:10.1007/BF00337113

Wessberg, J., Stambaugh, C. R., Kralik, J. D., Beck, P. D., Laubach, M., & Chapin, J. K. (2000). Real-time prediction of hand trajectory by ensembles of cortical neurons in primates. *Nature*, *408*(6810), 361–365. doi:10.1038/35042582

Wolpaw, J. R., & McFarland, D. J. (2004). Control of a two-dimensional movement signal by a noninvasive brain-computer interface in humans. *Proceedings of the National Academy of Sciences of the United States of America*, *101*(51), 17849–17854. doi:10.1073/pnas.0403504101

Yamada, T., & Meng, E. (Eds.). (2010). *Practical guide for clinical neurophysiologic testing: EEG*. Philadelphia, PA: Lippincott Williams & Wilkins.

ADDITIONAL READING

Abeles, M., Bergman, H., Gat, I., Meilijson, I., Seidemann, E., Tishby, N., & Vaadia, E. (1995). Cortical activity flips among quasi-stationary states. *Neurobiology*, *92*, 8616–8620.

Buzsáki, G., & Draguhn, A. (2004). Neuronal oscillations in cortical networks. *Science*, *304*(5679), 1926–1929. doi:10.1126/science.1099745

Classen, J., Gerloff, C., Honda, M., & Hallet, M. (1998). Integrative visuomotor behaviour is associated with interregionally coherent oscilations in the human brain. *Journal of Neurophysiology*, *79*, 1567–1573.

Coenen, A. M. L. (1995). Neuronal activities underlying the electroencephalogram and evoked potentials of sleeping and waking: Implications for information processing. *Neuroscience and Biobehavioral Reviews*, *19*, 447–463. doi:10.1016/0149-7634(95)00010-C

Damasio, A. R. (1989). The brain binds entities and events by multiregional activation from convergence zones. *Neural Computation*, *1*, 123–132. doi:10.1162/neco.1989.1.1.123

del R. Millán, J., Renkens, F., Mouriño, J., & Gerstner, W. (2004). Non-invasive brain-actuated control of a mobile robot by human EEG. *IEEE Transations on Biomedical Engineering*, *51*, 1–2.

Durstewitz, D., Seamans, J. K., & Sejnowski, T. J. (2000). Neurocomputational models of working memory. *Nature Neuroscience*, *3*, 1184–1191. doi:10.1038/81460

Engel, A. K., Fries, P., & Singer, W. (2001). Dynamic predictions: Oscillations and synchrony in top-down processing. *Nature Reviews. Neuroscience*, *2*(10), 704–716. doi:10.1038/35094565

Fuster, J. (2000). Cortical dynamics of memory. *International Journal of Psychophysiology*, *35*, 155–164. doi:10.1016/S0167-8760(99)00050-1

Fuster, J.M., (1984). Behavioral electrophysiology of the prefrontal cortex. *Trends in Neurosciences*, *7*, 408–414. doi:10.1016/S0166-2236(84)80144-7

Gat, I., Tishby, N., & Abeles, M. (1997). Hidden Markov modelling of simultaneously recorded cells in the Associative cortex of behaving monkeys. *Network (Bristol, England)*, *8*(3), 297–322. doi:10.1088/0954-898X/8/3/005

Georgopoulos, A. P., Langheim, F. J. P., Leuthold, A. C., & Merkle, A. N. (2005). Magnetoencephalographic signals predict movement trajectory in space. *Experimental Brain Research*, *167*(1), 132–135. doi:10.1007/s00221-005-0028-8

Gevins, A., Smith, M. E., McEvoy, L., & Yu, D. (1997). High resolution EEG mapping of cortical activation related to working memory: Effects of task difficulty, type of processing and practice. *Cerebral Cortex*, *7*(4), 374–385. doi:10.1093/cercor/7.4.374

Goldberg, R. R. (1976). *Methods of real analysis*. New York, NY: John Wiley and Sons Inc.

Howard, M. W., Rizzuto, D. S., Caplan, J. B., Madsen, J. R., Lisman, J., & Aschenbrenner-Scheibe, R. (2003). Gamma oscillations correlate with working memory load in humans. *Cerebral Cortex*, *13*(12), 1369–1374. doi:10.1093/cercor/bhg084

Huxter, J. R., Senior, T. J., Allen, K., & Csicsvari, J. (2008). Theta phase-specific codes for two-dimensional position, trajectory and heading in the hippocampus. *Nature Neuroscience*, *11*(5), 587–594. doi:10.1038/nn.2106

Jensen, O. (2005). Reading the hippocampal code by theta phase-locking. *Trends in Cognitive Sciences*, *9*(12), 551–553. doi:10.1016/j.tics.2005.10.003

Jensen, O., & Lisman, J. E. (2005). Hippocampal sequence-encoding driven by a cortical multi-item working memory buffer. *Trends in Neurosciences*, *28*(2), 67–72. doi:10.1016/j.tins.2004.12.001

Kahana, M. J., Seelig, D., & Madsen, J. R. (2001). Theta returns. *Current Opinion in Neurobiology*, *11*, 739–744. doi:10.1016/S0959-4388(01)00278-1

Kim, J., Biggs, S. J., Srinivasan, M. A., & Nicolelis, M. A. L. (2000). Real-time prediction of hand trajectory by ensembles of cortical neurons in primates. *Nature*, *408*(6810), 361–365. doi:10.1038/35042582

Klimesch, W., Doppelmayr, M., Schimke, H., & Ripper, B. (1997). Theta synchronization and alpha desynchronization in a memory task. *International Journal of Psychophysiology*, *34*(2), 169–176. doi:10.1111/j.1469-8986.1997.tb02128.x

Kopp, F., Schroger, E., & Lipka, S. (2004). Neural networks engaged in short-term memory rehearsal are disrupted by irrelevant speech in human subjects. *Neuroscience Letters*, *354*(1), 42–45. doi:10.1016/j.neulet.2003.09.065

Kramer, M. A., Roopun, A. K., Carracedo, L. M., Traub, R. D., Whittington, M. A., & Kopell, N. J. (2008). Rhythm generation through period concatenation in rat somatosensory cortex. *PLoS Computational Biology*, *4*(9), e1000169. doi:10.1371/journal.pcbi.1000169

Latham, P. E., & Lengyel, M. (2008). Phase coding: Spikes get a boost from local fields. *Current Biology*, *18*(8), R349–R351. doi:10.1016/j.cub.2008.02.062

Lebedev, M. A., & Nicolelis, M. A. L. (2006). Brain-machine interfaces: past, present and future. *Trends in Neurosciences, 29*(9), 536–546. doi:10.1016/j.tins.2006.07.004

Lin, C. J. (1997). Siso nonlinear system identification using a fuzzy-neural hybrid system. *International Journal of Neural Systems, 8*(3), 325–337. doi:10.1142/S0129065797000331

Lisman, J. (2005). The theta/gamma discrete phase code occuring during the hippocampal phase precession may be a more general brain coding scheme. *Hippocampus, 15*(7), 913–922. doi:10.1002/hipo.20121

Mellinger, J., Schalk, G., Braun, C., Preissl, H., Rosenstiel, W., Birbaumer, N., & Kübler, A. (2007). An MEG-based brain-computer interface (BCI). *NeuroImage, 36*(3), 581–593. doi:10.1016/j.neuroimage.2007.03.019

Mormann, F., Fell, J., Axmacher, N., Weber, B., Lehnertz, K., Elger, C. E., & Fernandez, G. (2005). Phase/amplitude reset and theta-gamma interaction in the human medial temporal lobe during continuous word recognition memory task. *Hippocampus, 15*(7), 890–900. doi:10.1002/hipo.20117

Neuper, C., & Pfurtscheller, G. (2001). Event-related dynamics of cortical rhythms: Frequency specific features and functional correlates. *International Journal of Psychophysiology, 43*(1), 41–58. doi:10.1016/S0167-8760(01)00178-7

Nicolelis, M. A., Baccala, L. A., Lin, R. C., & Chapin, J. K. (1995). Sensorimotor encoding by synchronous neural ensemble activity at multiple levels of the somatosensory system. *Science, 268*(5251), 1353–1358. doi:10.1126/science.7761855

Pfurtscheller, G., Woertz, M., Supp, G., & Lopes da Silva, F. (2003). Early onset of post-movement beta electroencephalogram synchronization in the supplementary motor area during self-paced finger movement in man. *Neuroscience Letters, 339*(2), 111–114. doi:10.1016/S0304-3940(02)01479-9

Rakuša, M., Hribar, A., Koritnik, B., Belič, A., & Zidar, J. (2009) Cortical activity during reaching preparation. In B. Koritnik & D. Osredkar (Eds.), *Sinapsa Neuroscience Conference '09, Book of Abstracts* (pp. 59-60). Ljubljana, Slovenia: Sinapsa, Slovenian Neuroscience Association.

Sarnthein, J., Petsche, H., Rappelsberger, P., Shaw, G. L., & von Stein, A. (1998). Synchronization between prefrontal and posterior association cortex during human working memory. *Proceedings of the National Academy of Sciences of the United States of America, 95*(12), 7092–7096. doi:10.1073/pnas.95.12.7092

Seidemann, E., Meilijson, I., Abeles, M., Bergman, H., & Vaadia, E. (1996). Simultaneously recorded single units in the frontal cortex go through sequences of discrete and stable states in monkeys performing a delayed localization task. *The Journal of Neuroscience, 16*(2), 752–768.

Sternberg, S. (1966). High-speed scanning in human memory. *Science, 153*, 652–654. doi:10.1126/science.153.3736.652

von Stein, A., & Sarnthein, J. (2000). Different frequencies for different scales of cortical integration: From local gamma to long range alpha/theta synchronization. *International Journal of Psychophysiology, 38*(3), 301–313. doi:10.1016/S0167-8760(00)00172-0

Wang, L. X., & Mendel, J. M. (1992). Fuzzy basis functions, universal approximation, and orthogonal least-squares learning. *IEEE Transactions on Neural Networks, 3*(5), 807–814. doi:10.1109/72.159070

Whittington, M. A., Traub, R. D., Kopell, N., Ermentrout, B., & Buhl, E. H. (2000). Inhibition-based rhythms: Experimental and mathematical observations on network dynamics. *International Journal of Psychophysiology*, *38*(3), 315–336. doi:10.1016/S0167-8760(00)00173-2

Wolpaw, J. R., McFarland, D. J., Neat, G. W., & Forneris, C. A. (1991). An eeg-based brain-computer interface for cursor control. *Electroencephalography and Clinical Neurophysiology*, *78*(3), 252–259. doi:10.1016/0013-4694(91)90040-B

Ying, G. H. (1997). Necessary conditions for some typical fuzzy systems as universal approximators. *Automatica*, *33*, 1333–1338. doi:10.1016/S0005-1098(97)00026-5

KEY TERMS AND DEFINITIONS

Artificial Neural Networks (ANNs): Artificial intelligence methods for the modelling of non-linear relations derived exclusively from data. The ANN model represents an input-output relation that is described with the data. The structure of the ANN is derived from simplified neural networks of the brain, with biases and sinapse connection weights as the model parameters.

Brain Computer Interface (BCI): An interface that detects the brain activity and controls the computer actions based exclusively on the measured brain activity.

Electroencephalography (EEG): A technique for measuring electrical potentials on the scalp, usually with a large number of surface-mounted electrodes (16-128) and with different electrode-positioning systems. The EEG system consists of the EEG cap that positions the electrodes on the scalp, amplifiers that amplify the signals, and a computer system for logging and data analysis.

Fuzzy Models: An artificial intelligence method for the modelling of non-linear relations derived exclusively from data. The model structure resembles human reasoning, where numbers are first converted into fuzzy categories in a fuzzy-fication process; next, the reasoning is applied in the form of rules that apply for the relation; and finally, the reasoning result is converted into a number with a de-fuzzyfication process. The model parameters are the divisions of the input-variable space into suitable sub-spaces and the co-responding fuzzy rules.

Independent Component Analysis (ICA): A method that separates independent components from the variable set. It starts with a PCA and then optimises the eigenvector compositions to create the components with distinguishable distributions of values, while the variances of all the components are equal.

Phase Demodulation: A technique used in signal transmission for the separation of the carrier wave and the information signal if the information has been coded with a phase-modulation process.

Phase modulation: A technique for the coding of information signals in the phase characteristics of the carrier wave. The technique is used in signal transmission and enables several independent information signals to be sent through the same channel, using unique frequencies of carrier waves.

Principal Component Analysis (PCA): A method for analyzing the dimensionality of a variable set with respect to the eigenvalues of the variable set covariance matrix. The components are sorted on the basis of eigenvalues. The number of the largest eigenvalues whose sum is larger than 95% of the total eigenvalues sum estimates the dimensionality of the variable set.

Chapter 12
Visual Data Mining in Physiotherapy Using Self-Organizing Maps:
A New Approximation to the Data Analysis

Yasser Alakhdar
University of Valencia, Spain

José M. Martínez-Martínez
University of Valencia, Spain

Josep Guimerà-Tomás
University of Valencia, Spain

Pablo Escandell-Montero
University of Valencia, Spain

Josep Benitez
University of Valencia, Spain

Emilio Soria-Olivas
University of Valencia, Spain

ABSTRACT

The basis of all clinical science developments is the analysis of the data obtained from a particular problem. In recent decades, however, the capacity of computers to process data has been increasing exponentially, which has created the possibility of applying more powerful methods of data analysis. Among these methods, the multidimensional visual data mining methods are outstanding. These methods show all the variables of one particular problem on the whole allowing to the clinical specialist to extract his own conclusions. In this chapter, a neural approximation to this kind of data mining is shown by means of the valuation analysis of the knee in athletes in the pre- and post-surgery of the anterior cruciate ligament, studying variables of force and measurements at different distances of the knee.

INTRODUCTION

Clinical data provide information that enables us to establish new and better diagnoses and treatments for certain pathologies. In physical therapy the analysis of clinical data is of particular significance because of its wide range of research options in relation to patients, pathologies and their treatment, and the important number of variables that can influence the evolution of an injury and its recovery. A complete and accurate analysis of the data can contribute to the development of more effective therapies and treatments for the

DOI: 10.4018/978-1-4666-1803-9.ch012

patient. It should be noted that data in the clinical area (and specifically in physiotherapy) have a set of special characteristics compared to other kinds of data (DeMets et al., 2006):

1. The human body and its interaction with its environment is one of the most complex systems that exist. Therefore, it is logical to consider these relationships as non-linear, that is, an increase of one cause does not lead to a proportional increase of its effects.
2. There are many variables that define the evolution of an injury. We understand that the more the problem is simplified the greater the number of errors that are contained in model. Consequently, there is a non-linear problem owing to a large number of uncorrelated variables.
3. The patients' data collection sheets of a particular pathology or disease may be incomplete or contain errors of measurement.
4. The clinical data increase gradually over time, so the best models to apply are those that can take into account new data reliably.

These characteristics entail that the use of classical statistical models (multivariate regression, logistic regression, clustering algorithms) is not the most suitable given that these models do not highlight the subjectivity and the noise that, in many cases, affect these data. An alternative for the knowledge extraction from data is visual data mining. In this case a multidimensional visualization of the variables on the whole is considered (Chun et al., 2008).

In this way, the clinical specialist could extract his own conclusions with no need of learning the underlying of the models that the data specialist develops. As an example, if the results of a logistic regression are exposed, it is necessary to know what is understood by confidence intervals for the parameters, which are the initial hypothesis of the model as well as the interpretation of the model output. A visual approximation to the data

analysis avoids all these problems since the clinical specialist observes the different behaviours that include his data in a direct way.

One of the most powerful multidimensional data visualization tools is the self-organizing map, a kind of neural model, which is described in the next section. Later is shown the application of these neural networks in a physiotherapy problem showing the potential of these methods. Finally the conclusions of the work are exposed.

SELF-ORGANIZING MAPS

The Self-Organizing Map (SOM) is a neural network proposed by Teuvo Kohonen in 1984 (Kohonen, 2000; Haykin, 2008). Neurons are arranged in two layers, Figure 1: an input layer, formed by n neurons (one neuron for each input variable) and an output layer in which information is processed; this second layer is usually arranged in a two-dimensional structure.

Neurons of the output layer are characterised by a weight vector with the same dimension as the input vector. For instance, neuron i,j (i-th row, j-th column) is characterised by the weight vector $w_{ij} = \left[w_{ij}^1 \; w_{ij}^2 .... w_{ij}^n \right]$. Similar input patterns are mapped close each other in the output layer (Kohonen, 2000). Algorithm procedure can be summarized, as follows (Haykin, 2008; Kohonen, 2000:

1. Weight initialisation.
2. Choice of an input pattern
   $x = \left[x_1 \; x_2 .... x_n \right]$.
3. Measurement of the similarity between weights and inputs. If the Euclidean distance is taken into account, then the similarity measure is given by

$$d(w_{ij}, x) = \sum_{k=1}^{M} (w_{ij}^k - x_k)^2.$$

4. The most similar neuron to the input pattern is called Best Matching Unit (BMU).

Figure 1. Self-organizing map scheme

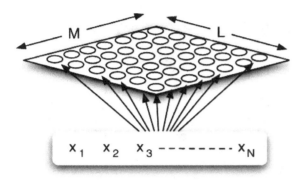

Figure 1. Self-organizing map scheme

5. Synaptic weights are updated as $w_{st} = w_{st} + \alpha \cdot h(BMU, w_{st}) \cdot (x - w_{st})$, where α(n) is the learning rate and h(n) is known as neighbourhood function. The value of this function depends on the distance between the BMU and the neuron to be updated, the closer the two neurons the higher the value of this function. Moreover, this function is the responsible of preserving the topological relationships among input patterns (Kohonen, 2000).

6. The previous steps are performed a predetermined number of iterations. When this number is reached, the learning algorithm is stopped. While the number of iterations is lower than the predetermined value, go to step 2.

The key issue of how the network works is that similar input patterns are mapped closed to each other in the output layer (Kohonen, 2000). Once the map is obtained, the visualization of the two-dimensional map provides qualitative information about how the input variables are related to each other for the data set used to obtain the map. SOM is a visualization tool rather than a clustering tool, although it is possible to obtain clusters of similar patterns from the two-dimensional map.

As an example, a synthetic problem is presented in which more than three variables are represented on the whole. A set of data has been generated containing the following variables: weight, height, body mass index, cholesterol index, and finally the fat level of the patient. By implementing this database model, we have managed to gather information from 900 patients. Once this model has been obtained, it provides us with enough information to show the following figure results:

Figure 2 is known as components' map, and it is the most powerful representation of a self-organizing map because it enables us to establish relationships among the variables of our problem. In order to work with this representation, bi-dimensional map areas are chosen to observe which values the variables in these areas take by using the colour code that appears next to each component. For example, two of these areas would be:

1. **Left-Down Corner**: In this area patients with low height (second component) and who weighs over 90 kg (first component) are located. This corresponds to a high body mass index (third component in the same area). These patients have high fat index (last component) and high cholesterol level (fourth component). Therefore, these patients are placed among high-risk patients (patients at risk).

2. **Up-Right Corner**: In this case we have placed patients who are about 1.75 meters tall but have very low weight (second component). This leads to a low body mass index and low fat index as well; therefore, these patients have low cholesterol levels.

By using this model, we observe that it is extremely easy to obtain immediate information in a relatively complex database, according to the number of variables and patterns that contains the database.

Figure 2. Components' map obtained with SOM algorithm for the synthetic problem

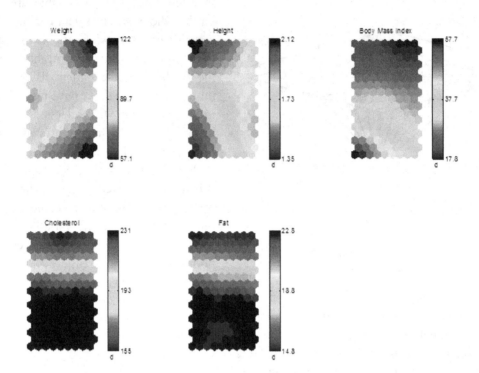

ANALYZED PROBLEM

Anterior Cruciate Ligament injury (ACL) is the most frequent lesion in the knee joint (Ageberg, 2002) and the most of torn ligaments occurs during the participation in sports activities (Gotlin and Huie, 2000). The main function of the anterior cruciate ligament is to avoid the anterior displacement of the tibia on femur. Likewise, it limits the tibial rotation and hyperextension, being considered as the first stabilizer of the knee joint in the sagittal (Imran and O'Connor, 1998). The injury risk of the ACL increases with high momentum strength that is generated when the corporal movements locate the knee joint in varus or valgus (Lloyd et al., 2005). Nevertheless, the movements that entail tibial rotation are which cause about 70% of the torn ACL.

As consequence of the torn ACL, it is produced a mechanical insufficiency that is manifested with synovial changes and arthrokinetics restrictions. A functional insufficiency also appears due to the affectation of the neuromuscular, and postural control of the propioception, and the strength of the musculature that surrounds the articulation. All the foregoing, causes static and dynamic instability that produces alterations in the movement patterns due to the deficient behaviour of the implied mechanisms, as well as due to the fear associated with an aggravation of the lesion. In short, symptoms with alterations at a biomechanical level are produced.

Among the different surgical techniques, most authors consider the intra-articular reconstruction techniques, which consist in the replacement of the injured ACL (Matsumoto and Seedhom, 1994), as the most successful for avoiding the pivot and restoring the biomechanical normality of the knee. Nowadays, the most used intra-articular reparation procedures are the autografts and allografts. At the moment the most used plasties are patellar tendon and ischiotibial. In this study the semitendinosus tendon graft was used.

After surgery, the subject must undergo a period of rehabilitation. This period is considered as important as the surgery or even more (Menetrey et al., 2008). Thus, in order to facilitate the functional recovery of the affected knee, it is crucial a monitoring, a control and an evaluation of the patient..

Accordingly, it is of vital importance to evaluate the strength levels, muscular measurements. Thus, the aim of the present work is to evaluate the efficiency of a rehabilitation protocol after an ACL reconstruction beside an ischiotibial tendon autograft. With this aim we will study the thigh contour at 5 cm representing the volume of the vastus medialis muscle, at 10 cm representing the vastus lateralis muscle, at 20 cm representing the rectus femoris. Also we will study the two-legs jump in the take off moment and the routing of the knee joint at the flexion and extension. Our goal is to check if the analysis of these variables permits to know if the recovery process has satisfied its final aim. Together with the measurements of the thigh contour and the muscle strength, in the SOM analysis it is also included the age, weight and height of each patient. Table 1 shows the mean and standard deviation of the employed variables.

RESULTS

The SOM algorithm basically depends on three parameters: kind of initialization (random or linear), neighbourhood function (Gaussian, cut gauss, bubble, Epanechnikov) and the kind of training (batch or sequential). For obtaining the best SOM it is carried out a sweep of parameters in order to train the maps with all the possible combinations. For the case of random initialization there have been carried out 100 different random initializations for every combination of the other parameters (neighbourhood function and kind

Table 1. Mean and standard deviation of the variables employed in the SOM analysis

	Mean	Standard deviation
Age (years)	28.0500	8.9647
Weight (Kg)	76.1650	9.0028
Height (cm)	174.9000	7.9067
Measurement5 (cm)	0.0027	0.0738
Measurement10 (cm)	0.0097	0.0468
Measurement20 (cm)	0.192	0.0459
Strength_Z	0.0090	0.0978
Strength_isqui	-0.8148	1.2776
Strength_quadriceps	-0.1152	0.5450

of training). The best network has been selected considering the best as the minimum topologic error. In this case the best training algorithm was batch and the best neighbourhood function was Gaussian.

Once the best map has been selected according to the minimum topologic error, the winners' map was represented in Figure 3. In this representation the number of patients that represent each neuron is shown. The hexagons totally filled black represent 3 patients, the medium filled represent 2 patients and the less filled represent 1 patients. This figure has to be used with the components' map in order to establish how many patients follow a particular behaviour.

The map has been separated in 6 different zones as Figure 1 shows. These zones have been chosen according to which zones of the map represented an interesting or particular behaviour to study.

The components' map obtained after training the algorithm is shown in Figure 4. In general terms it can be seen that the variables "measurement5" and "strength_ischio" are highly correlated, because they have a very similar behaviour since the upper left corner shows low values and the rest of the map shows high values. It is to note that, in fact, the high values in "strength_ischio"

Figure 3. Winners map of the obtained SOM

winners map

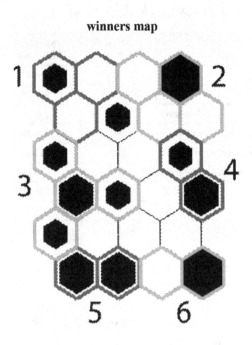

are negatives, so in this strength there was no recovery for any of the patients in the study, but it can be affirmed that the decrement is higher or lower depending on the "measurement5". However, the variable "measurement5" indicates the recovery of all the patients in the study except one. Along with this it can be observed that this two variables are inversely related to the variable "measurement10".

Below, the relationship between each of the variables in each of the selected areas of study is explained.

- **Zone 1:** In this zone there is only one patient. It has been selected as relevant zone because this pattern is far from the others (it is an outlier) and it represents an abnormal or strange behaviour. It is a medium age patient, medium weight and low height, as it can be seen on the components' map. It can be observed too that this patient has been recovered in measurements 10 and 20, in the first further, and that measure-

ment 5 has not been recovered. Regarding forces it can be observed that this patient recovers strength Z but the same does not happen in "ischio" and "quadriceps".

- **Zone 2:** In this zone, young patients and with heavy weight and height are found. It can be seen that these patients have been recovered in every measurement, being the 20 which has a lesser extent, in fact it has not incremented with respect to its initial value, it is about the same (note that the increment between the initial and final instants, that is what the SOM really represents, is about 0). Regarding the forces, it should be noted that in all of them, except in "strength_ischio", there is a noticeable increment, so not only strength has been recovered but also it has been augmented. This group of patients represents a good enough group, the best of the study, because they have reached an excellent recovery regarding strengths and measurements, except in "strength_ischio", that is not totally recovered, but it is near.

- **Zone 3:** This zone represents the older patients, medium-high weight and medium-low height. It can be observed in Figure 2 that in this zone of the map only the measurement 5 is recovered, the rest of the measurements have not recovered or this has been not significant. Regarding the forces, in all of them the increment between the initial and final instants is negative, so there is no recovery in any case. This group of patients is not very desirable because they do not have a good recovery in general terms. This fact could be closely linked to these are the most aged patients in the study.

- **Zone 4:** This zone applies to young patients, low weight and medium-high height. In this zone it can be seen that there is a recovery of the measurements 5 and 20, while the measurement 10 has not been recovered

Figure 4. Components' map obtained with SOM algorithm for the considered problem

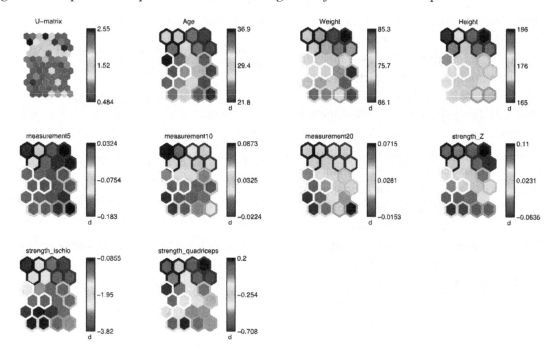

or it has a negligible recovery. Regarding forces, there is a recovery in "strengthZ" and "strength_quadriceps"; and as in all the cases of the study, "strength_ischio" has not recovered although this zone of the map represents one of the best zones of all the map in this type of force. Definitely, the recovery of the patients group belonging this zone have a positive recovery given that there is an increment in two of their forces and measurements.

- **Zone 5:** In this zone, patients of medium-high age, high weight and medium height are allocated. These patients have a very good recovery of the measurement 5 while the same does not happen for the other measurements, in which the worst values of the map are found. Regarding forces, the only one recovered is "strength_quadriceps" although "strength_ischio", that is not recovered, shows the best values of the

map. In general these patients do not have a good recovery.

- **Zone 6:** In this zone are represented the youngest patients with low weight and height. It can be observed that in these patients the measurements 5 and 20 are considerably recovered while the measurement 10 is more or less the same. Although they can recover or remain equal, which is positive, it can be observed that only the "strength_quadriceps" has augmented.

CONCLUSION

In this work visual data mining, which supposes a new approach in the massive database knowledge extraction, is presented in the physical therapy field. With this approximation the clinic expert does not need the data specialist in order to interpret those models. According with the presented visualization the clinical specialist is able to extract the data trends.

One of the most extended neural models, self-organizing maps (SOM), has as a mission the visual data mining. In those structures a correspondence between the N-dimensional input space and a bi-dimensional space, where the relationship among the variables could be visually represented, is done. Its operation is described by a synthetic example that entails the simultaneous representation of five variables for later apply it to a physiotherapy problem. In the case of thigh muscle contours, and the measuring between the different times, there were significant negative changes (decrease of the contour) on the vastus lateralis, but there is a final improvement of the overall thigh muscle contours at six months, due to the fact that a proper rehabilitation program is applied.

In this field the data gathered might provide further information about the patients and, also, help us to improve certain injuries treatment. Thus, we understand that it is necessary to consider the use of new models, which are more powerful than the others that have over a century of life and, at that time arose from the lack of computing elements to develop more powerful models.

REFERENCES

Ageberg, E. (2002). Consequences of a ligament injury on neuromuscular function and relevance to rehabilitation using the anterior cruciate ligament-injured knee as model. *Journal of Electromyography and Kinesiology*, *12*(3), 205–212. doi:10.1016/S1050-6411(02)00022-6

Arbib, M. (2002). *The handbook of brain theory and neural networks*. MIT Press.

Bishop, C. M. (1996). *Neural networks for pattern recognition*. Clarendon Press.

Bishop, C. M. (2007). *Pattern recognition and machine learning*. Springer.

Chun, C., Hurdle, W., & Unwin, A. (2008). *Handbook of data visualization*. Springer.

DeMets, D. L., Furberg, C., & Friedman, L. (2006). *Data monitoring in clinical trials: A case studies approach*. Springer. doi:10.1007/0-387-30107-0

Gotlin, R. S., & Huie, G. (2000). Anterior cruciate ligament injuries. Operative and rehabilitative options. *Physical Medicine and Rehabilitation Clinics of North America*, *11*(4), 895–928.

Haykin, S. (2008). *Neural networks and learning machines* (3rd ed.). Prentice Hall.

Imran, A., & O'Connor, J. J. (1998). Control of knee stability after ACL injury or repair: Interaction between hamstrings contraction and tibial translation. *Clinical Biomechanics (Bristol, Avon)*, *13*(3), 153–162. doi:10.1016/S0268-0033(97)00030-2

Kohonen, T. (2000). *Self-organizing maps*. Springer.

Lloyd, D. G., Buchanan, T. S., & Besier, T. F. (2005). Neuromuscular biomechanical modeling to understand knee ligament loading. *Medicine and Science in Sports and Exercise*, *37*(11), 1939–1947. doi:10.1249/01.mss.0000176676.49584.ba

Matsumoto, H., & Seedhom, B. B. (1994). Treatment of the pivot-shift intraarticular versus extraarticular or combined reconstruction procedures. A biomechanical study. *Clinical Orthopaedics and Related Research*, *299*, 298–304.

Menetrey, J., Duthon, V. B., Laumonier, T., & Fritschy, D. (2008). "Biological failure" of the anterior cruciate ligament graft. *Knee Surgery, Sports Traumatology, Arthroscopy*, *16*(3), 224–231. doi:10.1007/s00167-007-0474-x

Chapter 13
Kernel Generative Topographic Mapping of Protein Sequences

Martha-Ivón Cárdenas
Universitat Politècnica de Catalunya, Spain

Alfredo Vellido
Universitat Politècnica de Catalunya, Spain

Iván Olier
The University of Manchester, UK

Xavier Rovira
Institut de Neurociències, Universitat Autònoma de Barcelona, Spain

Jesús Giraldo
Institut de Neurociències and Unitat de Bioestadística, Universitat Autònoma de Barcelona, Spain

ABSTRACT

The world of pharmacology is becoming increasingly dependent on the advances in the fields of genomics and proteomics. The –omics sciences bring about the challenge of how to deal with the large amounts of complex data they generate from an intelligent data analysis perspective. In this chapter, the authors focus on the analysis of a specific type of proteins, the G protein-coupled receptors, which are the target for over 15% of current drugs. They describe a kernel method of the manifold learning family for the analysis of protein amino acid symbolic sequences. This method sheds light on the structure of protein subfamilies, while providing an intuitive visualization of such structure.

INTRODUCTION

It has been just over 10 years since the publication of the first draft of the human genome decoding. The detailed description of the human genome is a milestone for science in general and for medicine in particular. It has opened the doors to new approaches to the investigation of pathologies that hold the promise of the advent of truly personalized medicine. Through these doors, though, a new challenge for intelligent data analysis has also entered.

DOI: 10.4018/978-1-4666-1803-9.ch013

Over the last decade, medicine has become a data-intensive area of research. One in which new data-acquisition technologies and a wider variety of investigative goals coalesce to make it one of the most important challenges for intelligent data analysis (Lisboa *et al.*, 2004). The *-omic's* sciences have contributed the most to this data deluge, stemming from microarrays in genomics, protein chips and tissue arrays in proteomics, etc. As very explicitly reported in (Kahn, 2011): "[...] *the need to process terabytes of information has become the rigueur for many labs engaged in genomic research.*"

Arguably, drug research has contributed more to the progress of medicine during the past century than any other scientific factor (Drews, 2000). One of the main areas of drug research is related to the analysis of proteins. The function of the proteins depends directly on their 3D structure, which is embodied in their amino acid sequence. Such 3D structure is difficult to unravel, though. Alternatively, protein sequences can be the direct object of our analysis, and they are easy to acquire. The analysis of the gene-family distribution of targets by drug substance reveals that more than 50% of drugs target only four key gene families, from which almost the 30% correspond to the G protein-coupled receptors (GPCRs) family. This family regulates the function of most cells in living organisms and is the focus of the work reported in this chapter. The grouping of GPCRs into types and subtypes based on sequence analysis may significantly contribute to helping drug design and to a better understanding of the molecular processes involved in receptor signaling both in normal and pathological conditions.

The challenge of managing the complexity of these types of data invites us to go one step further than traditional statistics and resort to intelligent pattern recognition approaches. In particular, statistical pattern recognition and machine learning methods bear the potential to both scale well to large databases and to deal with non-trivial types of data. Sound statistical principles are essential

to trust the evidence base built with any computational analysis of medical data (Lisboa, 2002). Statistical machine learning methods are already establishing themselves in the more general field of bioinformatics (Baldi, 2001).

This work is specifically motivated by the need of defining a robust probabilistic method for grouping and visualizing symbolic protein sequences. As mentioned in (Schölkopf, Tsuda & Vert, 2004), there is no biologically-relevant manner of representing the symbolic sequences describing proteins using real-valued vectors. This does not preclude the possibility of assessing the similarity between such sequences. Kernel methods can be used to this purpose if understood as similarity measures.

In the following sections, we report our work on grouping and visualization of GPCR protein sequences using a kernel variant of a nonlinear model of the manifold learning family. A suitable kernel for this type of data is described. The visualization of the sequence data and the grouping results can be a useful tool in the quest for interpretability. The reported results reinforce the veracity of this statement.

FROM PROTEINS TO DRUGS

Introduction

As stated in (Overington, Al-Lazikani, & Hopkins, 2006), there is a paradox in the fact that an industry such as pharma that spends yearly more than US $50 billion on R+D, has not been able to generate enough knowledge about the set of molecular targets that are the object of its products. That is why drug target discovery has of late received much attention in different areas of biochemistry-related drug research.

Lately, drug target discovery has received much attention from different areas of biochemistry-related drug research contributing more to the progress of medicine than any other factor. This is the result of advances in chemistry, pharmacology, and the clinical sciences. Molecular biology and genomics are now at the forefront on drug research. This has been exponentially amplified by developments in information, communication, and computation technologies. Genomics, proteomics, and the bioinformatic tools that support them, can provide us with knowledge of suitable targets for medicines yet to be designed and, therefore, with a more proactive leverage on the process of drug design.

Receptors

In biochemistry, a receptor is a protein embedded in either the membrane, the cytoplasm or the nucleus of a cell, to which signalling molecules may attach. Certain types of receptors are the targets with the most number of drugs approved. Receptors play an important role in physiological functions such as mental functions: attention, learning, and memory. These functions decline in the course of natural aging and accelerated deficit of cognitive functions is a typical symptom of Alzheimer's disease. GPCRs, the biological system of the present study, are membrane receptors that modulate biochemical functions by coupling to and activating G proteins.

The idea of a receptor as a selective binding site for chemotherapeutic agents and its pharmacological characterization in almost all organs, including the brain, has provided the basis for a large number of very diverse drugs. Cell membrane receptors, largely GPCRs, constitute the largest subgroup with 45% of all targets. They represent very attractive drug targets in the quest for new medicines.

GPCRs as Pharmacological Targets

GPCRs constitute the most abundant family of membrane-bound receptors and one of the largest in the whole human genome (Pin, Galvez & Préseau, 2003). They have been the subject of a vast research effort in the pharmaceutical industry due to their ubiquity and involvement in a broad spectrum of physiological functions. Moreover, drugs do not need to have the ability to cross the cell membrane to stimulate these receptors, thus increasing the size of the drug discovery space and the possibility of success. Some examples of therapeutic indications for drugs acting on GPCRs are: antihistamines, anaesthetics, antidepressants, antipsychotics, anxiolytics, anti-ulcer, hypertension controllers, asthma, heart failure, Parkinson's, schizophrenia, migraines and cancer.

In this chapter, we focus on metabotropic glutamate receptors (mGluRs), a main GPCR class that has generated a wealth of publications over the last few years, which shows that these receptors are very attractive as a pharmacological target for innovative drugs in neurological and psychiatric disorders.

GPCRs: Structure, Function, and Classification

GPCRs consist of a single protein chain that crosses the membrane seven times (Horn *et al.*, 1998). They constitute the most abundant family of membrane receptors and one of the largest in the whole human genome (Pierce, Premont & Lefkowitz, 2002). The name is derived from their association with heterotrimeric G proteins, which have GTPase activity and act as intermediary components, activating or inhibiting several intracellular effectors. GPCRs have an extracellular amino terminus and an intracellular carboxyl terminus. The most variable structures among the family of GPCRs are the carboxyl terminus, the intracellular loops and the amino terminus.

GPCRs were discovered in 1970 by Martin Robdell, who determined the link between the activity of glucagon peptide and a molecule called guanosine triphosphate (GTP). At the same time, Alfred G. Gilman corroborated these results by finding the same trend in adrenergic receptors. The molecule responsible for the signal transduction was called G-protein (Gilman, 1987). These discoveries allowed both researchers to share the Nobel Prize in 1994.

The great importance of the GPCR family comes from its ubiquity in terms of location and function. Nearly a thousand GPCRs exist, mediating a host of molecular physiological functions by serving as receptors for hormones, neurotransmitters, cytokines, lipids, small molecules, and various sensory signals (such as light and odors), to name a few. Their stimulation leads to activation of specific G-proteins that transduce extracellular mediator messages to specific intracellular signalling pathways.

All GPCRs share a common general protein structure. The seven transmembrane helices are connected between them by three intracellular and three extracellular loops with varying lengths for each receptor subtype.

The heptahelical transmembrane domain is largely hydrophobic, whereas the extracellular and intracellular segments, or loops, are generally hydrophilic. According to GPCR database (Horn *et al.*, 1998), the principal GPCR classes are:

- **Class A:** Rhodopsin-like receptors
- **Class B:** Secretin receptors
- **Class C:** Metabotropic glutamate/pheromone receptors
- **Class D:** Fungal mating pheromone receptors
- **Class E:** Cyclic AMP receptors
- **Class F:** The "Frizzled/Smoothened" receptors

mGluRs (GPCRs Class C) Offer New Possibilities for Drug Discovery

The mGlu receptors are activated by glutamate, the major excitatory neurotransmitter in the central nervous system (CNS), and play important roles in regulating cell excitability and synaptic transmission. The mGlu receptors are widely distributed throughout the CNS, and a whole range of neuro-

logical and psychiatric disorders might be treated using drugs that act directly on these receptors. There are eight types of mGlu receptors (8 genes encoding for mGlu1 to mGlu8 in human) divided into three groups based on structure, pharmacology and mechanism of signal transduction (Rondard, Goudet, Kniazeff, Pin & Prézeau, 2011).

This chapter pays special attention to mGluRs, which play central roles in regulating synaptic transmission and represent relevant therapeutic targets for a number of neurological and psychiatric diseases. Class-C GPCRs have become an increasingly important target class for new therapies, particularly in areas such as pain, anxiety, neurodegenerative disorders and as antispasmodics, but also potentially for the treatment of hyperthyroidism and osteoporosis. Both positive and negative allosteric modulators have been identified against many targets in this class and can be particularly therapeutically active because they tend to be highly selective towards the targeted receptors.

Furthermore, they often have useful attributes such as the ability to cross the blood brain barrier whilst having fewer side effects than agonists. In contrast to other GPCRs classes, class C receptors are composed of three main structural domains, not including the C-terminal tail which can be very long and where a multitude of intracellular scaffolding and signalling molecules bind. These domains are the Venus flytrap domain (VFT), which contains the agonist binding site, the cysteine-rich domain (CRD) and the heptahelical domain (HD) involved in G-protein activation. Class C GPCRs have been shown to be constitutive dimers and therefore represent a good model for studying the functional relevance of GPCR dimerization.

Thanks to their modular structure, it has been possible to clearly identify two distinct domains, one containing the orthosteric site (the VFT module) and the other the allosteric site (the heptahelical domain). This offers several new possibilities to identify drugs able to modulate the activity of these receptors.

The Amino Acid Sequence Provides Fundamental Information of the Structure and Function of the Protein

The function of the proteins depends directly on their 3D structure, which is embodied in their amino acid sequence. GPCRs are membrane proteins, and this environment makes their 3D structure difficult to unravel through nuclear magnetic resonance or X-ray crystallography. Knowledge about the three-dimensional structure of a GPCR is crucial for the understanding of its function and for the design of drugs. Modern molecular biology methods, though, make their sequences easy to acquire. The grouping of GPCRs into types and subtypes based on sequence analysis may significantly contribute to helping drug design and to a better understanding of the molecular processes involved in receptor signalling both in normal and pathological conditions (Cobanoglu, Saygin & Sezerman, 2010).

Due to the lack of high resolution structural data, theoretical research on GPCRs relies on the availability and easy accessibility of all available data in an information system that allows for the four basic data dissemination functions: browsing, retrieval, querying and inference.

ANALYZING PROTEIN SEQUENCES USING KERNEL METHODS

Protein Classification: Comparisons between Amino Acid Sequences

The grouping of GPCRs into types and subtypes based on sequence analysis may significantly contribute to helping drug design and to a better understanding of the molecular processes involved in receptor signalling both in normal and pathological conditions (Cobanoglu, Saygin & Sezerman, 2010). Fortunately, the importance of the GPCR as physiological agents and drug targets more than justifies our efforts in addressing this challenge.

In order to group GPCR sequences, we need a measure of similarity between them. Pattern recognition and machine learning techniques can help us in this task. Unsupervised data analysis using clustering algorithms provides a useful tool to explore data structures. Broadly speaking, the aim of clustering methods is to group patterns on the basis of similarity (or dissimilarity) criteria where groups or clusters are set of similar patterns. Unsupervised methods that were capable of providing simultaneous grouping and visualization of sequence data would be especially adequate for the problem at hand, as visualization can help us to intuitively interpreting the grouping and classification results. The visualization of the high-dimensional GPCR sequences would indeed considerably help understanding their global grouping structure. In the following sections, we provide details on one such method.

Kernel Generative Topographic Mapping

The Generative Topographic Mapping (GTM) (Bishop, Svensén & Williams, 1998) is a nonlinear latent variable model of the manifold learning family, with sound foundations in probability theory. It could be understood as a probabilistic counterpart to the well-known Self-Organizing Maps (SOM) (Kohonen, 2001). It performs simultaneous vector quantization and visualization of the observed data, through a nonlinear and topology-preserving mapping from a visualization latent space in $\Re^L$ (with L being usually 1 or 2 for visualization purposes) onto the $\Re^D$ space in which the observed data reside. The mapping that generates the embedded manifold takes the form:

$$y = W\phi(u) \qquad (1)$$

where u is an L-dimensional point in latent space, W is the matrix that generates the mapping, and ϕ consists of S basis functions (radially symmetric Gaussians in the standard model for continuous data).

199

To achieve computational tractability, the prior distribution of u in latent space is constrained to form a uniform discrete grid of M centers, analogous to the layout of the SOM units, in the form:

$$p(u) = \frac{1}{M} \sum_{i=1}^{M} \delta(u - u_i) \qquad (2)$$

where M is the number of nodes in the grid.

Since the data do not necessarily lie in an L-dimensional space, it is necessary to make use of a noise model for the distribution of the data points x. The integration of this data distribution over the latent space distribution, gives Equation 3 in Box 1, where D is the dimensionality of the data space, and $m_i = W\varphi(u_i)$ for the discrete node representation (2), according to expression (1). Using the SOM terminology, m_i can be considered as reference vectors, each of them the centre of an isotropic Gaussian distribution in data space (Bishop, Svensén & Williams, 1998). A log-likelihood can now be defined as:

$$L(W, \beta) = \sum_{n=1}^{N} \ln \ p(x^n \mid W, \beta) \qquad (4)$$

for the whole input data set x_n. The distribution (3) corresponds to a constrained Gaussian mixture model, hence its parameters can be determined using the Expectation-Maximization (EM) algorithm (Dempster, Laird & Rubin, 1977), details of which can be found in (Bishop, Svensén & Williams, 1998b). As part of the Expectation step, the mapping from latent space to data space,

defined by (1), can be inverted using Bayes theorem so that the posterior probability of a GTM latent space node i, given a data-space point x_n, can be calculated. We can also add a regularization term to control model complexity, so that the log-likelihood becomes:

$$L'(W, \beta) = \sum_{n=1}^{N} \left\{ \ln \ p(x^n \mid W, \beta) \right\} + \frac{\alpha}{2} \|w\|^2 \qquad (5)$$

where w is a vector shaped by concatenation of the different column vectors of the weight matrix W and α is a regularization coefficient. This regularization term is effectively preventing the GTM to fit the noise in the data and is used under the assumption that there exists an underlying data generator which is a combination of the density functions for each of the segments.

The optimum values for all these complexity-controlling parameters should ideally be evaluated in a continuous space of solutions. Given that the GTM is formulated within a probabilistic framework, this can be accomplished using the Bayesian formalism and, more specifically, the evidence approximation (Mackay, 1992). The application of this methodology produces update formulae for the regularization coefficient α and for the inverse variance of the noise model β (Olier, Vellido & Giraldo, 2010). Once the parameters α and β have been adaptively optimized, the best GTM model (in the sense that it reaches the best compromise between fitting the data and representing the underlying distribution from which the data were generated) can be obtained by experimenting with different combina-

Box 1.

$$p(x \mid W, \beta) = \int p(x \mid u, W, \beta) \, p(u) = \frac{1}{M} \sum_{i=1}^{M} \left(\frac{\beta}{2\pi} \right)^{\frac{D}{2}} \exp \left\{ -\frac{\beta}{2} \|m_i - x\|^2 \right\} \qquad (3)$$

tions of the number of Gaussian basis functions and its width, σ.

The main advantage of the GTM over the SOM model is that the former generates a density distribution in the input data space so that the model can be described and developed within a principled probabilistic framework. An example of development of the GTM is the use of a Bayesian approach to automatic regularization and smoothing of the resulting mapping. As part of this process, the GTM learning parameters calculation is grounded in a sound theoretical basis. The GTM also provides the well-defined objective function (4), whereas the SOM training does not involve the minimization of any error function; its maximization using either standard techniques for non-linear optimization or the EM-algorithm has been proved to converge, unlike in the case of the SOM.

Let's consider the problem of embedding GPCR sequences in a high-dimensional space in such a way that their relative distance in that space reflects their similarity and that the inner product between their images can be computed efficiently. The first decision to be made is what similarity notion should be reflected in the embedding, or in other words what features of the sequences are informative for the task at hand. Are we trying to group sequences by length, composition, or some other properties? What type of patterns are we looking for? (Shawe-Taylor & Cristianini, 2004).

The meaning of similarity in biological applications is related to both functional similarity and sequence similarity, measured by the number of insertions, deletions and symbol replacements. Measuring sequence similarity should therefore give a good indication about the functional similarity that bioinformatics researchers would like to capture.

A kernel function can be thought of as a measure of similarity between sequences. Different kernels correspond to different notions of similarity, and can lead to discriminative functions with different performance. Kernelization is a method

originally defined for Support Vector Machines (SVM), which could be used to develop generalizations of any algorithm that could be cast in dot product terms.

Kernels have been developed to compute the inner product between images of strings in high-dimensional feature spaces using dynamic programming techniques. Any kernel methods solution comprises two parts: a module that performs the mapping into the embedding or feature space and a learning algorithm designed to discover linear patterns in that space.

A method formulated in terms of kernels can use the one that best suits the problem and data type at hand. Probably the most important data type after vectors and free text is that of symbol strings of varying lengths. This type of data is commonplace in bioinformatics applications, where it can be used to represent proteins as sequences of amino acids, genomic DNA as sequences of nucleotides, promoters and other structures.

With this purpose, the kernel-GTM (KGTM) was recently defined (Olier, Vellido & Giraldo, 2010). It takes advantage of the original GTM functionalities to achieve vector quantization and visualization of a wider variety of data types. KGTM also builds on previously described similar models such as Kernel PCA (KPCA) (Schölkopf, Smola & Müller, 1997) and Kernel SOM (KSOM) KPCA is the application of Principal Component Analysis in a kernel-defined feature space, making use of the dual representation. This method makes possible to detect nonlinear relations between variables in the data by embedding the data into a kernel-induced feature space, where linear relations can be found by means of PCA. Also, KPCA can be seen as a way of inferring a low-dimensional explicit geometric feature space that best captures the structure of the data. KPCA provides a method according to which we can visualize GPCR sequences in a representation space (e.g. spanning only two PCs) but, unfortunately, this visualization through projection is not accompanied by a grouping of the sequences through vector quantization. This limitation is overcome by recently defined kernel versions of the SOM vector quantization technique (Andras, 2002; MacDonald & Fyfe, 2000). KSOM can be understood as a kernelization of the k-means clustering algorithm, but with added neighbourhood learning. Although KSOM makes the standard Kohonen map much more flexible, it still inherits the limitations of SOM outlined above.

The kernel trick allows the observed data X to be implicitly mapped into a high-dimensional feature space H via a nonlinear function: $x \rightarrow \psi(x)$. A similarity measure can then be defined from the dot product in space H as follows:

$$K\left(x, x'\right) = \left\langle \psi\left(x\right), \psi\left(x'\right) \right\rangle \tag{6}$$

K is a kernel function that should satisfy Mercer's condition (Schölkopf & Smola, 2002). It allows us to deal with learning algorithms using linear algebra and analytic geometry. In general, this method deals with data in the high-dimensional dot product space H, usually known as feature space. This use of the feature space avoids expensive computation costs by employing the kernel function K instead of directly computing the dot product in H, so we don't need to know explicitly the mapping ψ.

The kernelization of GTM can be implemented by redefining equation (3) in feature space as

$$p(\psi(x) \mid u_m, \Theta) = \left(\frac{\beta}{2\pi}\right)^{\frac{D}{2}} \exp\left\{-\frac{\beta}{2}\left\|\psi(x) - y_m\right\|^2\right\} \tag{7}$$

Note that the prototypes y_m are now defined in the feature space and not in data space, as originally. Consequently, D is now the dimension of the feature space, which is usually unknown. In most cases, the term $\left\|\psi(x) - y_m\right\|^2$ cannot be directly evaluated, given that the function $\psi(\cdot)$ is usually unknown. However, this term can be also expressed as follows:

$$\left\|\psi(x) - y_m\right\|^2 = \left\langle \psi(x), \psi(x) \right\rangle + \left\langle y_m, y_m \right\rangle - 2\left\langle \psi(x), y_m \right\rangle \tag{8}$$

Here, we assume that, as in KPCA, y_m can be expanded on the training data in the feature space. That is, $y_m = \Psi w_m$, where Ψ is a $D \times N$-matrix of vector columns $\Psi\left(x_n\right)$, $n = 1..N$, and w_m a weight vector. With the aim of preserving the topology, we correlate the weight vector to the latent space by $w_m = \Lambda \varphi_m$, where Λ is an adaptive weight matrix and $\varphi_m = \varphi\left(u_m\right)$ is the set of radial basis functions typically used by GTM. Therefore, Equation (8) becomes:

$$\left\|\psi(x_n) - y_m\right\|^2 = K_{nn} + \left(\Lambda \varphi_m\right)^T K \Lambda \varphi_m - 2k_n \Lambda \varphi_m \tag{9}$$

where K is a kernel matrix with elements $K_{nn}' = \left\langle \psi\left(x_n\right), \psi\left(x_{n'}\right) \right\rangle$, and row vectors k_n. Thereby J_{mn} is expressed in terms of the kernel matrix, making the definition of function $\psi(.)$ unnecessary. The adaptive parameters of the model are now Λ and β, which can be optimized by ML using EM, as in GTM. The likelihood of the model is formulated as follows:

$$L\left(\Lambda, \beta\right) = \prod_{n=1}^{N} \frac{1}{M} \sum_{m=1}^{M} p\left(\psi\left(x_n\right) \mid u_m, \Lambda, \beta\right) \tag{10}$$

Following the usual EM algorithm, we are specially interested in one of the results of the expectation step of EM, namely the estimation of the posterior distribution $R_{mn} = p\left(u_m \mid \psi\left(x_n\right), \Lambda, \beta\right)$, defined as:

$$R_{mn} = \frac{p\left(\psi\left(x_n\right)\middle|\ u_m, \Lambda, \beta\right)}{\sum_{m'=1}^{M} p\left(\psi\left(x_n\right)\middle|\ u_{m'}, \Lambda, \beta\right)} \qquad (11)$$

R_{mn} measures the degree of responsibility (probability) of a point u_m in the latent space for the generation of a $\psi\left(x_n\right)$ GPCR data subsequence. In turn, each R_{mn} is an element of a $M \times N$ responsibility matrix R.

In the maximization step we use Equation (10) as the optimization function to determine the parameters Λ and β, which results in the following expressions:

$$\Lambda^T = \left(\Phi^T G \Phi\right)^{-1} \Phi^T R \qquad (12)$$

$$\frac{1}{\beta} = \frac{1}{ND} \sum_{n=1}^{N} \sum_{m=1}^{M} R_{mn} J_{mn} \qquad (13)$$

Starting with a random initialization of these parameters, steps E and M of EM are sequentially repeated until convergence of the likelihood function is reached.

RESULTS

The dataset analyzed with the KGTM algorithm consists of 232 protein sequences obtained from GPCRDB (Horn *et al.*, 1998), corresponding to family C. Each position in a sequence is called a residue, which in turn may be one of 20 possible amino acids. Each amino acid has a standard one-letter code, and a sequence is therefore represented by a combination of these letters. The number of residues by sequence in the dataset is 253 (data dimensionality). In our experiments, we built the kernel function as a quantitative measure of similarity between two GPCR sequences.

The kernel function designed to analyze such data with KGTM is a variation on that in (Olier,

Vellido & Giraldo, 2010), based on the mutations and gaps between sequences:

$$K\left(x, x'\right) = \exp\left\{\nu \frac{\pi\left(x, x'\right)}{\sqrt{\pi\left(x, x\right)\pi\left(x', x'\right)}}\right\} \qquad (14)$$

where x and x' are two sequences and ν is a prefixed parameter; $\pi\left(.\right)$ is a score function commonly used in bioinformatics and expressed as: $\pi\left(x, x'\right) = \sum_r s\left(x_r, x_r'\right) - \gamma$, where x_r and x_r' are the rth residue in the sequences. The value of $s\left(x_r, x_r'\right)$ can be found in a mutation matrix (Durbin, Eddy, Krogh & Mitchison, 2004) and is a gap penalty (usually the number of gaps in sequences). A normalization factor, defined as the geometric mean of the maximum scores for each of the sequences, is used in the kernel function instead of the sum of them as used in (Olier, Vellido & Giraldo, 2010). Results are expected to remain almost invariant using either of both kernel functions, former and new one. Nevertheless, the modified kernel function has a proper delimitation of its range.

The KGTM does not use the labels of types and subtypes, even if known, as part of model generation, because it is an unsupervised model. Labelling is accomplished *a posteriori*, in order to assess the visualization of the sequences.

The basic visualization results with KGTM are shown in Figure 1. Seven subtypes of class C have been modelled. There is a quite clear separation between many of the GPCR subtypes, which are visualized in the latent space using the mode-projection, defined as: $m_{mode} = \arg\max_m R_{mn}$

Many subtypes occupy a rather differentiated area on the map, showing little overlapping. A few of them, though, have overlapping representations. Both cases could be the source of insight on the peculiarities of subtype structure. Metabotropic glutamate (subtype 1), GABA-B (3), and

Figure 1. Data visualization on a 10 × 10 representation map using the mode- projection as described in the text. Left) Pie charts represent latent points and their size is proportional to the ratio of sequences assigned to them. Each portion of a chart corresponds to the percentage of sequences belonging to each subtype. Right) The same map without sequence ratio size scaling, for better visualization. Labels: 1: Metabotropic glutamate, 2: Calcium sensing, 3: GABA-B, 4: Vomeronasal, 5: Pheromone, 6: Odorant, 7: Taste.

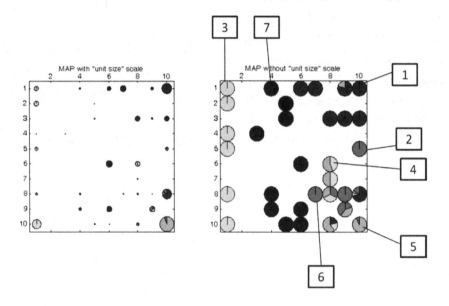

Figure 2. CR_c representation maps for all GPCR class C subtypes. Labels: 1: Metabotropic glutamate, 2: Calcium sensing, 3: GABA-B, 4: Vomeronasal, 5: Pheromone, 6: Odorant, 7: Taste. Subtype 1 (Metabotropic glutamate), the most populated, is well-defined on the top-right corner of the map; subtype 3 (GABA-B), also isolated and unmixed in the left hand-side of the map; subtype 5 (Pheromone), strongly focused on the bottom right corner of the map, but partially overlapping with right: subtype 6 (Odorant). The layout corresponds to that of Figure3 although with its viewpoint slightly displaced to the left, to provide some perspective.

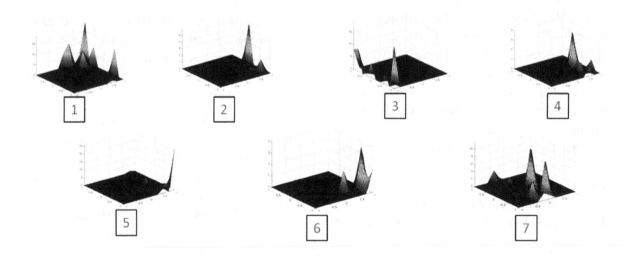

Figure 3. Visualization of the global CR (on the vertical axis) of the data set in the representation map. Layout as in Figure 2

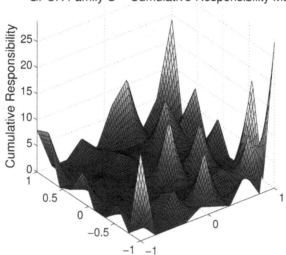

GPCR Family C – Cumulative Responsibility Map

Taste (7) are clearly differentiated from the rest of subtypes, which show significant overlapping between them.

The mode-projection is an intuitive form of visualization that sacrifices detail in favour of clarity. By using only the maximum of the responsibilities in R, though, it disposes of much of the rich information that might be contained in this matrix of probabilities. There are different ways of visually representing this information. One of them is the display of maps of probability R_i, for a given sequence i. Sequences clearly ascribed to a subtype are likely to have their responsibilities concentrated in only a few modes (latent points), whereas the probabilities of sequences without clear subtype ascription may be more evenly spread across the map. We may be also interested in the responsibilities of all sequences of a given subtype at once. In this case, we would aim to assess if each subtype has its responsibilities located in a well-defined area of the map or not. The cumulative responsibility of the sequences that belong to a given subtype c

is defined as a vector $CR_c = \sum_{\{n \in c\}} R_{mn}$, for $m = \{1, ..., M\}$. Figure 2 provides the visualization of the CR_c for all subtypes of the C family.

This takes us to the possibility of displaying the cumulative responsibility of all sequences in the database, defined as vector. With this map of probability, the existence of CR peaks and valleys can be explored. The latter are likely to define the boundaries between subtypes. The global CR is displayed in Figure 3. Consistent with the subtype specific representations in Figure 2, several local maxima are shown to correspond to each subtype, which could be an indication of heterogeneity within the subtypes. Some deep valleys of probability can be seen in the central parts of the map, drawing clear boundaries between subtypes represented in the periphery of the map and those around its center. Some amongst the latter are the ones with a higher level of mixing and would merit further investigation.

Our results are consistent with early classification studies using other techniques such as Hidden

Figure 4. Mode projection of the type 1 mGlu subtypes. Labels: 1: mGluR1, 2: mGluR2, 3: mGluR3, 4: mGluR4, 5: mGluR5, 6: mGluR6, 8: mGluR8, 9: Like. Our dataset has no mGluR7 subtypes. Also, there is a visible separation of the subtypes in three main groups, according to the amino acid sequence similarity, agonist pharmacology and the signal transduction pathways to which they couple: group I (mGluR1, mGluR5), group II (mGluR2, mGluR3, Like) and group III (mGluR4, mGluR6, mGluR8)

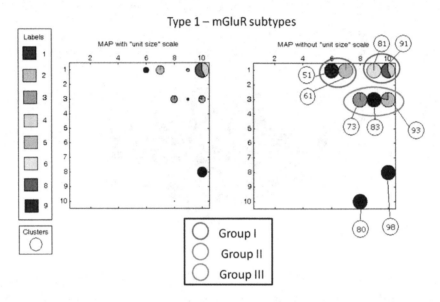

Figure 5. General KGTM visualization of mGluRs types and the type 1 mGluRs subtypes

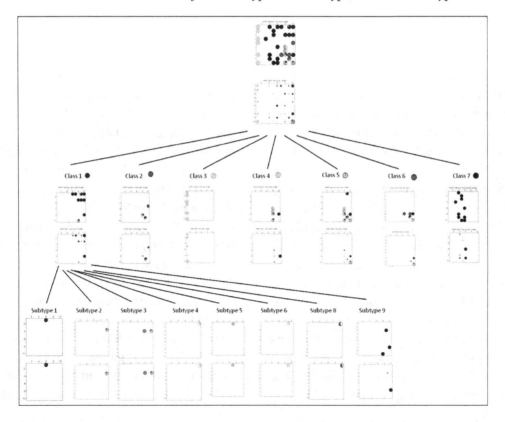

Markov Models, thereby validating the present methodology. Importantly, the method herein presented reveals mixing between some receptor subtypes, suggesting its possible applicability to the study of heterodimerization between receptors. Receptor heterodimerization has been confirmed experimentally for a number of receptors. This finding paves the way for new strategies in drug discovery research providing a conceptual framework for the rational combination of drugs. KGTM may help in the exploration of receptors susceptible of heterodimerization and thus be useful in the quest of more potent and safer drugs.

According to the results of Figures 4 and 5, the examples of subtype 9 corresponding to *Like*, assigned to cluster 83 are very homogeneous. They include the subsubtypes *Like2* and *Like3* and are well-located between mGluR2 and mGluR3. On the other hand, the *Like* group assigned to clusters 98 and 80 is quite far from Type 1- mGluRs but very close to the Types 4 (*Vomeronasal*), 5 (*Pheromone*) and 6 (*Odorant*) (See Figure 5 for the complete detail), taking into account their neighbourhood.

CONCLUSION

The world of pharmacology is pointedly veering towards research based on the data generated by pharmacogenomics and proteomics. More than half of the existing drugs target just a handful of protein families and, due to data availability, much research in the area is currently devoted to analyzing protein amino acid sequences.

In this chapter, we have shown a kernel method of the manifold learning family that is capable of simultaneously revealing the grouping structure of GPCRs while making the intuitive visualization of such structure possible.

Future research will relate the KGTM mapping of sequences with phylogenetic trees, in order to explore whether the structure revealed by the KGTM is revealing the evolutionary differentia-

tion of proteins. These trees are branching graphs that visually indicate the inferred evolutionary path of protein development within a family.

REFERENCES

Andras, P. (2002). Kernel-Kohonen networks. *International Journal of Neural Systems*, *12*, 117–135. doi:10.1016/S0129-0657(02)00108-4

Baldi, P., & Brunak, S. (2001). *Bioinformatics: The machine learning approach*. MIT Press.

Bishop, C. M., Svensén, M., & Williams, C. K. I. (1998). GTM: The generative topographic mapping. *Neural Computation*, *10*(1), 215–234. doi:10.1162/089976698300017953

Bishop, C. M., Svensén, M., & Williams, C. K. I. (1998b). Developments of the generative topographic mapping. *Neurocomputing*, *21*(1-3), 203–224. doi:10.1016/S0925-2312(98)00043-5

Cobanoglu, M. C., Saygin, Y., & Sezerman, U. (2010). Classification of GPCRs using family specific motifs. *IEEE/ACM Transactions on Computational Biology and Bioinformatics*, *8*(6).

Dempster, A. P., Laird, N. M., & Rubin, D. B. (1977). Maximum likelihood from incomplete data via the EM algorithm. *Journal of the Royal Statistical Society. Series B. Methodological*, *39*(1), 1–38.

Drews, J. (2000). Drug discovery: A historical perspective. *Science*, *287*, 1960. doi:10.1126/science.287.5460.1960

Durbin, R., Eddy, S. R., Krogh, A., & Mitchison, G. (2004). *Biological sequence analysis: Probabilistic models of proteins and nucleic acids*. Cambridge, UK: Cambridge University Press.

Gilman, A. G. (1987). G proteins: Transducers of receptor-generated signals. *Annual Review of Biochemistry*, *56*, 615–649. doi:10.1146/annurev. bi.56.070187.003151

Horn, F., Weare, J., Beukers, M. W., Horsch, S., Bairoch, A., & Chen, W. (1998). GPCRDB: An information system for G protein-coupled receptors. *Nucleic Acids Research, 26*, 275–279. doi:10.1093/nar/26.1.275

Kahn, S. D. (2011). On the future of genomic data. *Science, 331*(6018), 728–729. doi:10.1126/science.1197891

Kohonen, T. (2001). *Self-organizing maps* (3rd ed.). Berlin, Germany: Springer-Verlag.

Lisboa, P. J. G. (2002). A review of evidence of health benefit from artificial neural networks in medical intervention. *Neural Networks, 15*, 9–37. doi:10.1016/S0893-6080(01)00111-3

Lisboa, P. J. G., Vellido, A., Tagliaferri, R., Napolitano, F., Ceccarelli, M., Martin-Guerrero, J. D., & Biganzoli, E. (2004). Data mining in cancer research. *IEEE Computational Intelligence Magazine, 5*(1), 14–18. doi:10.1109/MCI.2009.935311

MacDonald, D., & Fyfe, C. (2000). The kernel self organising map. In *Proceedings of the 4th International Conference on Knowledge-Based Intelligent Engineering Systems and Allied Technologies*, Vol. 1, (pp. 317-320).

MacKay, D. J. C. (1992). A practical Bayesian framework for back-propagation networks. *Neural Computation, 4*(3), 448–472. doi:10.1162/neco.1992.4.3.448

Olier, I., Vellido, A., & Giraldo, J. (2010). Kernel generative topographic mapping. In *Proceedings of the 18th European Symposium on Artificial Neural Networks* (ESANN 2010), (pp. 481-486).

Overington, J. P., Al-Lazikani, B., & Hopkins, A. L. (2006). How many drug targets are there? *Nature Reviews. Drug Discovery, 5*, 993–996. doi:10.1038/nrd2199

Pierce, K. L., Premont, R. T., & Lefkowitz, R. J. (2002). Seven-transmembrane receptors. *Nature Reviews. Molecular Cell Biology, 3*, 639–650. doi:10.1038/nrm908

Pin, J. P., Galvez, T., & Prézeau, L. (2003). Evolution, structure and activation mechanism of family 3/C G-protein-coupled receptors. *Pharmacology & Therapeutics, 98*(3), 325–354. doi:10.1016/S0163-7258(03)00038-X

Rondard, P., Goudet, C., Kniazeff, J., Pin, J.-P., & Prézeau, L. (2011). The complexity of their activation mechanism opens new possibilities for the modulation of mGlu and GABAB class C G protein-coupled receptors. *Neuropharmacology, 60*, 82–92. doi:10.1016/j.neuropharm.2010.08.009

Schölkopf, B., & Smola, A. (2002). *Learning with kernels*. Cambridge, MA: The MIT Press.

Schölkopf, B., Smola, A., & Müller, K. R. (1997). Kernel principal component analysis. In *Proceedings of the 7th International Conference on Artificial Neural Networks* (ICANN 1997), (pp. 583-588).

Schölkopf, B., Tsuda, K., & Vert, J.-P. (2004). *Kernel methods in computational biology*. Cambridge, MA: The MIT Press.

Shawe-Taylor, J., & Cristianini, N. (2004). *Kernel methods for pattern analysis*. Cambridge, MA: The MIT Press. doi:10.1017/CBO9780511809682

Chapter 14
Medical Critiquing Systems

Ian Douglas
Florida State University, USA

ABSTRACT

Computer Science has traditionally focused on the functional aspects of design, underemphasizing the human element in the success of any technology. The failure of technologies and the accidents that happen during use require the consideration of the user and the technologies as symbiotic parts of a whole systems approach to improving diagnosis and treatment. This chapter provides an overview of the history of the critiquing approach to knowledge systems that illustrates a more human-centered approach. It is an approach that, unlike traditional knowledge-based systems, aims to provide a check on human reasoning, rather than a replacement for it. The chapter will also discuss future possibilities for research, in particular the use of social networking and recommender systems, as a means to enhance the approach.

INTRODUCTION

The human factors issues in medical applications of computing are often overlooked. Computing experts often focus solely on the functionality of the technology, rather than its integration with the user and their working environment. In the nineteen seventies and eighties there was a large investment in AI-based systems to support clinical decision-making. These largely failed, not because these systems could not be made to

function and provide accurate advice, but because doctors had no desire to use them. Consulting a machine during diagnosis did not fit in with the way doctors worked. It affected the patient's view of the doctor's status and expertise and therefore not surprisingly, it met resistance despite proven effectiveness.

One solution that emerged for this problem was the idea of expert critiquing systems. This approach did not tell the doctor what to diagnose, nor did it determine treatment selection. It required that the doctor take the lead in decision making, and

DOI: 10.4018/978-1-4666-1803-9.ch014

acted only as an independent review and check on the decision made. The system served to identify possible slips or errors in the recommendations, rather than to make the recommendations itself. It is estimated that there are up to 100,000 deaths a year from medical errors in the USA. Even a minimal amount of additional checking of medical staff's actions could help prevent some of these deaths.

This chapter will discuss some of the human factors issues in medical decision support systems and review work on the expert critiquing approach to medical AI. The underlying technology in the critiquing approach is similar to other medical AI-based systems (production rules, databases); it differs mainly in its user interaction model. Unlike the nineteen eighties when these systems were first developed, the fact that more treatment and diagnosis notes are being recorded digitally provides a new impetus to the development and success of critiquing systems.

KNOWLEDGE-BASED SYSTEMS IN MEDICINE

In the thirty-five years or more that knowledge-based (expert) systems have been part of computer science, there have been a number of developments in the architectures used. The earliest expert systems, for example MYCIN (Shortliffe, 1976) and DENDRAL (Buchanan 1969) had three basic components; knowledge base, user interface and inference engine. There are now several new approaches that exist as alternatives to the basic architecture, for example neural networks (Zurada, 1992), and agent-based systems (Foster et al, 2006).

Within the traditional architecture there have been many changes in the back end operation of the tools. The first expert systems primarily had a database (or knowledge base) in the form of knowledge production rules and an inference engine, which given inputs of initial informa-

tion would chain through the rules to produce a diagnosis. In relation to the knowledge base, production rules were complimented with the full range of knowledge representation techniques (van Harmelen, Lifschitz, & Porter, 2008). Research has also focused on improving inference engines with new approaches and developing better user interfaces (Pandey & Mishra, 2009).

It is on the change in the approach to the user interface, that we will focus in this chapter. There are a number of ways in which decisions support and knowledge-based systems can support medical practice. Wright & Sittig conducted a review and synthesis of the history of clinical decision support systems since 1959. From this they developed a four-phase model of various architectures for integrating decision support systems with clinical systems. The four phases are: standalone decision support systems, decision support integrated into clinical systems, standards for sharing clinical decision support content and service models for decision support. The authors claim this fits with the chronological history of clinical decision support, and note that the trend is towards better integrating decision support systems into clinical workflows and other clinical technology.

One aspect missed from this analysis is the decision support system configured as a tutor. A knowledge-based system can be used to provide the performance knowledge of an "expert" to a student. Thus the knowledge present in the expert system is not used just to solve a problem, but is in some way imparted to the user. From the earliest days of the field, various ways have been conceived for adapting decision support systems for learning.

The standalone decision support system was the predominant model for expert systems interaction established in one of the first medical expert systems MYCIN and adopted by many subsequent systems. In this traditional model, users must first recognize they have a problem and be aware that the system has an ability to solve it. The problem is then entered into the system, which initiates a series of questions derived from the chaining of its inference rules. Once a conclusion is reached it is presented to the users. At various points in the dialogue users can access explanation of the system's reasoning. In the move towards integration with clinical systems the development of critiquing systems was an important step.

CRITIQUING BASED SYSTEMS

Critiquing systems operate by either asking the users how they are planning to do a particular task, or if the task is computerized, monitoring the users while they actually carry out the task. A critiquing expert system assesses a user's actual or planned actions in comparison with knowledge of an expert approach to the task. This allows the initiation of a dialogue on the advantages and disadvantages of the user's approach. The essential point about critiquing systems from the user's perspective is that it does not tell them what to do, but rather helps them to evaluate their own approach. The critiquing approach will use a similar back-end process but in the user interface it can work in the background provided the user has some digital representation of their intended diagnosis and/or treatment plan.

There are several advantages of critiquing when compared to the more traditional modes of expert system interaction.

Acceptability

There are two reasons why critiquing systems may be more acceptable than the more traditional systems. Firstly, they act to help develop the user's own thinking, rather than just delivering poorly justified conclusions in relation to the user's queries. Secondly, in many cases they do not require a change of working practices, in that they operate along with someone doing a task. They collect the information they need without

having to ask. In conventional systems, users are required to halt what they are doing and actively consult the expert system. They have to supply much basic information about the current situation before they can derive advice.

Explanation

This is related to acceptability in that good explanation facilities are likely to lead to more confidence in any conclusion given by a knowledge-based system. From the earliest work this has been found to be particularly true in relation to medical computing (Young, 1984; Teach and Shortliffe, 1981). In the more traditional systems, explanation is predominantly of the HOW-WHY type, i.e. the user can ask why a question is being asked or how a conclusion was reached. In each case they are presented with the inference rule from which the question/conclusion was derived.

The initial approaches to explanation were much criticized as being too far removed from the explanation provided by real experts (Rogers and Leiser, 1987) and studies showed user dissatisfaction (O'Neill and Morris, 1989). More recently there have been a number of new approaches to explanation, including the use case-based explanation (Nugent, Doyle & Cunningham, 2009).

In critiquing, explanation has the potential to be much more effective, as the explanation dialogue is based around the actions of the user, rather than the action of the system. The user's own actions or plans provide an indication of the knowledge that is important to the user, which can then be used to guide explanation.

Responsibility

The critiquing approach forces the user to confront any difficult problems before turning to the computer. The users are the primary decision makers and cannot sit back and let the knowledge system do the work. The critiquing expert system works from the user's attempts to solve problems, rather than from the problems themselves. The user is thus forced to some extent to consider the problem at hand. Cooley (1987) noted that the traditional expert consultant approach to knowledge systems leads to a cognitive de-skilling of the user. In using the expert system, the user is relegated to providing information for the machine's work. They are not required to use cognitive skills such as categorizing, evaluation or decision-making. With traditional expert systems, users can go into cognitive autopilot, allowing the expert system to do all the work. Morris (1987) cites the inflexibility of the expert system dialogue facilities as a reason for their relative lack of impact.

Inherent Variation

In many domains there is no one correct way of dealing with a problem, although each approach may have its advantages and disadvantages. Critiquing approaches do not force a particular style of dealing with a problem, although they mold their advice around the style a user has chosen. There is the possibility for more than one style of problem solving to be included, allowing for critiques to be presented from different perspectives with the user making a choice.

System Does Not Have to be Complete

In order to be effective, a traditional expert system needs to be reasonably complete. It requires knowledge to deal with all the expected problems within a domain. A critiquing system may still be useful even if it has knowledge relating to only some of the problems in a domain. A critiquing expert system can go into use without a comprehensive knowledge base; new knowledge can be added at a later date. An example of this might be a medical critiquing system, which does not

have knowledge concerning the optimal treatment, but does have knowledge about combinations of drugs in a treatment plan that may be dangerous to the patient.

Such problems in medical treatment are not uncommon due the bewildering array of possible treatments available. In observations of epilepsy treatment specialists by Douglas (1986) one case had been referred to them where the patient had been given two separate doses of the same drug, one under its generic name, the other under a manufacturer's brand name. If treatment records were entered into a computer, a critiquing expert system might easily have prevented such confusion.

Is More Useful in an Educational Role

This is related to the fact that the critiquing system cannot take away all the responsibility for problem solving from the user. It is often argued that traditional knowledge systems are useful in education because they have the knowledge to solve certain problems. It is suggested that by posing problems and observing their behavior, users learn to recognize the patterns of problem solution (Dixon, 1988). Learning by this method appears somewhat haphazard, requiring motivated and observant users.

In the critiquing approach, the users cannot rely on the system to do all the work for them. They must perform some of the problem solving tasks for themselves. The critiquing expert system gets the users to confront what they have done and why they have done it. It highlights their mistakes and can reinforce good practice.

The operating mode of critiquing expert systems is consistent with what happens in many expert-novice dialogues. While working on a medical expert system (Gotts, Hunter and Sinnhuber, 1984), the author noted that medical consultants would almost never give a straight answer to a question asked by more junior staff. The junior doctor would instead be hit by a barrage of questions such as 'Did you check x?', 'What did you deduce from finding y?', 'Tell me what you know of how aspect z of the particular organ works.' It was clear that the approach of the experts was to get the novices to do more thinking on the problem, to relate the problem to classroom learning, to consider underlying mechanisms and to refine their problem solving strategies. The aim was to refine the skills of the junior doctors rather than provide the immediate solution to the problem at hand.

Disadvantages of Critiquing

Of course, there are some disadvantages to the approach. There are situations in which a user might like to be provided with a decision quickly, rather than have to generate their own solution for a critique. Automated decision-making is sometimes proven to be more accurate than human decision-making. In cases where human expertise is short or not available, and time is critical, the traditional approach may be better. There is also a potential annoyance factor in having workflow interrupted by a critiquing system. An extreme example was the infamous "clippy" that would pop-up to assist Microsoft office users. Clippy was an intelligent agent that monitored the users actions and when it detected that there may be a better way of doing things would pop-up with advice. Many users found it to be unhelpful and intrusive, although a case can be made that for new users the approach is potentially helpful. The experience with Clippy highlights the need to carefully plan when critiques are provided and ensure that the critique is well timed and relevant and constructive. Getting a good balance in automated assistance between being helpful without being distracting has become the focus of research, particularly in relation to mobile computing e.g. Inbar, Lavie & Meyer (2009).

CRITIQUING SYSTEMS RESEARCH ISSUES

In order to conform to the critiquing approach, a knowledge system must be designed to overcome several problems.

Access Users' Plans or Actions

The starting point for a critiquing system is the user's own attempt to solve a problem. It is therefore necessary for the system to gain access to a computer representation of the users' actions. A representation is obtained from one of two sources; if the task is computerized (for example, electronic form filling) the users' actions can be directly accessed by the critiquing expert system. The link can be achieved by either passing information to the critiquing system through a network, or having the expert system embedded within the data gathering main program. If the task is not computerized, some conversion process will be necessary, for example, selecting from a series of menus to input the planned actions of the users.

Analysis of the Plan or Action

Fischer et al (1990), identifies two approaches to this problem within critiquing systems. The first approach is differential critiquing where the representation of the users' actual or intended actions is compared with a representation of the actions that would form part of the system's own solution. Thus if the user decided on the steps A-B-D-F in solving a problem and the knowledge-based system would have used the steps A-B-C-F, then the critiquing system would focus on why step C was more appropriate than step D.

Differential critiquing has an advantage in identifying all differences between the users' and the system's expert derived solution, although this can present problems in domains where there may be a number of valid solutions to a problem. The differential solution focuses on the differences between two approaches, rather than looking for good or bad aspects of the users' solution.

The second approach to this problem is analytical critiquing. This involves checking the users' actual or planned actions for the presence of notable items. In medical critiquing systems analytical critiquing will involve some analysis of the risk involved in different actions, for example, the risk of certain items may increase if a patient is very old or very young. Analytical approaches do not have to solve the problem themselves and they do not require a complete understanding of the problem area. The approach involves pattern matching the user's solution against a set of identified constraints within the area, e.g. certain treatments should not be given to certain categories of patient.

Response Generation

This is perhaps the most difficult part of the process in that the system's analysis of the user's approach must be converted into an informative and readable critique. There is a range of possible techniques in response generation available to the developers of critiquing expert systems. The techniques range from the production of canned text to methods derived from natural language generation research (Rankin et al 1989). Most practical systems rely on some development of canned text.

As well as the mechanics of generating a response to the users, it is also important for a critiquing system to have a strategy of how and when to respond. A decision on strategy depends on the task involved, for example, when monitoring a doctor's treatment plan it may be important to immediately alert the users when a potentially harmful treatment is recommended. As opposed to this, an educational critiquing system may allow users to make a number of errors uninterrupted, in order that they can learn from making mistakes.

There is also likely to be a delicate balance in terms of how often the critiquing system is activated; this will depend on the users and the complexity of the task. The critiquing system could interrupt too much and be disruptive to the task or fail to interrupt enough and thus not give the required help at crucial parts of the problem solving process. There is a choice between making the critiquing system passive and only invoked by the users, or constantly active where there is a danger of the system becoming too intrusive.

Most critiques tend to operate negatively by looking for deficient aspects of user's actions. It may also be important to offer positive criticism that reinforces good practice and helps to maintain a user-positive attitude toward the system.

CRITIQUING SYSTEMS RESEARCH

Although the approach has been applied to wide variety of domains, the pioneering work in critiquing systems was carried out primarily in medicine (Miller, 1986). The following section give some examples of the kinds of problem tackled and approach used. It is by no means exhaustive and tends to highlight both the earliest and latest examples of work done in the medical domain. A point made by Silverman (1992) is that a number of programs exist that are essentially critiquing systems but are not acknowledged as such. An example here would be the grammar checker used in Microsoft Word, which uses rules of grammar to check for potential errors and suggests alternative phrasing.

The pioneering work in critiquing was often undertaken by medical doctors with an interest in computers. A system called "Attending" was one of the first programs to use the critiquing approach. Before surgery the anesthetist must develop a plan of management, which involves a number of different decisions. For example, should a general or a local anesthetic be used? Some techniques have benefits in certain situations, for example intubation (passing a tube down the patient's throat) may prevent patients from choking on their own vomit. Some techniques have risks, for example if a patient has eye damage certain drugs should not be used.

Attending begins by getting the users to input their plan by selecting from a series of menu choices. This is then converted into a tree-structured form. The main knowledge representation used in the system is an augmented transition network ATN (Woods, 1970), which encapsulates most of the possible choices an anesthetist is faced with. In addition, a series of data tables hold risk information on illnesses that have implications for the use of the techniques available.

The basic approach of Attending is to take the tree representing the anesthetic plan and input it to an ATN analyzer, which uses the ATN of the domain to identify possible alternatives to the user's plan. The output of the analyzer is an augmented tree, which includes the original plan, and any alterative identified.

It is from the augmented tree that the critiquing text is generated. It should be noted that the domain in which Attending operates is relatively constrained compared with many other medical problems. The ATN approach would have proved much more difficult to implement in a less constrained domain.

Attending examines which arc of the network a physician has proposed in the plan tree and evaluates the risks associated with it. Attending then examines the alternative arcs evaluating the risks associated for each one. If they are more risky they are discarded, otherwise they are noted for the augmented tree and critique.

The risk analysis in Attending is performed by the application of heuristic rules, which will determine the risk of the various courses of action (arcs of the network) in relation to the circumstance of the case. An example of a typical rule would be "if the patient has a full stomach and intubation is not carried out then there is a possibility of aspiration of stomach contents into the lungs, which is often fatal."

The same architecture was also used to develop VQ-Attending (Miller, 1985), which critiques a physician's ventilator management plan when treating patients receiving mechanical respiratory support.

HT-Advisor (Clyman et al, 1989) uses the Attending approach for the treatment of hypertension. It differs from Attending in that it performs a deeper internal analysis and deals with a broader set of issues in the prose discussions. As part of the study the significance of the comments given to the user was determined by use of a ten-category classification scheme. Eight categories contained advice that was in some way critical. The remaining two were either supportive or neutral.

The benefit of the system was demonstrated when an analysis of data from 224 actual cases revealed that at least one critical comment was generated in 87% of cases and in 28% of cases a drug regime was identified that did not conform to accepted practice.

Essential-Attending (E-Attending) was the first shell for building critiquing expert systems. It was used to build CORSAGE, a critiquing system for coronary care by a group of doctors in Los Angeles (Powell et al, 1989). It is noted in this study, that despite the perceived success in medical AI (Clancey and Shortliffe, 1984), few consultation systems are actually used in clinical practice. The implementation of CORSAGE in clinical practice was evaluated and the high level of user acceptance found was attributed to the critiquing approach.

ICON critiques radiological diagnosis. It uses four diagnostic strategies in order to structure coherently its prose output. The strategies used were developed from the questioning strategies used in the well-known medical expert consultant system INTERNIST (Miller et al, 1984). In order to select which of the strategies is most appropriate for critiquing the user diagnosis, every relevant diagnosis is first ranked using a scoring system determined by the rule base. A *pursue* strategy is used if one diagnosis has a high score compared with others. A *conflict* strategy is used where a diagnosis is scored both high and low on different findings. A *rule-in-rule-out* strategy is used if findings do not highlight a single diagnosis but support several. A *not-enough-information* strategy is used when the findings do not suggest any diagnosis confidently.

The main difference in the use of these strategies between ICON and INTERNIST is that INTERNIST uses the strategies to direct questioning aimed at getting a particular diagnosis while ICON uses the strategies to suggest various alternatives within its critique. ICON also has a simpler weighting system due to having a more constrained domain.

ONCOCIN (Langlotz and Shortliffe, 1983) is a system that combines the data management for the routine care of cancer patients with a critiquing expert system. This addresses a reason cited by Wright and Sittig (2008) as to why clinical decision support systems in general are not widely used, the reason being that it is relatively difficult to integrate such systems in clinical workflows and existing computer systems. In ONCOCIN the data input was handled by computer-generated versions of paper forms that the physicians previously had to fill in as part of their normal routine. The input to computer generated forms gave a number of time saving advantages to the physicians, for example, automatic report generation, and at the same time gave the critiquing expert system the information it required without having to engage the physician in a dialogue.

The critiquing expert system has knowledge of cancer treatment protocols and develops its own recommendation for a treatment plan for a given patient. A comparison is then made between each component of the system and the user's treatment planning and when a significant difference is discovered the system explains the reason for its decision. The explanation is derived from the fact that each time ONCOCIN concludes the value for a parameter, it stores a justification. Natural language translations of the system's production rules are used in this process.

Roundsman, reported in Rennals et al (1989), represents a joint effort between the two pioneering centers for research into critiquing expert systems (Yale and Stanford). Roundsman will produce patient specific analyses of breast cancer management options based on a number of structured representations of clinical literature relating to the area. It will take representative factors of a patient (e.g. age, cancer type) and pattern match them against appropriate factors in the structured representations of case studies and clinical trials. The appropriate studies can be used to highlight potential problems with the proposed management.

HELP (Pryor et al, 1983) is a system designed to alert doctors to possible problems in the treatment plans. Such systems are of great use within medicine with the vast range of possible drug treatments available and the often complex drug interactions that can occur. HELP, which has 4,500 knowledge modules, has an average of 80,000 executions a day.

ILIAD (Cundick et al, 1989) is aimed at improving medical students' questioning strategies and decision making. The system is based around a patient case simulator. Once a case has been generated the user is presented with standard information about the patient (for example, age, sex) and must then indicate a hypothesis to pursue and pose questions about specific findings.

The user's hypotheses and questioning strategies are compared with the expert knowledge in ILIAD and an efficiency score is calculated. The efficiency score acts as a crude critique to the performance. A notable deficiency of this system from a learning point of view is the lack of textual feedback to the user giving the reasons for any change in efficiency.

RaPiD (Hammond et al, 1993) describes ongoing work to develop a design assistant to assist in prosthetic dentistry. In RaPiD, the users manipulate icons representing false teeth and instruments for a design, which is then critiqued using a logic database of design components. When design rules in the system go against a design, or proposed design alteration, a critique is generated and presented to the users.

In the mid nineteen nineties there was a reduction of interest in critiquing systems research, which corresponds to a more general reduction of interest in Artificial Intelligence research. As other areas of computing research became more prominent, the funding levels for AI research reduced. The research may also have been held back by more basic computing development problems in medical practice. The success of the critiquing approach to a certain extent depends on automated record keeping. There has been a recent re-discovery of the approach by several researchers.

Critiquing relies on good modeling of what is best practice in order to compare this with what physicians do. Groups of researchers in the Netherlands have investigated basing critiques on comparisons with formal models. Groot et al, (2007, 2008) use a formal model of clinical guidelines that use temporal logic. They have tested their model in a system to critique the diagnosis and treatment of breast cancer. Sips, Braun & Roos (2006) worked on the development of a formal language for describing recommended medical protocols in conjunction with a national electronic patient records (EPR) database in the Netherlands. The formal language is based on a BDI (beliefs, desires and intentions) approach, which they believe will overcome skepticism about critiquing being applied on a national scale to medical records. Marcos et al (2002) constructed fully formal knowledge models of realistic medical protocol in daily use for treating jaundice in new born babies, which they claim has improved the medical knowledge by providing machine-assisted proofs that determine the strength and weaknesses of a given protocol.

Formal approaches may have some limitations and assume a level of infallibility in the official guidelines and protocols. Marcos et al (2001) also investigated formal models based around common protocols. In a small test of 7 cases that compared pediatricians solving a set of test cases, they discovered many mismatches between the actions performed by the expert and the official protocol recommendations, which suggested a need for improvements in the protocol. Knowledge about best practice is often fluid, controversial and dependent on context (Quaglini, 2008).

In addition to using formal models, another recent approach is to make use of development in agent-based systems (Foster et al, 2006). In traditional expert systems there is a single intelligent processor (inference engine). Multi-agent systems have multiple processors, which collaborate to solve a problem. Bosansky & Lhotska (2009), describe architecture for an agent–based system making use of medical guidelines. The architecture has five collaborating agents. An environment agent models the specific medical environment the system is used in. An execution agent models the decision making of human experts (doctors, nurses). A role agent describes the roles in the environment and can determine the appropriate execution agent. A process agent manages the processes that occurs, e.g. treatment planning. Finally, a process director agent manages agent communication throughout the processes and accesses formal process guidelines. To demonstrate how the architecture would work, they describe a critiquing system that can monitor the progress of patients' treatment and alert a physician in case of inconsistencies.

FUTURE RESEARCH DIRECTIONS

The fact that the medical profession has been slow to adopt standards for digitization of medical records and treatment plans has been a barrier to critiquing. Even in 2011 many people are required to fill out paper-based forms providing essentially the same information every time they visit any medical facility. The advent of touch based mobile computing devices such as the iPad promise to make the data entry for both patient information, consultations and treatment plans easier to effect. iPads and similar devices are beginning to have a significant impact on medical practice (Evans, 2011) The system to critique breast cancer treatment, referred to above (Groot et al, 2007, 2008), was made possible by digital registry of patients in the Netherlands that contain 269 variables, including information on diagnosis and treatment.

Another technology area that provides the potential for greatly improved critiquing systems, is the work done on recommender systems (Adomavicius and Tuzhilin, 2005). Recommender systems come in many forms, but were pioneered by e-commerce sites such as Amazon. Each option for a purchase in the system comes with attached ratings and review based on crowd sourcing. Additionally, other useful information is provided, such as a list of products viewed and ultimately purchased by those who viewed the user's current choice. Further rating of the raters and reviews enhances such systems. Users may not just consider the highest rated items. For example, a history book on Amazon may be highly rated by a majority, as it is "a good read". However, the viewer may decide not to buy it if he sees a review by a historian who provides lengthy explanations of gross historical inaccuracies and a suggestion of an alternative book that is both a good read and historically accurate.

Recommender systems are a potential way of building better explanations and advice into critiquing systems. Although they are primarily dealing with recommendations for products, a similar set of trade-off properties might be identified for diagnostic and treatment alternatives. Recommender systems can now integrate with social networking sites such as Face book, so that users can rely on the recommendations of peers and trusted friends, rather than the open network (Bonhard & Sasse, 2006). Thus, recommendations in the medical domain can be restricted groups of

professionals who are members of online communities controlled by professional associations.

As most such systems are open for anyone to contribute to, there is an issue of trust involved in such ratings. A hotel on a travel site can be highly rated and have good reviews because a hotel owner and their employees and friends have entered high ratings and glowing comments, not because guests liked it. Pu and Chen (2007) note trust is a major issue in such recommenders and is dependent on the users' perception of the recommenders' competence and ability to explain their ratings. They build a model for recommender agents grouping results according to their trade-off properties. In a test it was shown to be significantly more effective in building user trust than the traditional approach.

Pu & Chen (2007) note that trust is more likely to be invested in the recommendations in the community of peers than it is in a computer. Recommenders can be restricted to closed groups and not made anonymous in order to increase trust. Many medical associations and private online medical services exist that could provide recommendations that add trust to alternative options a critiquing system identified, in reaction to a user's plan. When an alternative approach is recommended, comments from real doctors saying why they used the alternative approach and how it turned out, may provide crucial information not easily captured and catalogued by the creators of a critiquing system.

In Wright and Sittig's (2008) four phase model, the last phase: sharing content and services models, coincides with recent general developments in information technology towards the concepts of cloud computing and software as a service. A good example of this is the Google maps API that allows Google maps and interaction mechanisms to be relatively easily integrated into a whole host of information services (e.g. Douglas, 2009). Most critiquing systems exist as standalone software that runs on a local machine. Creating new critiquing systems as a software service that can be called on by different systems that have different interfaces to suit local need, may provide a mechanism for achieving more widely used systems.

CONCLUSION

This chapter has introduced the critiquing approach to decision support systems in medicine. A number of systems that come under the general descriptive term of critiquing have been identified and the design approaches of these systems discussed. The critiquing approach has been noted to have a number of advantages over the traditional approach to knowledge-based systems, including better acceptability, better explanation, not taking all the responsibility for problem solving, not having to be complete and being adaptable to problems with different approaches to the solution.

The critiquing approach as shown in this chapter, is supported by a number of systems and has a number of points in its favor. Despite this, it is generally less well known and used than more traditional approaches to knowledge systems and decision support, where the general goal is to provide the "right answer". From the point of view of education, critiquing has a clear advantage in not taking the responsibility of problem solving away from the user. Critiquing systems promote active learning by reacting to attempted problem solving by novices, rather than demonstrating solutions to passive observers.

The primary barrier to the success of critiquing as an approach has been the difficulty of integrating it into medical practice. The development of greater digitization for medical records, diagnosis and treatment protocol models, together with developments in mobile computing and recommender systems (to provide trusted alternatives as part of critiques), provide new opportunities for enhancing the approach and creating systems which are more widely used.

REFERENCES

Adomavicius, G., & Tuzhilin, A. (2005). Toward the next generation of recommender systems: A survey of the state-of-the-art and possible extensions. *IEEE Transactions on Knowledge and Data Engineering, 17*(6), 734–749. doi:10.1109/TKDE.2005.99

Bonhard, P., & Sasse, M. A. (2006). Knowing me, knowing you - Using profiles and social networking to improve recommender systems. *BT Technology Journal, 25*(3), 84–98. doi:10.1007/s10550-006-0080-3

Bosansky, B., & Lhotska, L. (2009). Agent-based process-critiquing decision support system. In *2nd International Symposium on Applied Sciences in Biomedical and Communication Technologies*, (pp. 1-6).

Braham, N., Le Beux, P., & Fontaine, D. (1987). An experimental knowledge-based system for simulation in hematology. *Proceedings of the third International Expert Systems Conference* (pp. 459-466).

Buchanan, B. G., Sutherland, G. L., & Feigenbaum, E. A. (1969). Heuristic Dendral: A program for generating explanatory hypotheses in organic chemistry. In Meltzer, B., & Michie, D. (Eds.), *Machine intelligence (Vol. 4)*. Edinburgh University Press.

Clancey, W. J., & Shortliffe, E. H. (1984). *Readings in medical AI: The first decade*. Reading, MA: Addison-Wesley.

Clyman, J. I., Black, H. R., & Miller, P. L. (1989). Assessing practice conformance for hypertension management using an expert system. *Computer Applications in Medical Care: Proceedings of the Thirteenth Annual Symposium*, Washington DC, USA, November 5-8.

Cooley, M. (1987). Human centered systems: An urgent problem for systems designers. *AI & Society*, *1*(1), 21–43. doi:10.1007/BF01905888

Cundick, R., Turner, C. W., Lincoln, M. J., Buchanan, J. P., Anderson, C., Homer, R., & Bouhaddou, O. (1989). ILIAD as a patient case simulator to teach medical problem solving. *Symposium on Computer Applications in Medical Care*, (pp. 902-906). Washington, DC: IEEE Computer Society.

Douglas, I. (2009). Global mapping of usability labs and centers. *Proceedings of Computer Human Interaction Conference, CHI 2009*, April 4 – 9, Boston, MA, USA, (pp. 4393-4398).

Douglas, I. W. (1986). *Medical expert systems: The problem of epilepsy*. M.Sc. Dissertation, University of Warwick.

Evans, J. (2011). In medicine, iPad today means a Mac tomorrow. *Computerworld*, April. Retrieved July 20, 2011, from http://blogs.computerworld.com/18134/collected_in_medicine_ipad_today_means_a_mac_tomorrow

Fischer, G., Lemke, A. C., & Mastaglio, T. (1990). Critics: An emerging approach to knowledge-based human-computer interaction. *Proceedings of Computer Human Interaction Conference, CHI 90*, April 1-5.

Foster, D., McGregor, C., & El-Masri, S. (2006). A survey of agent-based intelligent decision support systems to support clinical management and research. In G. Armano, E. Merelli, J. Denzinger, A. Martin, S. Miles, H. Tianfield, & R. Unland (Eds.), *Proceedings of MAS BIOMED '05*, Utretch, Netherlands.

Gotts, N. M., Hunter, J. R. W., & Sinnhuber, R. K. (1984). *An intelligent model based system for diagnosis in cardiology- A research proposal. AIM-7 Research Report of the AI in Medicine Group*. University of Sussex.

Groot, P., Hommersom, A., Lucas, P., Merk, R. J., ten Teije, A., van Harmelen, F., & Serban, R. (2008). Using model checking for critiquing based on clinical guidelines. *Artificial Intelligence in Medicine*, (n.d), 19–36.

Groot, P., Hommersom, A., Lucas, P., Serban, R., ten Teije, A., & van Harmelen, F. (2007). The role of model checking in critiquing based on clinical guidelines. *Lecture Notes on Artificial Intelligence*, 411-420.

Hammond, P., Davenport, J. C., & Fitzpatrick, F. J. (1993). Logic-based integrity constraints and the design of dental prostheses. *Artificial Intelligence in Medicine*, *5*(5), 431–446. doi:10.1016/0933-3657(93)90035-2

Inbar, O., Lavie, T., & Meyer, J. (2009). Acceptable intrusiveness of online help in mobile devices. In *Proceedings of the 11th International Conference on Human-Computer Interaction with Mobile Devices and Services* (MobileHCI '09), (p. 26). New York, NY: ACM.

Langlotz, C. P., & Shortliffe, E. H. (1983). Adapting a consultation system to critique user plans. *International Journal of Man-Machine Studies*, *19*, 479–496. doi:10.1016/S0020-7373(83)80067-4

Marcos, M., Balser, M., ten Teije, A., & van Harmelen, F. (2002). From informal knowledge to formal logic: A realistic case study in medical protocols. In *Proceedings of the 13th International Conference on Knowledge Engineering and Knowledge Management*. New York, NY: Springer-Verlag.

Marcos, M., Berger, G., van Harmelem, F., & ten Teije, A. Roomans, H., & Miksch, S. (2001). Using critiquing for improving medical protocols: harder than it seems. *Proceedings of the Eighth European Conference on Artificial Intelligence in Medicine (AIME '01), LNAI, vol. 2101*, (pp. 431-441). New York, NY: Springer-Verlag.

Miller, P. L. (1985). Goal-directed critiquing by computer: Ventilator management. *Computers and Biomedical Research, an International Journal, 18*, 422–438. doi:10.1016/0010-4809(85)90020-5

Miller, P. L. (1986). *Expert critiquing systems: Practice-based medical computing*. New York, NY: Springer Verlag.

Miller, R. A., Pople, H. E., & Myers, J. D. (1984). An experimental computer based diagnostic consultant for general internal medicine. In Clancey, W. J., & Shortliffe, E. H. (Eds.), *Readings in medical AI: The first decade*. Reading, MA: Addison-Wesley. doi:10.1056/NEJM198208193070803

Morris, A. (1987). Expert systems - Interface insight. In Diaper, D., & Winder, R. (Eds.), *People and Computers, 3* (pp. 307–324). Cambridge University Press.

Nugent, C., Doyle, D., & Cunningham, P. (2009). Gaining insight through case-based explanation. *Journal of Intelligent Information Systems, 32*(3), 267–295. doi:10.1007/s10844-008-0069-0

O'Neill, M., & Morris, A. (1989). Expert systems in the United Kingdom: An evaluation of development methodologies. *Expert Systems: International Journal of Knowledge Engineering and Neural Networks, 6*(2), 90–99. doi:10.1111/j.1468-0394.1989.tb00082.x

Pandey, B., & Mishra, R. B. (2009). Knowledge and intelligent computing system in medicine. *Computers in Biology and Medicine, 39*(3), 215–230. doi:10.1016/j.compbiomed.2008.12.008

Powell, L. T., Diamond, G. A., Prediman, K. S., & Ferguson, J. G. (1989). CorSage: A critiquing system for coronary care. *Computer Applications in Medical Care: Proceedings of the Thirteenth Annual Symposium*, November 5-8, Washington, D.C., USA, (pp. 152-156).

Pryor, T. A., Gardner, R. M., Clayton, P. D., & Warner, H. R. (1983). The HELP system. *Journal of Medical Systems, 7*(2), 87–102. doi:10.1007/BF00995116

Pu, P., & Chen, L. (2007). Trust-inspiring explanation interfaces for recommender systems. *Knowledge-Based Systems, 20*, 542–556. doi:10.1016/j.knosys.2007.04.004

Quaglini, S. (2008). Compliance with clinical practice guidelines. In Lucas, P. (Ed.), *Computer-based Medical Guidelines and Protocols: A Primer and current Research Trends* (pp. 160–179). Amsterdam, The Netherlands: IOS Press.

Rankin, I. (1989). Deep generation of a critique. *Second European Natural Language Generation Workshop*, Edinburgh, April, (pp. 39-44).

Rennals, G. R., Shortliffe, E. H., Stockdale, F. E., & Miller, P. L. (1989). Reasoning from the clinical literature: The Roundsman system. In Salmon, R., Blum, B., & Jorgenson, M. (Eds.), *MEDINFO 86*. New York, NY: Elsevier Science.

Rogers, Y., & Leiser, B. (1987). *What do you mean by that? Designing user requirements for expert system explanation. Colloquium on Man-Machine Interfaces for Intelligent Knowledge-Based Systems, 27 November*. London: IEEE Computer and Control Division.

Shortliffe, E. H. (1976). *Computer-based medical consultations: MYCIN*. New York, NY: North Holland.

Silverman, B. G. (1992). Survey of expert critiquing systems: practical and theoretical frontiers. *Communications of the ACM, 35*(4), 107–127. doi:10.1145/129852.129861

Sips, R. J., Braun, L., & Roos, N. (2008). *Enabling medical expert critiquing using a BDI approach.*

Sips, R. J., Braun, L. M. M., & Roos, N. (2006). Medical expert critiquing using a BDI approach. In P-Y. Schobbens, W. Vanhoof, & G. Schwanen (Eds.), *Proceedings of the 18th Belgium-Netherlands Conference on Artificial Intelligence* (BNAIC 06) (pp. 283-290). Namur, Belgium.

Teach, R. L., & Shortliffe, E. H. (1981). An analysis of physician's attitudes regarding computer-based medical consultation systems. *Computers and Biomedical Research, an International Journal, 14*, 542–558. doi:10.1016/0010-4809(81)90012-4

van Harmelen, F., Lifschitz, V., & Porter, B. (2008). *Handbook of knowledge representation.* Amsterdam, The Netherlands: Elsevier.

Van Melle, W. (1979). A domain-independent production rule system for consultation programs. *Proceedings of the Sixth International Joint Conference on Artificial Intelligence*, Tokyo, (pp. 923 -925).

Woods, W. A. (1970). Transition network grammars for natural language analysis. *Communications of the ACM, 13*, 591–606. doi:10.1145/355598.362773

Wright, A., & Sittig, D. F. (2008). A four-phase model of the evolution of clinical decision support architectures. *International Journal of Medical Informatics, 77*, 641–649. doi:10.1016/j.ijmedinf.2008.01.004

Young, D. W. (1984). What makes doctors use computers? *Journal of the Royal Society of Medicine, 77*, 663.

Zurada, J. M. (1992). Applications of neural algorithms and systems. In *Artificial neural systems.* St. Paul, MN: West Publishing.

Chapter 15

Learning Probabilistic Graphical Models:
A Review of Techniques and Applications in Medicine

Juan I. Alonso-Barba
University of Castilla-La Mancha, Spain

Jens D. Nielsen
University of Castilla-La Mancha, Spain

Luis de la Ossa
University of Castilla-La Mancha, Spain

Jose M. Puerta
University of Castilla-La Mancha, Spain

ABSTRACT

Probabilistic Graphical Models (PGM) are a class of statistical models that use a graph structure over a set of variables to encode independence relations between those variables. By augmenting the graph by local parameters, a PGM allows for a compact representation of a joint probability distribution over the variables of the graph, which allows for efficient inference algorithms. PGMs are often used for modeling physical and biological systems, and such models are then in turn used to both answer probabilistic queries concerning the variables and to represent certain causal and/or statistical relations in the domain. In this chapter, the authors give an overview of common techniques used for automatic construction of such models from a dataset of observations (usually referred to as learning), and they also review some important applications. The chapter guides the reader to the relevant literature for further study.

DOI: 10.4018/978-1-4666-1803-9.ch015

INTRODUCTION

Probabilistic Graphical Models (PGMs) have been used quite often to model complex problems where there is considerable uncertainty associated. The increased use of these models is due to two main reasons:

A. Its graphical representation is very attractive because dependencies between domain variables are represented explicitly, thus it is a powerful tool to describe real phenomena or complex domains.

B. Once the probabilistic graphical model is built it is usually relatively easy and efficient to perform the reasoning processes of various types such as predictive reasoning, abductive or diagnostic, backward and forward reasoning, etc.

The problem of learning a PGM from a database of observations has received an enormous amount of attention in the past two decades, and in this chapter we will give an overview of the most common approaches to this problem. We will focus our attention on learning Bayesian Network models, as they comprise the class of models that without doubt has received the most attention in the literature and also those models with the most intuitive interpretation.

Finally, we will give an overview of successful applications in Medical, Bioinformatics and Health fields. Those related to use PGMs as the core representation of the problems, as also by using learning methods to construct such model representation.

BACKGROUND: PROBABILISTIC GRAPHICAL MODELS

The focus of this section is how to represent and manage graphical representations of conditional independencies and dependencies in a domain of random variables. We expect the reader to have basic knowledge of conditional and joint probabilities and basic statistics. For a quick review of basic probabilistic and statistical themes, the reader is referred to (DeGroot, 1986).

We will build a graph over a set of random variables by considering each variable as a unique vertex in the graph, and no more vertices are included in the graph. Then, in this graph, the absence of an edge connecting variables A and B represents (marginal or conditional) independence between A and B.

A probabilistic statement of conditional independence is usually denoted as $I(A, B \mid \mathbf{S})$, where A and B are two random variables and S in the condition or context making A and B independent. Usually S is a subset of the rest of the variables in the domain. In the probabilistic framework we have that:

$I(A, B \mid \mathbf{S}) \Leftrightarrow \Pr(A \mid B, \mathbf{S}) = \Pr(A \mid \mathbf{S})$, where $\Pr(A \mid B, \mathbf{S})$ is the conditional probability distribution over variable A given the state of variable B and context $\mathbf{S}$. In a graph, an edge connecting two variables A and B can be directed $(A \rightarrow B)$ or undirected $(A - B)$, where undirected edges are also typically referred to as links. Directed edges can represent a causal relation where A is the cause and B the effect of A (e.g. A represents "rain" and B represents "wet grass"). But we can use that representation without any causal interpretation but only the direct relation between the variables. If we have an undirected link connecting the variables we do not suppose in advance any causal or ordered relation between the variables but only a relation "without direction" between the variables.

We can use several types of graphs to represent conditional independencies in a set $\mathbf{V}$ of random variables. We can have Directed Acyclic Graph (DAG), where we use only directed edges and without directed cycles. We can use only undirected links yielding an Undirected Graph (UG).

It is also possible to use a mixed representation with both kinds of edges, directed an undirected, but again with the constraint of avoiding both directed and semi-directed cycles. Such graphs are usually called Chain Graphs (CG).

In the case of using a DAG, we annotate it with a quantitative part to obtain a (Causal) Bayesian Networks. This model will be the focus of the rest of this chapter.

Bayesian (Causal) Network Models

A Bayesian (causal) Network (BN) consists of a set of a DAG over a set of random variables and a set of local conditional probability distributions. The DAG constitutes the quantitative part of a BN, while the set of local distributions constitute the quantitative part of the BN.

A random variable can be seen as representing a set of mutually exclusive and jointly exhaustive events, e.g. random variable "Rain?" could represent the events "rain" and "no rain". A random variable of this type will be denoted as discrete as it represents a finite (discrete) set of possible events. Another random variable could be "Millimeters of rain today" representing all values in the interval $[0...\infty)$. Such a variable will called continuous as it represents an infinite (and continuous) domain of possible events.

As previously stated, the absence of edges in the DAG of a BN has the semantics of some conditional independence between pairs of variables. In induced sub-graphs over triples of variables, we can have the following 3 important connections in a BN: serial connections $A \rightarrow B \rightarrow C$ or $A \leftarrow B \leftarrow C$; diverging connection $B \leftarrow A \rightarrow C$; and converging connection $B \rightarrow A \leftarrow C$.

In the first case, serial connections, we have a causal chain: A has an influence on B, and B has an influence on C, so A has also influence on C through B. If the value of B is known then the reasoning chain will be blocked, and we will say that A and C are conditional independent given

B. We say that A and C are *d-separated* given B (where "d" stands for "directed"). For example, if we have the following causal network: Smoking $\rightarrow$ Bronchitis $\rightarrow$ Dyspnea (all variables binary "yes"/"no"), and it is known that a person is a smoker, then the belief of both having bronchitis and dyspnea will increase. But once we know that the patient has bronchitis (Bronchitis="yes") then the fact of a person being a smoker will have no influence on our belief of whether this same person is also having dyspnea.

In the second case, diverging connections, the causal chain is that A is the common cause of two effects B and C, that is, knowledge on the state of A will influence our belief of both B and C. Without knowledge on the state of A, knowledge on the state of B will have influence on our belief of the state of A, which in turn will have influence on the other child C, and thus B will have indirect influence on C when the state of A is unknown. When the state of A is known, observing the state of B does not change our belief of C, and thus B is d-separated from C given A. For example the following causal network: Lung Cancer $\leftarrow$ Smoking $\rightarrow$ Bronchitis. Smoking is a common cause of having Lung Cancer and Bronchitis. So if we have a patient with Bronchitis (and no other information is provided) our belief of the patient being a Smoker will increase and therefore so will our belief of the patient having Lung Cancer. But once we know if the patient is a smoker or not, our belief of the patient having Lung Cancer will not be influenced by the observation of the patient having or not having Bronchitis.

In the last case, converging connections, the rules of reasoning are different. We have a common effect of two possible causes, so firstly we will have that A and C are marginally independent. But, once we have knowledge of B (the common child), A and C become conditionally dependent, that is, to know something about A will have influence on our belief of C. A causal example could be two diseases sharing a common symptom. Once the symptom is known, certainty of the absence

Figure 1. An example Bayesian network model and one example of the conditional probability distribution for variable X_5 given variables X_2 and X_4

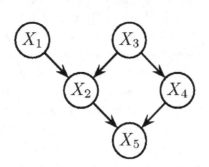

X_2	X_4	$\Pr(X_5\|X_2, X_4)$	
		0	1
0	0	0.21	0.79
1	0	0.65	0.35
0	1	0.99	0.01
1	1	0.45	0.55

of one disease will usually increase our belief of the presence of the second disease. That is, we need an explanation or cause of the observed symptom, and if only two diseases can produce the symptom, by the method of exclusion at least one of those has to be present.

All the sentences of conditional independence codified by a BN can be induced from the concept of d-separation (Jensen, 2001; Pearl, 1988), and we can establish a semantic between the probabilistic conditional independencies found in a model and the graphical conditional independencies found in the graph using d-separation.

The quantitative part of the BN consists of a set of conditional probability distributions. For each variable, the conditional probability of the variable given its parents in the DAG is specified: $\Pr(X \mid pa_G(X))$ where $pa_G(X)$ is the set of parents of X in graph G. We can then recover the joint probability distribution over all random variables **V** in the domain by the product:

$$\Pr(\mathbf{V}) = \prod_{X \in \mathbf{V}} \Pr(X \mid pa_G(X)).$$

When all involved variables are discrete, $\Pr(X \mid pa_G(X))$ is usually represented as an n-dimensional table where n is the number of variables involved. The quantitative part of the BN is then represented as set of such tables (see Figure 1).

LEARNING IN PROBABILISTIC GRAPHICAL MODELS

In previous sections we have described the semantics of Bayesian Network models. In this section we will introduce some of the most popular approaches to automatic construction of PGMs and BNs from data, usually termed "learning". This area has received a lot of attention in the literature, and this section mainly serves as a brief introduction to the area. The interested reader is therefore referred to more comprehensive and exhaustive material for further details, e.g. (Cowell et al., 1999; Jordan, 1998; Koller & Friedman, 2009; Neapolitan, 2003; Spirtes et al., 2000a).

We will briefly introduce the two main branches of learning in BN models. We first present the framework of *score-and-search* learning, and especially focus on the problem of *scoring* a candidate model. We then take a look at the *constraint-based* approach to learning a graphical model from data. It has been shown that the two approaches are based on identical mathematical theory (see (Cowell)) and thus should not be thought of as fundamentally different. However, we still present them separately as they highlight two different ways to think about the problem of learning in probabilistic graphical models, while the result is often the same.

Score-and-Search Based Learning

The approach of *score-and-search* is based on the idea that the problem of learning a PGMs from observational data can be stated as follows:

*"Let **X** be a set of random variables and let P be a joint probability distribution over **X**. Given a database D of samples from P, construct a model M over variables **X** such that the joint probability distribution P^M defined by M is an accurate and "simple" approximation of P."*

Assessing the accuracy of a model M w.r.t. distribution P can be done by using some distance measure for probability distributions, e.g. the Kullback-Leibler divergence. By a "simple" model, we usually understand that the model is not excessively complex and does not contain unnecessary parameters. This principle of parsimony is typical in the development of new scientific theories, and in the setting of learning PGMs from data it has the following additional justification. When parameters are estimated from limited data, our estimates will be more stable for models with few (low-dimensional) parameters than models with many (high-dimensional) parameters. One last justification for preferring "simple" models is the question of inference complexity, as simple models will often allows for tractable inference.

Let us take a closer look at distance measures, and in particular the Kullback-Leibler (KL) divergence that is a fundamental measure in information theory. For discrete domains it is defined as follows:

$$D_{KL}(P \parallel Q) = \sum_{i \in I} P(i) \log \frac{P(i)}{Q(i)},$$

where P and Q are discrete probability distributions over the same finite discrete domain I. Please note that KL-divergence is non-symmetric (hence, not a metric) and that it is only zero when P and Q are equal. In information theory, KL-divergence is motivated by the fact that it measures the average number of extra bits that must be transmitted when transmitting words from a distribution of words P using a code that is optimal for distribution Q. In our setting, we will let Q be the distribution encoded by the model while P is the distribution from which data was sampled. It is usually the case that P is unknown and only a database of samples from P is available, then the standard approach is to use the empirical distribution PD, where each element in the domain is assigned a probability that is equal to its relative frequency of occurrence in the database, that is $P^D(i) = \frac{N_i}{N}$, where Ni is the number of occurrences of element i in data and N is the size of data, that is $N = \sum_{i \in I} N_i$. Substituting P for P^D and Q for P^M we get:

$$
\begin{aligned}
D_{KL}(P^D \parallel P^M) &= \sum_{i \in I} \frac{N_i}{N}\left(\log\left(\frac{\frac{N_i}{N}}{P^M(i)}\right)\right) \\
&= \sum_{i \in I} \frac{N_i}{N}\left(\log \frac{N_i}{N} - \log(P^M(i))\right) \\
&= -H(P^D) - \frac{1}{N}\sum_{i \in I} N_i \log P^M(i)
\end{aligned}
$$

where $H(P^D)$ is the entropy of the empirical distribution of data D. The sums are over all possible instances, but in an implementation one would iterate over just the unique instances that are actually observed in D, and this set is usually much smaller. Then the term $N^{-1}\sum_{i \in I} N_i \log P^M(i)$ is what is usually called the log-likelihood of data D under model M, and it is clear that given a fixed D maximizing the log-likelihood for model M will result in a minimal KL-divergence.

One strategy for finding a model M that has sufficiently low KL-divergence and at the same time is sufficiently simple consists of enumerating all possible models. This is of course only possible for very small domains or very restricted model types, so the usual approach is to define a search space over the possible models and employ some heuristic search in this space. In order to guide the search, some metric for scoring candidate models must be defined. A usual score is one that combines the above-mentioned two desired properties of accuracy and simplicity, e.g.:

$$S(M, D) = L(D \mid M) - size(M),$$

where $L(D|M)$ is the log-likelihood of data D given model M and $size(M)$ is some measure of complexity of model M. Scoring functions that has the general form of the before-mentioned function S is usually referred to as *penalized likelihood*-scores.

As the number of different DAG structures prohibits exhaustive search over even smaller domains, heuristic approaches are usually employed for finding optimal models. A simple but effective heuristic approach to constructing a simple and accurate BN model is to use hill-climbing in the space of DAG structures searching for a structure with local optimal penalized likelihood score. This can be effectively implemented as penalized likelihood scores most often decompose into local independent factors meaning that computing the score difference between two models that differ only locally (e.g. existence of one edge) only requires a simple local computation. The typical operators are then the addition, removal and reversal of a single edge in the current candidate model until no such operation results in a score improvement.

It is important to mention that some DAG structures are statistically indistinguishable and that we can therefore talk about equivalence classes of DAG models. Two DAGs are equivalent if they entail the same set of independence relations, and many *score-and-search* algorithms guaranteeing optimality relies on the use of a score-equivalent score metric. A score metric is score-equivalent if it guarantees to assign the same score to equivalent DAGs.

Constraint-Based Learning

While the *score-and-search* approach above was focused on finding a simple model that approximated the un-known data-generating distribution, the *constraint-based* approaches sets a somewhat different goal:

"Let $\mathbf{X}$ be a set of discrete random variables and let I be a set of statements of conditional independence over variables $\mathbf{X}$. We then wish to find the graph G that "best" encodes the statements from I."

This goal is somewhat different from the goal in the *score-and-search* based approach, as instead of computing a score from data, we need to estimate the validity of conditional independence statements. We will look at how the validity of such statements can be estimated from data shortly, but for now we will just assume that we have an oracle that answer yes or no to questions of the form "Are X and Y independent given $\mathbf{Z}$?", where X and Y are distinct members of $\mathbf{X}$ and $\mathbf{Z}$ is a subset of $\mathbf{X}$ not containing neither X nor Y. Before devising a strategy for building a model, let us think about in what ways a graph G can try to encode the statements in I. Let Ind(G) be the set of independence relations entailed by graph G and let A($\mathbf{X}$) be the set of all candidate statements of conditional independence that can be formed over the variables X. If I $\subseteq$ Ind(G), that is, all statements of independence that are entailed in graph G are included in I, then we say that G is an I-map (Independence-map) of I. On the other hand, if A(X)-Ind(G) $\subseteq$ A(X)-I, that is, non of the independence statements that are not entailed by G are in I, then we say that G is a D-map (Dependence-map) of I. If G is both an I-map and a D-map of I we say that G is a perfect-map of I. There exists a trivial I-map and D-map for any distribution, namely the empty graph $G^\varnothing$ with no edges that is the trivial D-map of any distribution (as Ind($G^\varnothing$)=A(X)) while the complete graph G^*

is the trivial I-map of any distribution (as Ind(G^*)= $\varnothing$). The trivial maps are usually not interesting, and one will usually search for either a minimal *I-map* or even a *perfect-map*.

If a DAG model that is a *perfect-map* for some set of independence relations I exists, then it can be reconstructed by starting with the full (undirected) graph G^* and iteratively remove edges between pairs of variables that are found to be conditionally independent given some subset of the variables. Here it should be clear that exhaustive search over subsets of even small sets of variables is not tractable as for a set with n elements there exists 2^n different subsets. One typical heuristic is therefore to start with small subsets and including more and more variables until such a set is either found or our subset reaches a max size allowed. Also, because of the Markov Property, it makes sense to search only over subsets of the adjacent variables of the two variables in question (see (Pearl, 1988)). Next, we need to direct the edges. This can be done by first considering all triples of variables $\{X, Y, Z\}$ that induce a sub-graph of the pattern X-Z-Y. If X and Y are not conditionally independent given Z, the edges should be oriented towards Z making a v-structure. After no more v-structures can be found, any remaining undirected edge is directed with arbitrary orientation without 1) introducing a cycle in the graph, nor 2) introducing a new v-structure in the graph. The strategy sketched in the above is what is usually referred to as the PC algorithm by (Spirtes, et al., 2000a).

Finally, to estimate conditional independence from data, statistical tests such as the χ^2-test can be used. For instance, when all variables are discrete, the marginal G^2-statistics for two random variables X_i and X_j is:

$$G_{ij}^2 = 2\sum_{a=0}^{r_i}\sum_{b=0}^{r_j} N_{ab} \log\left(\frac{N_{ab}}{E[N_{ab}|N_a,N_b]}\right)$$
$$= 2\sum_{a=0}^{r_i}\sum_{b=0}^{r_j} N_{ab} \log\left(N\frac{N_{ab}}{N_a N_b}\right),$$

where r_i is the number of discrete states of variable X_i, N_{ab} is the number of joint occurrences of $X_i=a$ and $X_j=b$ in data, N_a is the number of marginal occurrences of $X_i=a$ and N is the size of the data. The expectation $E[N_{ab} \mid N_a, N_b]$ is the expected joint counts given that Xi and Xj are independent and multinomial distributed with the observed marginal counts, so we have $E[N_{ab} \mid N_a, N_b] = N\frac{N_a}{N}\frac{N_b}{N} = \frac{N_a N_b}{N}$. In case the independence is true, the G^2 statistics is distributed as χ^2 with (ri-1)(rj-1) degrees of freedom. Using any statistical package, one can compute the probability that G^2 would be as extreme or more extreme as what was obtained from data and based on this probability one accepts or rejects the hypothesis of independence. Conditional versions of the statistics are straight forwardly derived, for details see (Neapolitan, 2003; Spirtes, et al., 2000a).

APPLICATIONS

Diagnostic Reasoning

Medical diagnosis is the process of determining and/or identifying a possible disease or disorder based upon a set of indirect observations from diagnostic tests. Diagnostic tests, however, generally include some uncertainty in their results. This uncertainty should be taken into consideration upon constructing a diagnostic hypothesis. Bayesian networks offer a natural way to deal with this kind of reasoning with uncertainty.

Formally, the problem is to estimate the most probable disease, D^*, given a set of symptoms, signs and test results, E:

$$D^* = \underset{D}{\operatorname{argmax}} \operatorname{Pr}(D \mid E).$$

Some network-based systems for medical diagnosis have been developed in the past. The MUNIN network (Muscle and Nerve Inference Network) (Andreasen et al., 1987) was one of the first hand-built networks applied to diagnostic. It was used for diagnosis of muscle and nerve diseases through analysis of bioelectrical signals from muscle and nerve tissue. The Pathfinder expert system (Heckerman et al., 1992; Heckerman & Nathwani, 1992) was developed during the early 1990s. The core of the system is a Bayesian Network and it is used to assists surgical pathologists with the diagnosis of lymph-node diseases.

In the last years, a growing number of networks have been developed. In (Antal et al., 2001; Heckerman, et al., 1992) a Bayesian Network is used in order to discriminate between benign and malignant ovarian masses. The network was built from the available prior knowledge from expert and literature in a hybrid way. The developed system allows them to classify 80% of the cases with a low misclassification rate and identify the remaining 20% as hard cases that need special considerations. In (McNaught et al., 2001) the authors develop a Bayesian Network to classify patients into one of three categories associated with lower back pain. Several hand-constructed BN models were considered and finally the authors selected the one that obtained the highest classification rate.

In (Antal et al., 2004), the authors explore the potential of the huge collection of information available on the World Wide Web as prior information for learning Bayesian networks. One of the problems that are often encountered upon learning Bayesian networks for clinical problems is that the available clinical data sets are too small to be exploited. As a consequence, it is usually necessary to extract information from various complementary sources. In the paper of (Antal et al., 2004), techniques developed in the area of information retrieval are used as a basis for finding relationships among variables from the Web. The applicability of these techniques is studied

with the construction of Bayesian networks for the classification of ovarian tumours in patients.

In (Felgaer et al., 2006) the authors used a hybrid method of learning that combines the advantages of the induction techniques of the decision trees (the C4.5 algorithm) with those of Bayesian networks. The authors use a set of standard datasets that include the task of predicting the type of a tumour based on the characteristics or the prediction of a cardiology disease based on symptoms. The results outperform the ones obtained by the C4.5 classifier that was used as baseline.

In (Fischer et al., 2004) the authors investigate network structure learning and probability estimation from mammographic feature data in order to classify breast lesions into different pathological categories. The purpose was classifying breast lesions as benign or malignant and invasive or non-invasive. They utilized the Markov Chain Monte Carlo structure-learning algorithm with the operations of adding, removing or reversing an arc. The learned networks did not perform significantly different than the naive networks.

In (Blanco et al., 2001) the network is constructed in a hybrid way. First, the expert specifies diseases and findings, their interconnections, and specifies marginal and conditional probabilities. Then, the system generates the Bayesian network by adding nodes collecting enhancing and inhibiting factors of each single disease. Next, the conditional probabilities of the nodes are calculated according to the structure.

Parameter learning has also been the focus of the attention of researchers in this area. In (Antal, et al., 2001; Peek, 2001) the authors considered the fact that the assessment of the conditional probability tables (CPT) is often a more difficult task than structural learning. In this work, the parameters are estimated by applying an algorithm that (locally) maximizes entropy when the structure of the network is fixed. Another approach was used in (Nikovski, 2000) to solve the problem of CPT learning when only incomplete statistics are available.

Prognostic Reasoning

Prognostic reasoning in medicine and health-care is a prediction of the likely outcome of an illness. In prognostic reasoning uncertainty is even more predominant than in diagnostic reasoning. Another important feature of prognostic reasoning is the exploitation of knowledge about the evolution of processes over time.

Prognostic Bayesian networks are a recent research topic and studies have focused mainly in the area of oncology. In (Nagl et al., 2006) an objective Bayesian network (Williamson, 2005) was learned in order to help in the prognosis of breast cancer. In this work, the authors had different sources of information: two molecular databases and a study. A Bayesian Network was learned for each one of the sources using the Hugin software (Hugin). Finally they combine the three graphs to form the final network by merging identical variables and integrate the conditional probability tables.

Infectious disease is another of the areas in which prognostic networks have been used. In (Andreassen et al., 1999) a network is used to help in the treatment of patients where bacteria or fungi have been found in the blood. The network is used to calculate a prognosis, dependent on the choice of antibiotics. In (Lucas et al., 2000) a system is developed in order to assist doctors from the University of California, Irvine (UCI) in prescribing antibiotics to patients who are mechanically ventilated and display symptoms and signs possibly related to the development of pneumonia.

Genetics

With the development of microarray technology, a large amount of data related to gene regulation has become available. In this field, Bayesian Networks have received increasing attention as a tool to infer both causal relationships between genes and genetic regulatory networks from such

data (Bernard & Hartemink, 2005; Friedman, Nir, 2004; Friedman, Nir et al., 2000; Spirtes et al., 2000b). There are several reasons that BNs are especially suitable for these purposes (Chen et al., 2006; Spirtes, et al., 2000b):

1. They explicitly relate the DAG model of the causal relations among the gene expression levels to a statistical hypothesis.
2. They implicitly represent many of the different models used so far to deal with this problem.
3. There are already well-developed algorithms for searching for BNs from observational data.
4. They allow explicit modeling of the process by which data are gathered.
5. BNs can handle incomplete or missing data and permit incomplete or uncertain knowledge.

Despite these advantages, BN models must deal with some problems that are inherent to the task of microarray analysis. In (Spirtes, et al., 2000b) a complete review of such problems is given. One of them is that datasets obtained from microarrays usually contain information of thousands of genes, but only from a few (dozens) of subjects. This leads to small sample sizes and, therefore, makes it difficult to estimate reliable models. Another important problem is hidden common causes external to the microarray information, which in some cases are necessary to explain the genetic mechanisms. As these causes cannot be inferred from datasets, algorithms must be capable of dealing with hidden variables or, parts of the Bayesian models must be explicitly modeled. Another problem mentioned in (Spirtes, et al., 2000b) are measurement error, averaging, the distributions used, feedback, and lack of synchronization.

There are some works where standard BN learning techniques are used to detect genetic interactions. In some cases, they learn a simple

Bayesian Network (Chen, et al., 2006), but due to the temporal nature of genetic regulatory networks, it is more common to use dynamic BNs (Bernard & Hartemink, 2005; Göransson & Koski, 2002; Perrin et al., 2003; Zou & Conzen, 2005). Nevertheless, most BN-based algorithms used for genetics are explicitly build for this purpose, and try to deal with the aforementioned problems.

In (Friedman, Nir, et al., 2000), for instance, a specific algorithm is build to find two types of features (Markov relations and order relations) and estimate the confidence of each feature found. In order to deal with the lack of data, this is done through a bootstrapping process as follows:

1. Generate N bootstrap-datasets by sampling with replacement from the original dataset.
2. For each bootstrap-dataset, learn a BN model.
3. Estimate the confidence of each candidate feature as the relative frequency with which it appears in the N learnt BN models.

In the specific setting of (Friedman, Nir, et al., 2000), N=200 and the network is learnt in step 2 by the Sparse Candidate algorithm (Friedman, N. et al., 1999), which is a *search-and-score* algorithm that bounds the search space by limiting the number of possible parents for each variable.

A different approach is followed in (Pournara & Wernisch, 2004), where the goal is to recover a causal structure. This work addresses the problem that when learning BN models from observational data, the resulting structure may be equivalent to many alternative structures, that is, structures that are statistically equivalent and therefore encodes the same independencies. Rather than a single structure, we learn an equivalence class, and some causal relations are therefore undefined. That is, a relation between X and Y is identified, but whether X is the cause of Y or vice versa or the relation is undirected is not clear. By clever use of experimental data where intervention or manipulations of some selected variables has been performed, the equivalence class can be refined and the number of networks which truly reflect data is reduced and more causal relationships can be established. This in turn allows the discarding of causal relations that are not present in data. In this work, this process is done by an iterative process that, at each step, chooses a variable to be manipulated based on the expected loss in size of the resulting equivalence class.

There are some other algorithms which do not aim at discovering relations in a whole set of genes, but focus on one of them, and try to discover those genes which are causally related to it. In (Pena et al., 2005), the aim of the proposed algorithm is to find those genes that depends on a reference gene. In order to do that, the number of genes that mediate in such dependence are limited, and

Table 1. Software packages for learning and/or inference

Software	Models	Learning	Inference	Open source	API	GUI
GeNIe&SMILE	BN and dynamic BN (Discrete/Continuous)	Yes	Yes	Yes	Yes	Yes
SamIam	BN (Discrete)	No*	Yes	No	Yes	Yes
Elvira	BN (Discrete/Continuous)	Yes	Yes	Yes	Yes	Yes
CaMML	BN (Discrete)	Yes	No	No	No	Yes
TETRAD	BN (Discrete/Continuous)	Yes	Yes	Yes	Yes	Yes
Hugin Expert	BN (Discrete/Continuous)	Yes	Yes	No	Yes	Yes
Netica	BN (Discrete/Continuous)	No*	Yes	No	Yes	Yes

*Only parameter learning

a network is built in an iterative process, initially considering the target gene, and then adding parent and children of those genes contained in the network. These are determined by chi-square tests in the discrete case or Fisher's Z tests in the continuous case.

Besides causal relationships between genes, there are other typical problems that can be tackled by means of probabilistic graphical models. One of them is heterogeneity, which is related with the averaging considered above. In some cases, information related to the same phenomena (cancer, for instance) can come from different subtypes (different types of cancer), each one presenting different features at the genetic level. In many cases, it is important to isolate such subtypes when learning the models. However, because of limited data, learned models cannot reflect such heterogeneity. Luckily, due to the fact that graphs representing the genetic process are still sparse, it is possible to use probabilistic models to carry out clustering. Thus, in (Mukherjee & Hill, 2011) heterogeneity is found by using a Sparse Gaussian Markov Random Fields to do L1-penalized network clustering.

AVAILABLE SOFTWARE PACKAGES

In this chapter we have discussed basic principles in learning probabilistic graphical models from data, and we have reviewed some important applications mostly in the field of medicine. For a research project to apply PGMs and their learning to some specific problem under study, it may seem that a lot of novel computer implementation is needed. This is not necessarily the case, as many of the authors of the papers referenced in this chapter offer basic prototype implementations of their algorithms in some conventional programming language free of charge from their webpages, and we encourage the interested reader to explore this option. We also wish to highlight

the following software packages as especially interesting (see Table 1):

- **GeNIe&SMILE**: Developed by the Decision Systems Laboratory at the University of Pittsburgh[1].
- **SamIam**: Developed by the Automated Reasoning group at the University of California[2].
- **Elvira:** Developed by the Elvira consortium that consists of researchers in Graphical Models and Artificial Intelligence at different universities in Spain[3].
- **CaMML:** Developed by the Monash Data Mining Center at Monash University, Australia[4].
- **TETRAD:** Developed by people at the Department of Philosophy at Carnegie Mellon University[5].

As another option, some commercial packages are available, of which the most popular are:

- **Hugin Expert**: Developed by Hugin Expert A/S[6].
- **Netica**: Developed by Norsys Software Corp.[7]

REFERENCES

Andreasen, S., Woldbye, M., Falck, B., & Andersen, S. K. (1987). *MUNIN: A causal probabilistic network for interpretation of electomyographic findings*. Paper presented at the 10th International Joint Conference on Artificial Intelligence, Los Altos, CA.

Andreassen, S., Riekehr, C., Kristensen, B., Schonheyder, H. C., & Leibovici, L. (1999). Using probabilistic and decision-theoretic methods in treatment and prognosis modeling. *Artificial Intelligence in Medicine, 15*(2), 121–134. doi:10.1016/S0933-3657(98)00048-7

Antal, P., Fannes, G., De Smet, F., Vandewalle, J., & De Moor, B. (2001). *Ovarian cancer classification with rejection by Bayesian belief networks.* Paper presented at the European Conference on Artificial Intelligence in Medicine.

Antal, P., Fannes, G., Timmerman, D., Moreau, Y., & De Moor, B. (2004). Using literature and data to learn Bayesian networks as clinical models of ovarian tumors. *Artificial Intelligence in Medicine, 30*(3), 257–281. doi:10.1016/j.artmed.2003.11.007

Bernard, A., & Hartemink, A. J. (2005). Informative structure priors: Joint learning of dynamic regulatory networks from multiple types of data. *Pacific Symposium on Biocomputing. Pacific Symposium on Biocomputing*, (pp. 459-470).

Blanco, R., Larrañaga, P., Inza, I., & Sierra, B. (2001). *Selection of highly accurate genes for cancer classification by estimation of distribution algorithms.* Paper presented at the European Conference on Artificial Intelligence in Medicine, workshop on Bayesian Models in Medicine, Cascais, Portugal.

Chen, X. W., Anantha, G., & Wang, X. (2006). An effective structure learning method for constructing gene networks. *Bioinformatics (Oxford, England), 22*(11), 1367–1374. doi:10.1093/bioinformatics/btl090

Cowell, R. G. (2001). Conditions under which conditional independence and scoring methods lead to identical selection of Bayesian network models. *Proceedings of the Seventeenth Conference on Uncertainty in Artificial Intelligence* (pp. 91-97). Morgan Kaufmann Publishers.

Cowell, R. G., Dawid, A. P., Lauritzen, S. L., & Spiegelhalter, D. J. (1999). *Probabilistic networks and expert systems.* Springer.

DeGroot, M. H. (1986). *Probability and statistics.* Addison-Wesley.

Felgaer, P., Britos, P., & García-Martínes, R. (2006). Predition in health domain using Bayesian networks optimization based on induction learning techniques. *International Journal of Modern Physics C, 17*(3), 447–455. doi:10.1142/S0129183106008558

Fischer, E. A., Lo, J. Y., & Markey, M. K. (2004). *Bayesian networks of BI-RADS TM descriptors for breast lesion classification.* Paper presented at the 26th Annual International Conference of the IEEE EMBS.

Friedman, N. (2004). Inferring cellular networks using probabilistic graphical models. *Science, 303*(5659), 799–805. doi:10.1126/science.1094068

Friedman, N., Iftach, N., & Pe'er, D. (1999). Learning Bayesian network structure from massive datasets: The "sparse candidate" algorithm. *Proceedings of the Fifteenth Conference on Uncertainty in Artificial Intelligence.* Morgan Kaufmann Publishers.

Friedman, N., Linial, M., Nachman, I., & Pe'er, D. (2000). Using Bayesian networks to analyze expression data. *Journal of Computational Biology, 7*, 601–620. doi:10.1089/106652700750050961

Göransson, L., & Koski, T. (2002). *Using a dynamic Bayesian network to learn genetic interactions.* Stockholm, Sweden: Royal institute of Technology.

Heckerman, D. E., Horvitz, E. J., & Nathwani, B. N. (1992). Toward normative expert systems: Part I. The Pathfinder project. *Methods of Information in Medicine, 31*(2), 90–105.

Heckerman, D. E., & Nathwani, B. N. (1992). Toward normative expert systems: Part II. Probability-based representations for efficient knowledge acquisition and inference. *Methods of Information in Medicine, 31*(2), 106–116.

Hugin. (2011). *Hugin expert.* Retrieved from http://www.hugin.com

Jensen, F. V. (2001). *Bayesian networks and decision graphs.* Springer. Jordan, M. I. (Ed.). (1998). *Learning in graphical models.* The MIT Press.

Koller, D., & Friedman, N. (2009). *Probabilistic graphical models: Principles and techniques.* The MIT Press.

Lucas, P. J., de Bruijn, N. C., Schurink, K., & Hoepelman, A. (2000). A probabilistic and decision-theoretic approach to the management of infectious disease at the ICU. *Artificial Intelligence in Medicine, 19*(3), 251–279. doi:10.1016/S0933-3657(00)00048-8

McNaught, K., Clifford, S., Vaughn, M., Fogg, A., & Foy, M. (2001). *A Bayesian belief network for lower back pain diagnosis.* Paper presented at the European Conference on Artificial Intelligence in Medicine.

Mukherjee, S., & Hill, S. M. (2011). Network clustering: probing biological heterogeneity by sparse graphical models. *Bioinformatics (Oxford, England), 27*(7), 994–1000. doi:10.1093/bioinformatics/btr070

Nagl, S., Williams, M., & Williamson, J. (2006). Objective Bayesian nets for systems modelling and prognosis in breast cancer. In Holmes, D., & Jain, L. C. (Eds.), *Innovations in Bayesian networks: Theory and applications.* Springer Verlag. doi:10.1007/978-3-540-85066-3_6

Neapolitan, R. E. (2003). *Learning Bayesian networks.* Prentice Hall.

Nikovski, D. (2000). Constructing Bayesian networks for medical diagnosis from incomplete and partially correct statistics. *IEEE Transactions on Knowledge and Data Engineering, 12,* 509–516. doi:10.1109/69.868904

Pearl, J. (1988). *Probabilistic reasoning in intelligent systems: Networks of plausible inference.* Morgan Kaufmann Publishers.

Peek, N. (2001). *The notion of diagnosis in decision-theoretic planning.* Paper presented at the Eorupean Conference on Artificial Intelligence in Medicine Workshop on Bayesian Models in Medicine.

Peña, J. M., Bjorkegren, J., & Tegner, J. (2005). Growing Bayesian network models of gene networks from seed genes. *Bioinformatics (Oxford, England), 21*(Suppl 2), ii224–ii229. doi:10.1093/bioinformatics/bti1137

Perrin, B. E., Ralaivola, L., Mazurie, A., Bottani, S., Mallet, J., & d'Alche-Buc, F. (2003). Gene networks inference using dynamic Bayesian networks. *Bioinformatics (Oxford, England), 19*(Suppl 2), ii138–ii148. doi:10.1093/bioinformatics/btg1071

Pournara, I., & Wernisch, L. (2004). Reconstruction of gene networks using Bayesian learning and manipulation experiments. *Bioinformatics (Oxford, England), 20*(17), 2934–2942. doi:10.1093/bioinformatics/bth337

Spirtes, P., Glymour, C., & Scheines, R. (2000a). *Causation, prediction, and search.* The MIT Press.

Spirtes, P., Glymour, C., & Scheines, R. (2000b). *Constructing Bayesian network models of gene expression networks from microarray data.* Paper presented at the The Atlantic Symposium on Computational Biology, Genome Information Systems & Technology.

Williamson, J. (2005). Objective Bayesian nets. In Artemov, S. (Eds.), *We will show them! Essays in honour of Dov Gabbay* (pp. 713–730). College Publications.

Zou, M., & Conzen, S. D. (2005). A new dynamic Bayesian network (DBN) approach for identifying gene regulatory networks from time course microarray data. *Bioinformatics (Oxford, England)*, *21*(1), 71–79. doi:10.1093/bioinformatics/bth463

ENDNOTES

[1]   GeNIe&SMILE webpage: http://genie.sis.pitt.edu/

[2]   SamIam webpage: http://reasoning.cs.ucla.edu/samiam/

[3]   Elvira webpage: http://www.ia.uned.es/~elvira/index-en.html

[4]   CaMML webpage: http://www.datamining.monash.edu.au/software/camml/

[5]   TETRAD webpage: http://www.phil.cmu.edu/projects/tetrad/index.html

[6]   Hugin webpage: http://www.hugin.com/

[7]   Netica webpage: http://www.norsys.com/

Chapter 16

Natural Language Processing and Machine Learning Techniques Help Achieve a Better Medical Practice

Oana Frunza
University of Ottawa, Canada

Diana Inkpen
University of Ottawa, Canada

ABSTRACT

This book chapter presents several natural language processing (NLP) and machine learning (ML) techniques that can help achieve a better medical practice by means of extracting relevant medical information from the wealth of textual data. The chapter describes three major tasks: building intelligent tools that can help in the clinical decision making, tools that can automatically identify relevant medical information from the life-science literature, and tools that can extract semantic relations between medical concepts. Besides introducing and describing these tasks, methodological settings accompanied by representative results obtained on real-life data sets are presented.

INTRODUCTION

Since its early beginnings, artificial intelligence research directed its interests towards the medical field. Expert systems are among the first applications that merged the two fields. Since the early 70's, when expert systems like MYCIN[1] were built, a lot has changed. Living in an information explosion era, a big emphasis is currently made on automatic ways to extract relevant medical information form huge amounts of various data types (data mining). Textual data is one of the most common ways of representing medical information and, with the recent trend of using digital medical records, this type of data becomes a valuable resource for both the medical and the computational linguistics field.

DOI: 10.4018/978-1-4666-1803-9.ch016

Achieving a superior medical practice most often correlates with having medical practitioners use automatic tools. This chapter presents work done on three major tasks in which the computerized world can help: assisted clinical decision making for obesity-related diseases, identification of relevant medical information for building systematic reviews on medical topics, and identification of important relations between medical concepts like disease, treatments, and tests.

The first task that we address, assisted clinical decision-making, is motivated by the fact that disease identification and profiling represents a challenging task in the medical domain. A valuable source of information for understanding the way medical conditions appear, progresses, and get cured is represented by clinical narratives. Besides scientific discoveries that get published in technical journals, new information that can be extracted from medical records becomes accessible to the research community, facilitating progress both in medicine and in computational linguistics. The fact that reliable and relevant information can help solve these paramount tasks motivated us to use natural language processing techniques combined with machine learning tools to solve these tasks.

Since obesity has become a major medical problem nowadays, we decided to focus our work on building clinical decision support systems capable to automatically identify obesity-related diseases in clinical data. The benefits of having such tools are in assisting with the clinical decision process (the believed rate of diagnostic error is between 15-20%), in identifying groups of patients (e.g., patients that belong to a specific type of disease, high-risk patients, patients suitable to participate in a specic clinical trial, etc.), and in extracting information that can be useful for disease prevention and therapy.

The second research issue that we address in this current work is the identification of relevant medical information from huge amounts of data. Identifying relevant information from the life-science literature can help in identifying the best medical evidence for a certain medical problem and, more importantly, can help in the process of building systematic reviews – summaries of research discoveries which represent fundamental tools for decision making in an evidence-based medicine practice. From a computerized point of view, this task entails a text-classication approach that automatically identifies relevant data to a specific medical problem. We focused our work on identifying relevant information that answers the issue of efficiency of medical care for elderly people.

The third task which we address in this current work is focused on identifying relations between medical concepts in technical and clinical data. Three types of concepts: diseases, treatments, and medical tests are included in the list of eight semantic relations that we try to automatically identify. The outcome of this task can help in the development of medical ontologies, question-answering systems on medical problems, in the creation of clinical trials, in stratifying patients by disease susceptibility and response to therapy, in reducing the size, duration, and cost of clinical trials, and ultimately in leading to the development of new treatments, diagnostics, and prevention therapies.

BACKGROUND

From the wealth of relevant research that has been done in the biomedical domain, we are going to present only representative work focused on the tasks that we address. Research on clinical data is less represented in the literature, due to lack of access to data.

The research endeavors that we followed in order to build a clinical decision support system that can assist in the diagnosis of obesity-related diseases builds on previous research that has been done on this topic. Some of the representative work on this topic uses lexical and domain knowledge resources: additional lexical resources such as precompiled dictionaries of disease, symptom, treatment, and medication terms, in order to find sentence matches with the training data (Yang, Spasic, Keane, & Nenadic, 2009), rule-based classifiers (Solt, Tikk, Gal, & Kardkovacs, 2009), regular expressions with additional keywords (Ware, Mullet & Jagannathan, 2009), and decision trees classifiers with features that included signs, symptoms, and medication names related to each disease (Patrick & Asgari, 2008). Chapman, Fizman, Chapman & Haugfound (2001) found that expert rules performed better than Bayesian networks or decision trees at automatically identifying chest X-ray reports that support acute bacterial pneumonia.

Pure machine learning approaches have also been used (Ambert & Cohen, 2009), (DeShazo & Turner, 2008). The machine learning systems use a combination of lexical, semantic, and domain specific knowledge. Uzuner, Zhang & Sibanda (2009) present the full overview of these systems.

The general observations regarding the work that has been done for the task of identifying obesity-related diseases in full discharge summaries is that the lexical knowledge is a valuable resource for both the rule-based systems and the machine learning-based systems. While rule-based systems are hard to build since they require human effort, the machine learning ones are at times more suitable to use.

The task of identifying relevant information to a medical problem from the large amounts of available published research is a natural application of the well-developed area of automatic text classification. Our ultimate goal is to identify relevant articles that will be part of a summary of research on a certain medical problem – a systematic review. Prior efforts to exploit text classification techniques for such reviews have been limited. The research done by Aphinyanaphongs & Aliferis (2005) appears to be the first such attempt. In that paper, the authors experimented with a variety of text classification techniques,

using the data derived from the ACP Journal Club[2] as their corpus. They found that support vector machines (SVM) was the best classifier according to a variety of measures, but could not provide a comprehensive explanation as to how SVM decides whether a given scientific abstract is relevant or not. The authors emphasized the difficulties related to the predominance of one class in the datasets (i.e., the number of relevant abstracts is only a small portion of the total number of abstracts), along with the difficulty of achieving both good recall and good precision. Further work was done by Cohen, Hersh, Peterson, & Yen (2006), who focused mostly on the elimination of non-relevant documents.

The third problem that we tackle because we believe that it can improve the medical practice is the automatic identification of relations between medical concepts. We have addressed this task both in technical published data and in clinical data. We decided to focus on both, types of data since each of them present research challenges. Medical technical data is challenging due to its vast vocabulary and due to lack of tools adapted to this domain. Clinical data is known to represent a challenge to natural language processing techniques due to high number of grammatical errors, ambiguous abbreviations, highly versatile vocabulary, etc.

There are three major approaches used in literature of extracting relations between entities: co-occurrences analysis, rule-based approaches, and statistical methods. The co-occurrences methods are simple and based only on occurrences of two entities in the same text. These methods are mostly based on lexical knowledge – words in context, and even though they tend to obtain good levels of recall, their precision is low. Good representative examples for this method were presented by Jenssen, Laegreid, Komorowski, & Hovig (2001) and Stapley & Benoit (2000).

Rule-based approaches have been used in the biomedical literature for solving relation extraction tasks. The main sources of information used by this technique are either syntactic: part-of-speech (POS) and syntactic structures; or semantic information in the form of fixed patterns that contain words that trigger a certain relation. The main drawback of a method based on rules is the fact that it requires a lot of human-expert effort. Representative work done using syntactic rule-based approaches for relation extraction is presented by: Thomas, Milward, Ouzounis, Pulman, & Carroll (2000), Yakushiji, Tateisi, Miyao, & Tsujii (2001), and Leroy, Chen, & Martinez (2003). A major drawback for semantic rule-based approaches is the fact that the lexicon changes from domain to domain and new rules need to be created each time.

Statistical methods are the ones that are most used in the community. They do not require human effort to build rules. These rules are automatically extracted by the learning algorithm when using statistical approaches to solve various tasks. Taking a statistical approach to solve the relation extraction problem, the most-used representation technique is bag-of-words. It uses the words in context to create a feature vector (Donaldson et al., 2003) (Mitsumori, Murata, Fukuda, Doi, & Doi, 2006). Other researchers combined the bag-of-words features with other sources of information like POS (Bunescu & Mooney, 2005). Giuliano, Lavelli, & Lorenza (2006) used two sources of information: whole sentences in which the relation appears and the local context where the entities are present, and showed that simple representation techniques bring good results.

Statistical methods used on clinical data to infer relations between medical entities were used by Roberts, Rink & Harabagiu (2010). Their system uses an SVM classifier for a 9-class classification task: the 8 relations in question and an additional one that shows that the pair of concepts stands in no relation.

A semi-supervised system that uses maximum entropy (ME) classifiers to infer relations was proposed by Bruijn, Cherry, Kiritchenko, Martin & Zhu (2010). The types of features they used

are based on parse trees information, Pointwise Mutual Information (PMI) between the concepts in a pair, and domain-specific resources. Grouin et al. (2010) used a systems that is a combination of rule-based and SVM classification techniques.

Our work differs from the ones mentioned above, since we use different representation techniques in combination with suitable classifiers.

TEXT MINING HELPS SOLVE MEDICAL PROBLEMS

In this section, we present in more details the three medical applications that we focus on. All methods that we propose are based on data analysis, more precisely textual-data analysis. Our work is guided by the fact that intelligent data analysis, in particular textual analysis, can help in solving important problems in the medical field. As solutions for the problems that we address, we propose domain-specific natural language processing techniques in combination with suitable machine learning algorithms.

Machine Learning, a field of empirical studies, gained its momentum in various domains due to its power of applicability. Off-the-shelf implementations of various algorithms are ready to be deployed to solve a large spectrum of computational problems. The real gain of using ML techniques, as viable solution for solving problems, stands in the ability to identify the right algorithm and the right data representation for a particular task and domain. The data and the way it is used in the process of training ML models represent the key factors that drive the strength of machine learning. The way the data is represented and fed to the algorithm is a fundamental step in achieving good results.

We have to bear in mind that there are at least two challenges that can be encountered while working with ML techniques. One is to find the most suitable model for prediction. The ML field offers a suite of predictive models (algorithms) that can be used and deployed. The task of finding the suitable one relies heavily on empirical studies and knowledge expertise.

The second one is to find a good data representation that undergoes feature engineering steps, since features strongly influence the performance. Identifying the right and sufficient features to represent the data, both when a huge and a small amount of data is available, represents a crucial aspect of research.

Using textual and domain specific representations in combination with suitable learning tools, we build solutions for the problems we address.

Clinical Decisions Support Systems Focused on Obesity-Related Problems

Disease profiling represents a challenging task that can benefit from the tremendous amount of available information. A valuable source of information for understanding the way medical conditions appear, progresses, and get cured is represented by clinical narratives. Besides scientific discoveries that get published in technical journals, new information that can be extracted from medical records becomes accessible to the research community, facilitating progress both in medicine and computational linguistics.

The task that we address is to build reliable models that can identify obesity-related diseases in clinical records. These types of systems, besides the fact that they can represent tremendous help in clinical decision making, can also help in clinical trials preparations by identifying past and current records that contain mentions of specific diseases.

The hypothesis that guides our research is that intelligent data analysis based on suitable natural language processing and machine learning techniques can build automatic models able to predict the presence of diseases in medical records. We propose models that are fully supervised and that use a variety of features that combine lexical, semantic, and domain-specific knowledge.

Identification of Relevant Articles for Building Systematic Reviews

Systematic reviews represent summaries of research on different medical topics and bring the best medical evidence to medical researchers and practitioners. For the evidence-based medicine practice they represent fundamental tools for decision making. The reviews contain relevant and high-quality research published on life-science topics. The process of building these reviews is a tedious process that requires human knowledge to curate thousands and thousands of documents and identify which articles are relevant and which are not. Automatic means that can help in the process of identifying articles to be included in the review would facilitate the human effort and reduce the time and cost of building the reviews. By having systems that are capable to automatically or semi-automatically identify relevant published data, the time a medical practitioner will need to spend to find this type of data will be tremendously reduced.

Summaries of the latest discoveries bring cutting-edge information to the desk of healthcare providers, and by building and using these types of tools we could transform the medical practice into a better-informed care.

Compared to previous research, our work is focused on developing a classifier for systematic review preparation, relying on characteristics of the data and on the task in question, by taking into account the following problems that need to be considered when using machine learning techniques.

- **Distribution of the Data**: In most systematic reviews, the number of relevant documents is much smaller than the number of non-relevant documents creating a class imbalance which can cause problems for the machine-learning algorithms.
- **Noise**: When reviewers are not sure from an abstract whether the article is relevant, a final decision will be made during the

second screening process where the entire document is reviewed. This "benefit of the doubt" approach will affect the quality of the data used to train the classifier, since a certain amount of "noise" is introduced, in that abstracts that are in fact non-relevant are often labeled as relevant in the first screening process.

- **Labeling Cost**: The labeling process is expensive both in human effort and money, so a key goal of the machine learning approach is to reduce the human effort required.
- **Misclassification Cost**: If an abstract does not pass the first level of screening, the article will not be examined for information extraction during the second level of screening. Failure to identify a relevant abstract in the first screening process can have a profoundly negative impact on the validity of systematic review results (Cohen, Hersh, Peterson, & Yen, 2006).
- **Representation**: Due to the vast number of abstracts in the medical domain repositories, the machine learning representation must take into account the huge number of possible attributes.

Relation Identification between Medical Concepts

As mentioned before, we believe that intelligent data analysis can help identify important medical relations that exist between medical concepts. The outcome of this task can help achieve a better medical practice by identifying better treatments for a particular medical case when looking at other cases that followed a similar clinical path, can help in the creation of clinical trials Groopman (2007), in stratifying patients by disease susceptibility and response to therapy by reducing the size, duration, and cost of clinical trials leading to development of new treatments, diagnostics, and prevention therapies. From the computational linguistics point

of view, the outcome of such tools can be used for developing medical ontologies and question-answering systems focused on medical problems.

The objective of this work is to show which natural language processing techniques, what type of textual representation, and which machine learning techniques are suitable to use for identifying and classifying medical relations in short texts. We focus on disease, treatment, and tests relation identification and classification. We believe that tools capable of identifying reliable information in the medical domain stand as building blocks for a healthcare system that is up-to-date with the latest discoveries.

The three problems that we decided to address are just a few of the multitudes of tasks that intelligent data analysis can help the medical field with. The models that we propose use a combination of reliable and domain-specific features in combination with suitable classifiers that take into account the specifics of the task.

Textual Representation and Classification Techniques

In this subsection we present the standard and customized representation techniques that we used.

The Bag-of-Words (BOW) representation is commonly used for text classification tasks. It is a representation in which features are chosen among the words that are present in the training data. Selection techniques are often used in order to identify the most suitable words as features, especially when we deal with very large amounts of data. We used as features in our experiments all the words extracted from the training data that are delimited by spaces and simple punctuation marks such as: (,), [,], ., ' . When we deal with large amounts of data we remove words that appear less than three times in the training data. After the feature space is identified, each training and test instance is mapped to this feature representation by giving values to each feature for a certain instance. Two most common feature value representations

Figure 1. Example of MetaMap system output

Inhibition	Inhibition	NN	B-NP	O
of	of	IN	B-PP	O
NF-kappaB	NF-kappaB	NN	B-NP	B-protein
activation	activation	NN	I-NP	O
reversed	reverse	VBD	B-VP	O
the	the	DT	B-NP	O
anti-apoptoctic	anti-apoptoctic	JJ	I-NP	O
effect	effect	NN	I-NP	O
of	of	IN	B-PP	O
isochamaejasmin	isochamaejasmin	NN	B-NP	O

for BOW representation are: binary feature values or frequency feature values. The feature values for the BOW representation should be chosen by taking into consideration the characteristics of the data. For example, when we used short texts we used a frequency value representation. We decided to use frequency values, because we believe that, if in a short text a feature appears more than once, it suggests that it is important, and also because the difference between a binary value representation and a frequency value representation is not large. When we work with long texts, we use binary representations, since they showed to be more reliable due to the huge amounts of data.

Manning and Shutze (1999) present a good overview of different representation techniques used for text classification.

Medical and biomedical concepts features are similar to multi-word expressions. Using these concepts, features are represented by a sequence of words. Unified Medical Language System[3] (UMLS) is a knowledge source developed at the U.S. National Library of Medicine (NLM) that contains a metathesaurus, a semantic network, and a specialist lexicon for the biomedical domain. The metathesaurus is organized around concepts and meanings; it links alternative names and views of the same concept and identifies useful relationships between different concepts. We extracted UMLS features using the MetaMap[4] tool.

Figure 1 presents an example of the output of the MetaMap system for the phrase "*to an increased risk*." The information present in the brackets, "Qualitative Concept, Quantitative Concept" for the candidate with the fit function value 861 is the concept used as feature in the UMLS representation.

For identifying biomedical concepts, we used the Genia[5] tagger tool. The tagger analyzes English sentences and outputs the base forms, part-of-speech tags, chunk tags, and named entity tags. The tagger is specifically tuned for biomedical texts, such as Medline[6] abstracts.

Additional representation features are based on syntactic information, such as verb-phrases and noun-phrases extracted from the textual data. We used the Genia tagger to extract these features.

Figure 2 presents an example of the output of the Genia tagger for the sentence: "*Inhibition of NF-kappaB activation reversed the anti-apoptotic effect of isochamaejasmin..*" The tag O stands for Outside, B for Beginning, and I for Inside.

As classification algorithms, we used an SVM implementation, a Naïve Bayes classifier specially tuned for imbalanced-data sets named Complement Naïve Bayes, and the AdaBoost classifier, all from the same Weka[7] package. These classifiers are well-known in the literature, to work well with sparse data sets and imbalanced class distribution and this is why we chose to work with them. The default settings of the classifiers

Figure 2. Example of Genia tagger output

Meta Candidates (6)
861 Risk [Qualitative Concept, Quantitative Concept]
694 Increased (Increased (qualifier value)) [Functional Concept]
623 Increase (Increase (qualifier value)) [Functional Concept]
601 Acquired (Acquired (qualifier value)) [Temporal Concept]
601 Obtained (Obtained (attribute)) [Functional Concept]
588 Increasing (Increasing (qualifier value)) [Functional Concept]

---

were used. We decided not to tune the parameters, since we want to better stress the importance of the methodology rather than the parameter tuning. We want to show that a suitable representation technique that takes into account the specifics and the domain of the tasks, in combination with reliable classification algorithms, can lead to a winning solution.

Methodology and Results

In this subsection, we present the specific methods and the results for each of the there tasks.

Identification of Obesity-Related Diseases

In the process of building our obesity-related decision support system, we use the data set distributed in the research challenges organized by the Informatics for Integrating Biology and the Bedside (i2b2), a National Center for Biomedical Computing[8]. In the second research challenge that took place in 2008, we participated in the task of identification of obese-related diseases (Frunza & Inkpen, 2008).

The data set that we used in this task consists in discharge summaries of patients, annotated with obesity and 15 related diseases, released in the second i2b2 challenge. The records were extracted from the Research Patient Data Repository (RPDR) using a query that drew records of patients who were evaluated for either obesity or diabetes. Each of the records in the data includes

from zero to more than ten occurrences of the stem "obes." Each patient record went through a process of de-identification.

The records were annotated at the document-level with obesity information and its co-morbidities. Two types of annotation were supplied for each record: *textual annotation* - judgments made only on texts, and *intuitive annotation* - judgments made on implicit information in the narrative text (e.g., computing the BMI (Body Mass Index) is considered part of an intuitive annotation process).

For the textual judgments, the possible classes are: "Y" that stands for "Yes, the patient has the co-morbidity," "N" that stands for "No, the patient does not have the co-morbidity," "Q" that stands for "Questionable whether the patient has the co-morbidity," "U" that stands for "the co-morbidity is not mentioned in the record." For the intuitive annotations, only the "Y," "N," and "Q" class labels are used; "U" is irrelevant as an intuitive judgment.

The data set was divided 60%-40% split between training and test sets. In average, 700 instances were used for training each class in the textual data set, and around 600 in the intuitive data set.

The representation techniques that we use in this task were BOW features after we remove features that appear less than three times in the training data, UMLS concepts, and noun-phrases that were extracted from each patient record. As classification algorithms, CNB and AdaBoost are used, with AdaBoost obtaining superior results.

Results

Table 1 and Table 2 present the results on the test data for the there representation techniques, when using the AdaBoost as classifier. We report recall, precision, and F-measure. For a classification with more than two classes, F-measures can be computed in two ways. Macro F-measure represents the per-class averaged F-measures, while the micro F-measure is calculated per overall instances and not per individual classes. We report macro F-measure because it is more commonly used.

Looking at the results obtained on the test set both for the intuitive and textual annotations, the simple BOW representation outperformed the other two representations. A possible improvement over the current results might have been obtained with a combination of representations. A possible explanation for the good performance of the BOW representation can be the fact that clinical and medical texts, in general, use a highly-versatile vocabulary. The same medical concept can be lexicalized in many ways. Due to this factor, the noun-phrase representation suffers from a high-sparsity problem, which in the end gets reflected in the algorithms' performance.

The UMLS concepts that get identified in the text are mapped into high-level medical concepts, giving rise to a representation that finds it hard to discriminate between classes. Due to the nature of the text, the MetaMap tool tends to annotate abbreviations with medical concepts, and in this way a lot of false positive annotations are part of the feature space.

When identifying obesity-disease mentions in clinical data, lexical features that capture the mention of the diseases performed well. Features that capture the lexical unit of a particular disease, e.g., "obese," "gout," etc., represent strong indicators for the classifiers that a particular disease is present.

Table 1. Results for the textual annotations

Features	Precision (%)	Recall (%)	F-Measure (%)
BOW	96.35	45.37	45.79
UMLS	94.45	43.39	43.84
NPs	83.03	31.96	32.24

Table 2. Results for the intuitive annotations

Features	Precision (%)	Recall (%)	F-Measure (%)
BOW	94.59	60.21	60.69
UMLS	92.60	56.74	57.76
NPs	78.86	43.82	44.33

Identification of Relevant Articles for Building Systematic Reviews

For identifying topic related medical abstracts, we used as data a set of 47,274 MEDLINE[9] abstracts that are part of a systematic review done by McMaster University's Evidence-Based Practice Center. The initial set of abstracts was collected using a set of Boolean search queries that were run for the specific topic of the systematic review which was "the dissemination strategy of health care services for elderly people of age 65 and over." A collection of 47,274 abstracts were obtained. 20,000 are used for the training data set and the remaining 27,274 for the test set.

Each of this abstracts were annotated by a set of reviewers that had to answer questions that helped identify which abstracts are relevant to the topic of the review. This process can happen several times, each time the remaining abstracts are questioned using a more detailed topic-specific set of questions. Both in the training and test data the class distribution is 1:5.6. The number of irrelevant abstracts retrieved from the Boolean query is much larger than the number of relevant abstracts.

Table 3. Representative results for identifying abstracts relevant to a medical problem

Global Method	Recall (%)	Precision (%)	F-measure (%)	Human-Machine Recall/Precision (%)
BOW	65.3	34.9	45.5	87.7/17.8
UMLS	67.8	23.8	35.2	88.6/16.9
BOW+UMLS	65.9	34.8	45.5	87.7/17.8
Domain-specific method				
BOW	77.2	24.1	36.8	91.6/17.0
UMLS	63.2	21.5	32.0	86.6/16.4
BOW+UMLS	79.7	23.4	36.2	92.7/17.0

For this task, we used two methods: one that it is a straight-forward global machine-learning application, and one that takes into consideration the specific protocol of building systematic reviews. The latter uses more domain- and task-specific information by means of the questions that the human judges have to answer in order to determine the relevance of an abstract. More details about the methodology used can be found in Frunza, Inkpen, Matwin, Klement & O'Blenis (2011).

For both methods we used BOW, UMLS, and a combination of both features as representation techniques. The CNB classifier obtains the most promising results.

Results

Table 3 presents representative results for the task of identifying relevant abstracts for building systematic reviews. The first set of results is representative for the global method, a method where the models were trained on the whole training data and evaluated on the test data. The first column shows what representation technique that it is used. For all the experiments, the CNB classifiers are used.

The second set of results represents the best results that we obtained with our second technique, the one that used the specific questions that are asked in the systematic review protocol. In this case, the model is an ensemble of classifiers that

are trained only the part of the training data that contains answers to a particular question. These parts correspond to particular answers that are given to some of the questions to which reviewers need to answer for deciding the relevance of the article to the systematic review.

Besides the standard evaluation measures that we report, we also present results for a possible scenario where the automatic model works together with a human judge to identify relevant abstracts.

The global method achieved good results in terms of precision, but its recall level was low and significantly outperformed by the per-question method. Overall, the best results are obtained by the second method including BOW representation with or without UMLS features. When we combine the features, we merge together the BOW and UMLS features to create the feature vector, in order to represent each instance.

When we combined the automatic classification system with one human reviewer, we obtained a major improvement in recall. In order to combine the classifier with the human judge, we take the classification output of the classifier and the human decision for a particular article, and decide the final inclusion or exclusion of an article. If the two decisions are in contradiction, and the human judge decides for inclusion, we consider the reviewer's decision to be the final one. The relative low level of precision is due to the fact that we work with abstracts and not with entire documents; therefore not enough information is available from some abstracts.

Relation Identification between Medical Concepts

For the task of identifying relations between medical concepts, we used both technical data, in form of sentences extracted from Medline articles, and clinical data, sentences extracted from discharge summaries of patients. The technical data that we used is the data set released by Rosario & Hearst (2004). The data consists in sentences that contain mentions of diseases and treatments and are annotated with 8 semantic relations. Our work is mostly focused on the three most represented and most important relations. Compared to this previous work, our research is focused on different representation techniques, different classification models, and most importantly in obtaining improved results with less annotated data.

For clinical data, we used the data set released in the forth i2b2 competition. The data set is annotated with 8 semantic relations between medical problems, treatments, and tests. Our work is focused on all 8 relations, even though some are very scarce in the data, since they all address important relations between these medical concepts.

For technical data, we focused our work on three most important relations: *Cure, Prevent, and Side Effect*. A total number of 616 sentences constituted the training data set, and another 307 the test set. The *Prevent* and *Side Effect* classes were highly under-represented, less than 1% in both the training and the test data set. Table 4 presents the distribution of the classes in the technical data set.

On clinical data, there were 8 relations, depending on the types of concepts involved. Table 5 presents the relations and their distribution in the data.

The models that obtained the best results on technical data for three relations of interest used a combination of BOW, verb phrases, UMLS, and biomedical concepts in combination with probabilistic classifiers Naïve Bayes and CNB. Similar results were obtained by the SVM classifiers as well. Table 6 presents F-measure results for the three classes of interest on the technical data. We achieve 100% F-measure for the *Prevent* class, and in the high 80's and 90's for the other two classes. More details about the methods that we used can be found in Frunza, Inkpen, and Tran (2011).

The methods that we used on the clinical data followed the same guidelines as the ones we used on the technical data: rich data-representation techniques in combination with suitable classifiers. On the clinical data, the task was significantly harder since one sentence can have more than two concepts, which was not the case with the technical data, and these concepts can exist in more than one of the 8 relations or in no relation. Besides the types of features that we mentioned in the previous sections, for these experiments we added more domain-specific information by using ConText (Chapman, Chu & Dowling, 2007), a system that provides three types of contextual information for a medical condition: *Negation, Temporality,* and *Experiencer.* We also added information about the correlation and the cosine distance between a pair of concepts and the corpus of one of the existing relations. We used the Semantic vectors[10] tool.

In the experiments that we performed on clinical data, we noticed that when using the entire sentence as an instance, as we did on the technical data, the results are not satisfactory. On technical data, we had only one single pair of concepts in a sentence, while in the clinical data, sentences there was more than one pair per sentence. The best results on clinical data were obtained when we used as instance the context, the words be-

Table 4. Medical technical data set

	Training Test			
	Positive	**Negative**	**Positive**	**Negative**
Cure	554	531	276	266
Prevent	42	531	21	266
SideEffect	20	531	10	266

Table 5. The number of sentences of each relation in the training and test data sets for the clinical data

Relation	Training	Test
PIP (medical problem indicates medical problem)	1239	1,989
TeCP (test conducted to investigate medical problem)	303	588
TeRP (test reveals medical problem)	1734	3,033
TrAP (treatment is administered for medical problem)	1423	2,487
TrCP (treatment causes medical problem)	296	444
TrIP (treatment improves medical problem)	107	198
TrNAP (treatment is not administered because of medical problem)	106	191
TrWP (treatment worsens medical problem)	56	143

Table 6. Results for the relation classification task on technical data

Relation	Method	Precision	Recall	F-measure
Cure	BOW+NPs+VPs+Biomed+UMLS-*NB*	98.55%	98.55%	98.55%
Prevent	BOW+NPs+VPs+Biomed+UMLS-*NB*	100%	100%	100%
SideEffect	BOW+NPs+VPs+Biomed+UMLS-*CNB*	100%	80%	88.89%

Table 7. Results on the clinical data

Method	Micro Precision	Micro Recall	Macro F-measure	Micro F-measure
BOW(sentence)+SemVect+VPs+ConceptType	34.23%	77.72%	43.64%	47.53%
BOW(context)+ SemVect+VPs+ConceptType	52.42%	75.72%	43.72%	61.95%

tween the concepts of the pair, and not the entire sentence. Table 7 presents these results. We report both macro and micro F-measure, because the latter one was the main evaluation measure in the fourth i2b2 competition (while in the second the former one was used).

For classifying relations between all pairs of concepts in a full sentence, including the no relation class, the best representation technique is the one that uses a combination of BOW, semantic vector cosine distance, verb phrases, the type of the concept, and the top 300 most representative words for each relation. This representation, in combination with the SVM classifier, achieves a macro and micro F-measure value of 43.64% and 47.53%, respectively. When we use only the context of the pair and not the entire sentence, we obtained a macro and micro F-measure value of 42.30% and 60.95%, respectively; this represents an increase of 13 percentage points in micro F-measure. These results suggest that using only the words between the concept pair represents a better choice than using the entire sentence.

If we are to use data that consists only of the 8 relations of interest without the no-relation pairs, the best micro F-measure result that we obtain is of 86.15% when using all the representation features in combination with SVM classifier. More detailed information about the results can be found in Frunza & Inkpen (2011).

FUTURE RESEARCH DIRECTIONS

With the tremendous growth of medical textual data, automatic tools that can analyze, synthesize, extract, and classify important medical information represent the tools of a better-informed medical practice.

We believe that the tasks that we addressed in this chapter and the methods that we used represent the basis of what will be the future tools of the medical practice. A medical practice focused on one's individual needs and characteristics – a personalized medicine, needs to use tools that can automatically mine information and extract the best knowledge to present to healthcare providers. These tools will be able to automatically answer important medical questions and assist the medical personnel in various tasks.

CONCLUSION

This chapter described three medical related tasks that can be successfully solved using intelligent textual data analysis. The emerging fields of natural language processing and machine learning have shown to be reliable tools that can be used in the medical domain.

We have developed models that can identify obesity-related diseases in clinical data. To build these models, we used various representation techniques based on lexical information (BOW representation), syntactic information (noun-phrase representation), and semantic information extracted from controlled vocabularies (UMLS concepts). These representation techniques are used in combination with suitable classifiers. The model that obtained the best results for both types of annotations is the BOW representation in combination with the Complement Naive Bayes (CNB) classifier. The results suggest that, at times, simple lexical representations in combination with the right algorithm achieve good results.

To automatically identify topic-relevant published information, we build two types of models. The first methodology is based on straight-forward machine learning approach, while the second one uses specific information from the protocol of building systematic reviews. The results suggest that it is beneficial to use additional specific knowledge, in order to obtain more robust results. Using a combination of lexical and medical concepts and the CNB classifier we show that good recall performance can be obtained on a real data set. The results also show that when we combine the classifier's output with judgments from one of the human experts, the best results are obtained.

Identifying and mining relations between medical entities represents valuable information for healthcare providers and consumers. The models used lexical, syntactic, and semantic information to represent the data, in combination with various learning algorithms. The results suggest that a richer representation technique in combination with suitable classifiers brings the best results on both technical and clinical data.

REFERENCES

Ambert, K. H., & Cohen, A. M. (2009). A system for classifying disease comorbidity status from medical discharge summaries using automated hotspot and negated concept detection. *Journal of the American Medical Informatics Association*, *16*(4), 447–458. doi:10.1197/jamia.M3095

Aphinyanaphongs, Y., & Aliferis, C. (2005). Text categorization models for retrieval of high quality articles. *Journal of the American Medical Informatics Association*, *12*(2), 207–216. doi:10.1197/jamia.M1641

Bruijn, B., Cherry, C., Kiritchenko, S., Martin, J., & Zhu, X. (2010). *NRC at i2b2: One challenge, three practical tasks, nine statistical systems, hundreds of clinical records, millions of useful features.* Paper presented at the i2b2 Workshop on Challenges in Natural Language Processing for Clinical Data, Washington, DC.

Bunescu, R., & Mooney, R. (2005). A shortest path dependency kernel for relation extraction. In *Proceedings of the Conference on Human Language Technology and Empirical Methods in Natural Language Processing (HLT/EMNLP)* (pp. 724–731). Morristown, NJ: ACL.

Chapman, W., Chu, D., & Dowling, J. N. (2007). ConText: An algorithm for identifying contextual features from clinical text. *In Proceedings of the Workshop on Biological, Translational, and Clinical Language Processing (BioNLP)* (pp. 81-88). Prague, Czech Republic.

Chapman, W. W., Fizman, M., Chapman, B. E., & Haug, P. J. (2001). A comparison of classification algorithms to automatically identify chest x-ray reports that support pneumonia. *Journal of Biomedical Informatics*, *34*(1), 4–14. doi:10.1006/jbin.2001.1000

Claudio, G., Lavelli, A., & Romano, L. (2006). Exploiting shallow linguistic information for relation extraction from biomedical literature. *In Proceedings of the 11th Conference of the European Chapter of the Association for Computational Linguistics*. Trento, Italy.

Cohen, A. M., Hersh, W. R., Peterson, K., & Yen, P. Y. (2006). Reducing workload in systematic review preparation using automated citation classification. *Journal of the American Medical Informatics Association*, *13*(2), 206–219. doi:10.1197/jamia.M1929

Deci, E. L., & Ryan, R. M. (1991). A motivational approach to self: Integration in personality. In R. Dienstbier (Ed.), *Nebraska Symposium on Motivation: Vol. 38, Perspectives on Motivation* (pp. 237-288). Lincoln, NE: University of Nebraska Press.

DeShazo, J. P., & Turner, A. M. (2008). *Hands-on NLP: An interactive and user-centered system to classify discharge summaries for obesity and related co-morbidities.* Paper presented at the i2b2 Workshop on Challenges in Natural Language Processing for Clinical Data, Washington, DC.

Donaldson, I. (2003). PreBIND and textomy: Mining the biomedical literature for protein-protein interactions using a support vector machine. *BMC Bioinformatics*, *4*, 11. doi:10.1186/1471-2105-4-11

Frunza, O., & Inkpen, D. (2008). *Representation and classification techniques for clinical data focused on obesity and its co-morbidities.* Paper presented at the i2b2 Workshop on Challenges in Natural Language Processing for Clinical Data, Washington, DC.

Frunza, O., & Inkpen, D. (2011). Extracting relations between diseases, treatments, and tests from clinical data. In *Proceedings of the 24th Canadian Conference on Artificial Intelligence*. St. John's, Canada.

Frunza, O., Inkpen, D., Matwin, S., Klement, W., & O'Blenis, P. (2011). Exploiting the systematic review protocol for classification of medical abstracts. *Artificial Intelligence in Medicine*, *51*, 17–25. doi:10.1016/j.artmed.2010.10.005

Frunza, O., Inkpen, D., & Tran, T. (2011). A machine learning approach for identifying disease-treatment relations in short texts. *IEEE Transactions on Knowledge and Data Engineering*, *23*(6). doi:10.1109/TKDE.2010.152

Groopman, J. (2007). *How doctors think*. Boston, MA: Houghton Mifflin Company.

Grouin, C., et al. (2010). *CARAMBA: Concept, assertion, and relation annotation using machine-learning based approaches.* Paper presented at the i2b2 Workshop on Challenges in Natural Language Processing for Clinical Data, Washington DC., DC.

Jenssen, T. K., Laegreid, A., Komorowski, J., & Hovig, E. (2001). A literature network of human genes for high-throughput analysis of gene expression. *Nature Genetics*, *28*(1), 21–28. doi:10.1038/ng0501-21

Leroy, G., Chen, H. C., & Martinez, J. D. (2003). A shallow parser based on closed-class words to capture relations in biomedical text. *Journal of Biomedical Informatics*, *36*(3), 145–158. doi:10.1016/S1532-0464(03)00039-X

Manning, C., & Schutze, H. (1999). *Foundations of statistical natural language processing*. Cambridge, MA: MIT Press.

Mitsumori, T., Murata, M., Fukuda, Y., Doi, K., & Doi, H. (2006). Extracting protein-protein interaction information from biomedical text with SVM. *IEICE Transactions on Information and Systems. E (Norwalk, Conn.)*, *89D*(8), 244–246.

Patrick, J., & Asgari, P. (2008). *A brief summary about the approach and explanation of the attributes of the developed system.* Paper presented at the i2b2 Workshop on Challenges in Natural Language Processing for Clinical Data, Washington, DC.

Roberts, K., Rink, B., & Harabagiu, S. (2010). *Extraction of medical concepts, assertions, and relations from discharge summaries for the fourth i2b2/VA shared task.* Paper presented at the i2b2 Workshop on Challenges in Natural Language Processing for Clinical Data, Washington, DC.

Rosario, B., & Hearst, M. A. (2004). Classifying semantic relations in bioscience text. *In Proceedings of the 42nd Annual Meeting on Association for Computational Linguistics*.

Solt, I., Tikk, D., Gal, V., & Kardkovacs, Z. T. (2009). Semantic classification of diseases in discharge summaries using a context-aware rule-based classifier. *Journal of the American Medical Informatics Association*, *16*(4), 580–584. doi:10.1197/jamia.M3087

Stapley, B. J., & Benoit, G. (2000). Bibliometrics: Information retrieval visualization from co-occurrences of gene names in MEDLINE Abstracts. *In Proceedings of the Pacific Symposium on Biocomputing*: Vol. 5. (pp. 526–537).

Thomas, J., Milward, D., Ouzounis, C., Pulman, S., & Carroll, M. (2000). Automatic extraction of protein interactions from scientific abstracts. *In Proceedings of the Pacific Symposium on Biocomputing*: Vol. 5. (pp. 538–549).

Uzuner, O., Zhang, X., & Sibanda, T. (2009). Machine learning and rule-based approaches to assertion classification. *Journal of the American Medical Informatics Association, 16*(1), 109–115. doi:10.1197/jamia.M2950

Ware, H., Mullet, C. J., & Jagannathan, V. (2009). Natural language processing framework to assess clinical conditions. *Journal of the American Medical Informatics Association, 16*(4), 585–589. doi:10.1197/jamia.M3091

Yakushiji, A., Tateisi, Y., Miyao, Y., & Tsujii, J. (2001). Event extraction from biomedical papers using a full parser. *In Proceedings of the Pacific Symposium on Biocomputing*: Vol. 6. (pp. 408–419).

Yang, H., Spasic, I., Keane, J. A., & Nenadic, G. (2009). A text mining approach to the prediction of a disease status from clinical discharge summaries. *Journal of the American Medical Informatics Association, 16*(4), 596–600. doi:10.1197/jamia.M3096

ADDITIONAL READING

Agichtein, E., & Gravano, L. (2000). Snow-ball: Extracting relations from large plaintext collections. In *Proceedings of the 5th ACM Internal Conference on Digital Libraries (ACMDL'00)* (pp. 85–94).

Ambert, K., & Cohen, A. (2009). A system for classifying disease comorbidity status from medical discharge summaries using automated hotspot and negated concept detection. *Journal of the American Medical Informatics Association, 16*, 590–595. doi:10.1197/jamia.M3095

Ananiadou, S., & McNaught, J. (2006). *Text mining for biology and biomedicine*. Norwood, MA: Artech House Inc.

Chen, E. S., Hripcsak, G., Xu, H., Markatou, M., & Friedman, C. (2008). Automated acquisition of disease-drug knowledge from biomedical and clinical documents: An initial study. *Journal of the American Medical Informatics Association, 15*, 87–98. doi:10.1197/jamia.M2401

Craven, M. (1999). Learning to extract relations from Medline. *In Proceedings of the AAAI-99 Workshop on Machine Learning for Information Extraction* (pp. 25–30).

Demner-Fushman, D., Chapman, W., & McDonald, C. J. (2009). Methodological review: What can natural language processing do for clinical decision support? *Journal of Biomedical Informatics, 42*, 760–772. doi:10.1016/j.jbi.2009.08.007

Erhardt, R. A., Schneider, R., & Blaschke, C. (2006). Status of text-mining techniques applied to biomedical text. *Drug Discovery Today, 11*, 315–325. doi:10.1016/j.drudis.2006.02.011

Giuliano, C., Lavelli, A., & Romano, L. (2006). Exploiting shallow linguistic information for relation extraction from biomedical literature. In *Proceedings of the 11th Conference of the European Chapter of the Association for Computational Linguistics* (pp. 401–409).

Haynes, R., Wilczynski, N., McKibbon, K., Walker, C., & Sinclair, J. (1994). Developing optimal search strategies for detecting clinically sound studies in medline. *Journal of the American Medical Informatics Association, 1*, 447–458. doi:10.1136/jamia.1994.95153434

Lean, M. E. J., Mann, J. I., Hoek, J. A., & Elliot, R. M., & Scho□eld, G. (2008). Translational research. *British Medical Journal, 337*, 705–706. doi:10.1136/bmj.a863

Moore, C., Wisnivesky, J., Williams, S., & McGinn, T. (2003). Medical errors related to discontinuity of care from an inpatient to an outpatient setting. *Journal of General Internal Medicine*, (n.d), 18.

Pestian, J. P., Brew, C., Matykiewicz, P., Hovermale, D. J., Johnson, N., Cohen, K. B., & Duch, W. (2007). A shared task involving multi-label classi□cation of clinical free text. In *Proceedings of the Workshop on BioNLP 2007* (pp. 97–104).

Pustejovsky, J., Castano, J., Zhang, J., Kotecki, M., & Cochran, B. (2002). Robust relational parsing over biomedical literature: Extracting inhibit relations. *Paci□c Symposium on Biocomputing* (pp. 362–373).

Roberts, A., Gaizauskas, R., & Hepple, M. (2008). Extracting clinical relationships from patient narratives. In *Proceedings of the Workshop on Current Trends in Biomedical Natural Language Processing*, Morristown, NJ, USA (pp. 10–18).

Sackett, D. L., Rosenberg, W. M. C., Gray, J. A. M., Haynes, R. B., & Richardson, W. S. (1996). Evidence based medicine: What it is and what it isn't. *British Medical Journal*, *312*, 71–72. doi:10.1136/bmj.312.7023.71

Sibanda, T. (2006). *Was the patient cured? Understanding semantic categories and their relationships in patient records*. Massachusetts Institute of Technology: Department of Electrical Engineering and Computer Science.

Srinivasan, P., & Rind〉esch, T. (2002). Exploring text mining from Medline. *In Proceedings of the American Medical Informatics Association Symposium* (pp. 722–726).

Szarvas, G., Farkas, R., & Almasi, A. (2009). Semi-automated construction of decision rules to predict morbidities from clinical texts. *Journal of the American Medical Informatics Association*, *16*, 601–605. doi:10.1197/jamia.M3097

Ware, H., Mullet, C., & Jagannathan, V. (2009). Natural language processing framework to assess clinical conditions. *Journal of the American Medical Informatics Association*, *16*(4), 585–589. doi:10.1197/jamia.M3091

Witten, I. H., & Frank, E. (2005). *Data mining: Practical machine learning tools and techniques*. Morgan Kaufmann.

Yang, H., Spasic, I., Keane, J., & Nenadic, G. (2009). A text mining approach to the prediction of a disease status from clinical discharge summaries. *Journal of the American Medical Informatics Association*, *16*, 596–600. doi:10.1197/jamia.M3096

Zweigenbaum, P., Demner-Fushman, D., Yu, H., & Cohen, K. (2007). Frontiers of biomedical text mining: current progress. In *Proceedings of the Brief Bioinformatics* (pp. 358–75).

KEY TERMS AND DEFINITIONS

Clinical Informatics: The task of solving various problems that uses clinical data.

Computational Linguistics: The theoretical aspects of natural language processing applications.

Evidence-Based Medicine: Medical practice that combines acquired experience with the latest research discoveries.

Information Extraction: The task of automatically extracting information from data.

Machine Learning: The automatic process of learning hypotheses from annotated data.

Natural Language Processing: The automatic process of representing, understanding, and generating natural text.

Systematic Reviews: Summaries of important information for specific medical topics, systematically collected from all the relevant publications.

Text Classification: The automatic task of classifying textual data in a set of predefined classes.

ENDNOTES

1   http://www.aaai.org/AITopics/pmwiki/
     pmwiki.php/AITopics/RuleBasedExpert-
     Systems

2   http://www.acpjc.org/

3   http://www.nlm.nih.gov/research/umls/

4   http://metamap.nlm.nih.gov/

5   http://www-tsujii.is.s.u-tokyo.ac.jp/GENIA/
     tagger/

6   http://www.nlm.nih.gov/databases/data-
     bases_medline.html

7   http://www.cs.waikato.ac.nz/ml/weka/

8   https://www.i2b2.org/NLP/Relations/Previ-
     ousChallenges.php

9   http://medline.cos.com

10   http://code.google.com/p/semanticvectors/

Chapter 17
Modeling Interpretable Fuzzy Rule–Based Classifiers for Medical Decision Support

Jose M. Alonso
University of Alcala, Spain

Ciro Castiello
University of Bari, Italy

Marco Lucarelli
University of Bari, Italy

Corrado Mencar
University of Bari, Italy

ABSTRACT

Decision support systems in Medicine must be easily comprehensible, both for physicians and patients. In this chapter, the authors describe how the fuzzy modeling methodology called HILK (Highly Interpretable Linguistic Knowledge) can be applied for building highly interpretable fuzzy rule-based classifiers (FRBCs) able to provide medical decision support. As a proof of concept, they describe the case study of a real-world scenario concerning the development of an interpretable FRBC that can be used to predict the evolution of the end-stage renal disease (ESRD) in subjects affected by Immunoglobin A Nephropathy (IgAN). The designed classifier provides users with a number of rules which are easy to read and understand. The rules classify the prognosis of ESRD evolution in IgAN-affected subjects by distinguishing three classes (short, medium, long). Experimental results show that the fuzzy classifier is capable of satisfactory accuracy results – in comparison with Multi-Layer Perceptron (MLP) neural networks – and high interpretability of the knowledge base.

DOI: 10.4018/978-1-4666-1803-9.ch017

INTRODUCTION

Interpretability of fuzzy systems is really appreciated in many applications, especially in those involving high interaction with humans. For instance, decision support systems in Medicine must be easily comprehensible, both for physicians and patients, with the aim of being widely accepted and successfully applicable. Thanks to its semantic expressivity close to natural language, fuzzy logic is acknowledged for its well-known ability for linguistic concept modeling. In consequence, fuzzy logic makes easier the knowledge extraction and representation phases when dealing with complex problems. In addition, the use of linguistic variables and rules (Zadeh, 1973) allows adopting the same formalism for both expert knowledge and knowledge automatically extracted from data (Alonso et al., 2008). Therefore, there are many applications regarding the use of fuzzy logic in Medicine and healthcare (Abbod et al., 2001; Nauck & Kruse, 1999).

In this chapter we describe the applicability of the fuzzy modeling methodology called HILK (Highly Interpretable Linguistic Knowledge) (Alonso et al., 2008; Alonso & Magdalena, 2011c) with the aim of building highly interpretable fuzzy rule-based classifiers (FRBCs) in the context of medical decision support problems. Namely, we tackle the case study of a real-world scenario concerning the development of an interpretable FRBC that can be used to predict the evolution of the End-Stage Renal Disease (ESRD) in subjects affected by Immunoglobin A Nephropathy (IgAN). It represents a renal disease whose impact is very relevant through the world since its progress gradually leads to chronic renal failure (with the consequent recourse to renal transplant). The role of a predictive model in such a context would be to assist the physician in providing a prognosis, consisting in the evaluation of a patient's risk to reach ESRD (namely, the pathology final stage) in a shorter or longer period. Of course, the added

value of this prediction should rely on the one hand on a timely information for the patient (i.e. prognosis should be available since from the initial contacts with the physician); on the other hand on the possibility to integrate the suggestions coming from the predictive system with the knowledge held by the expert (physician). This motivates the need of an interpretable predictive system. HILK enables the integration of expert knowledge with knowledge directly acquired from data, and it is implemented as a free software tool called GUAJE (Alonso & Magdalena, 2011a; Alonso & Magdalena, 2011b). Furthermore, the use of fuzzy logic let us dealing with the inherent imprecision of the predictive problem. In perspective, this may represent a relevant achievement since the obtained information could enable the discovery of new patterns underlying data, which could be useful for the physicians to propose targeted therapies.

The rest of the chapter is structured as follows. Next section provides the background regarding intelligent data analysis for medical decision support. It provides broad definitions and discussions considering not only fuzzy logic but also other techniques. Then, we go in deep with the main focus of the chapter. First, HILK methodology is sketched. Second, it is applied to solve the case study previously introduced, which is the prognosis of ESRD. Finally, the chapter ends pointing out future research directions and drawing main conclusions.

BACKGROUND

Current technology enables the acquisition and storage of large amounts of data, thus favoring the digital representation of complex phenomena in almost any field of human interest, being it scientific, commercial, engineering, etc. Medicine is one of such scientific fields where complex phenomena are most frequent, and a thoughtful comprehension of them is of prominent importance for the advance of knowledge at service of human health.

However, making sense of data is not a trivial task, especially when they describe complex phenomena. To this pursuit, Intelligent Data Analysis (IDA) is a methodology that prescribes a set of stages and techniques that can be applied for extracting useful knowledge from massive amounts of data. Nevertheless, IDA requires skillful application of the available techniques, which can only be accomplished by a careful intervention of human experts.

The objectives of IDA can be classified into three main categories (Berthold, 2010): finding patterns, finding explanations and finding predictors. Patterns are templates or prototypes that can be used to aggregate large quantities of data through simpler representations, like clusters, association rules, maps, etc. Finding patterns usually does not require the selection of a target variable, whose value could be explained in terms of observed features. This task is accomplished by explanations models, like decision trees, Bayes networks, rule-based systems, etc. Predictive models are also aimed at finding a relationship between the target variable and the observed value, but their structures need not to be transparent to the end-user. These models, which include neural networks, support vector machines or other model-free predictors like k-nearest neighbors, are usually more accurate than explanatory models, but they can be only used as black-box models, where users must rely on the model output without a full understanding of the inference carried out from the input values.

In Medicine, the use of predictive models is really useful only when their accuracy is so high that they can be reliably used without the intervention of the physician. However, this is rarely the case. Most often than not, phenomena (like diseases) are so complex that an accurate prediction of the target (e.g. the diagnosis) from observed value (e.g. symptoms, biometric data, subject's his-

tory) is not possible. In these cases, IDA models could be better used for decision support, i.e. as an aid for the physician in the determination of the diagnosis, the prognosis and the eventual therapies. Furthermore, explanatory models can be validated by physicians by a careful inspection of the knowledge base; this validation process can lead to an improvement of the predictive capabilities of the model or, more interestingly, can lead to the discovery of new relationships that were not known, in order to relate the target with the observed variables.

In consequence of these considerations, explanatory models can be deemed useful in fields, like Medicine, where decision support is of utmost utility. Alas, not every explanatory model can be actually of use in Medicine. In a great number of medical contexts, indeed, available data are imprecise, maybe because collected after interviews to the patients (thus relying on human memory and perceptions), or are derived by perception-based judgments (e.g. the reports of diagnostic imaging). Even more importantly, knowledge and experience of physicians are themselves imprecise, perception-based and without neat decision boundaries.

Based on these considerations, the use of explanatory models that ignore inherent imprecision of data and, at the same time, try to explain the target variable through sharp decisions, is not of great utility in medical applications. We claim that the knowledge base expressed by explanatory models should be highly co-intensive with the physician knowledge: it means that the form of the knowledge provided by the models should be similar to the way human mind defines concepts and infers knowledge, which is usually expressed in natural language.

This point of view is strictly connected with the "Comprehensibility Postulate" (CP) formulated by (Michalski, 1983). The postulate is a guidance for the design of intelligent systems, like those used in IDA:

"The results of computer induction should be symbolic descriptions of given entities, semantically and structurally similar to those a human expert might produce observing the same entities. Components of these descriptions should be comprehensible as single 'chunks' of information, directly interpretable in natural language, and should relate quantitative and qualitative concepts in an integrated fashion."

Explanatory models that use natural language terms to express their knowledge base are highly attractive since they are capable of simplifying the representation of complex relationships by highlighting the most essential information and hiding unnecessary details. This principle is at the base of the so-called "granular computing" paradigm, which enables the representation and processing of information granules, corresponding to the "chunks of information" involved in the CP.

Natural language is rich of terms that correspond to information granules. As an example, we may consider the following definition of "nephritic syndrome" from the Medical Encyclopedia of the U.S. National Library of Medicine, National Institute of Health (NIH)[1]:

"Nephritic syndrome is a group of symptoms including protein in the urine (more than 3.5 grams per day), low blood protein levels, high cholesterol levels, high triglyceride levels, and swelling."

The above definition uses five information granules, like the granule defined by the term "low blood protein level", which includes all the protein levels in blood that are below the normal values. It is immediate to notice that such an information granule does not have a sharp boundary, and the applicability of this information granule to a specific protein level is a matter of degree. Similarly, the information granule represented by the term "more than 3.5 grams per day [of protein in urine]" cannot be intended as sharply defined

since the amount of, say, 3.4 g/day cannot totally exclude a nephritic syndrome.

Imprecise information granules that do not have sharply defined boundaries can be formalized within the Fuzzy Set Theory (FST). FST is based on a simple yet effective idea: sets are extended so that partial membership is allowed. Fuzzy sets are hence sets where membership of elements is a matter of degree. The degree of membership can be defined so as to represent the degree of similarity with respect to a prototype, or the degree of preference of an item in a set of alternatives, or the possibility that a variable has a specific value. The latter case enables the use of fuzzy sets to represent possibility distributions, which are capable of representing uncertainty when the probabilistic constraints are too restrictive. FST extends the standard theory of sets by properly defining operations and relations among fuzzy sets. The logical counterpart of FST is fuzzy logic, where fuzzy propositions and rules are defined and partial truth is allowed. Within fuzzy logic, inference operations are extended allowing approximate reasoning, an inferential machinery that resembles human-like reasoning, while being faced with imprecise and gradual information and knowledge.

Representation of knowledge through fuzzy logic is mainly attained with fuzzy rules. Fuzzy rules are formal constructs defined by an antecedent and a consequent. When an antecedent is verified to a certain degree, the consequent is also verified to a degree that is established by the adopted implication operator. Antecedents and consequents are formal structures that are interpreted as soft constraints. Usually, the consequent defines a soft constraint on the target variable, while the antecedent defines a compound soft constraint on the observed variables. A soft constraint ties a variable to a fuzzy set: the degree of satisfaction of the soft constraint is defined by the degree of membership of the variable value to the fuzzy set. Composition of soft constraints is usually made up with logical connectives (conjunction, disjunction, negation), which are interpreted within FST with the corresponding set operations. A fuzzy rule-base is usually defined by several fuzzy rules: all of them simultaneously contribute in the determination of the target variable by aggregating the results of each rule (the type of aggregation depends on the implication operator used). Usually, the result is a soft constraint on the target variable: whenever a single value is required, a defuzzification process is carried out, which is highly application oriented.

Fuzzy rules are a powerful tool for designing explanatory models. They guarantee interpretability when knowledge experts formalize their own knowledge in fuzzy sets, soft constraints and fuzzy rules. In IDA, however, models are not designed by knowledge experts; they are rather acquired from data. In this case, the mere fact of using fuzzy rules to express the acquired knowledge is not enough to guarantee interpretability. Indeed, the acquired fuzzy sets may be defined in such a way that any interpretation in natural language is impossible. We must recall that FST extends sets with partial membership, but no other constraints are imposed on fuzzy sets in order to ensure that they can always be interpreted in natural language. As a result, a naïve application of data-driven techniques to derive fuzzy rules from data usually leads to unintelligible models that are not far away from other black-box models.

Fuzzy rules that are not interpretable pose a severe obstacle on the real utility of the corresponding explanatory models. We should recall that predictive (not explanatory) techniques are usually equipped with powerful learning algorithms that lead to highly accurate models. As a consequence, models with incomprehensible rules are poor in their explanatory ability and do not usually compete with black-box models in terms of predictive accuracy. This motivates the research in the direction of assessing the interpretability of fuzzy rules (and models), as well as to design

techniques for acquiring interpretable fuzzy rules from data.

The requirement of interpretability in fuzzy rules and fuzzy models is complex and multi-faceted. It involves the application context, the end users, the nature of data onto which models are built and so on. We restrict our discussion on the specific facet of rule representation and semantic interpretation. In this case, the objective of interpretability analysis is to verify how much it is plausible that a fuzzy rule-base can be expressed with natural language terms. This requires not only the formal attachment of linguistic labels to the involved fuzzy sets, but the assurance that the natural semantics of these linguistic labels corresponds to the semantics defined by the fuzzy sets. This latter requirement is hard, if not impossible, to formalize in a mathematical way, since it needs the definition of natural semantics, which is blur and subjective. Nevertheless, a number of approaches have been proposed to approximate these requirements by some formal or semi-formal constraints. These are called interpretability constraints and can be categorized in different ways. One type of categorization divides the interpretability constraints on the basis of the elements that are constrained (e.g. rules, partitions, etc.). Another type of subdivision splits constraints in structural (i.e. regarding the constitution of the fuzzy rule-base in terms of their elements) and semantical (i.e. concerning the ability of the rule-base to express sound knowledge) (Gacto et al., 2011). A well-known example of structural constraint is the number of rules in a rule-base, which should be kept reasonably small for interpretable fuzzy models; an example of semantic constraint evaluates the consistency of the rule-base with respect to logical inference (*modus ponens*).

The choice of interpretability constraints is subjective and sometimes application-dependent. Once a set of interpretability constraints has been chosen, data-driven techniques must be selected amongst those that satisfy these constraints.

BUILDING INTERPRETABLE FUZZY MODELS FOR MEDICAL PROGNOSIS

HILK Fuzzy Modeling Methodology

Medical prognosis is expected to be provided by physicians who may be successfully assisted by intelligent decision support systems with explanatory capabilities. The problem of drawing a right decision can be translated into a classification problem where objects to be classified are actually the most suitable decisions to be made. In consequence, we can use HILK (Highly Interpretable Linguistic Knowledge) (Alonso et al., 2008; Alonso & Magdalena, 2011c) with the aim of generating highly interpretable FRBCs, i.e., fuzzy rule-based systems able to carry out classification tasks, while satisfying several interpretability constraints, for medical prognosis.

HILK is a fuzzy modeling methodology that was conceived for carefully integrating expert and induced knowledge under the fuzzy logic formalism, producing compact and robust classifiers easily comprehensible by human beings. It enables the user to follow a step-by-step procedure in the generation of all elements involved in a fuzzy knowledge base, starting from the design of fuzzy partitions, going through the rule-based learning and ending up with a knowledge base improvement stage which iteratively refines both partitions and rules. For each step, HILK offers a number of alternative methods so that the user can make his/her best choice depending on each specific problem and on the available experimental data at hand.

To start with, the use of linguistic variables favors the readability of the model. Psychologists recommend to work with an odd number of terms (because it is easier to make reasoning around a central term) and a small number of terms (around 7 plus or minus 2 which is taken as a limit of human information processing capability). Moreover, the design of the related fuzzy partitions must be made carefully to guarantee readability. To do so, HILK advocates for the use of the so called Strong Fuzzy Partitions (SFPs) which satisfy Equation (1) and are proved to be the best ones from the interpretability point of view because they satisfy all the semantic constraints (distinguishability, normalization, coverage, overlapping, etc.) demanded to be comprehensible (Mencar & Fanelli, 2008). Figure 1 shows an example of SFP with five linguistic terms. VL stands for "Very Low", L means "Low", M is "Medium", H corresponds to "High", and VH is "Very High". Each linguistic term is characterized by a fuzzy set (A) which is described by a membership function $(\mu_A(x))$. It yields the membership degree of x to A. Satisfying Equation (1), for every point x in the universe of discourse (UD) that represents the range of feasible values the selected variable V can take, there are always at maximum only two fuzzy sets with membership degree $(\mu_A(x))$ greater than zero and their addition equals 1. Please notice that A represents one of the N defined linguistic terms (VL, L, etc.) which are ordered but their related fuzzy sets are not necessarily uniformly distributed.

$$\forall x \in UD, \sum_{i=1}^{N} \mu_A(x) = 1 \qquad (1)$$

We can state that working with SFPs is an essential prerequisite when looking for interpretable FRBCs. Fuzzy partition design involves first gathering expert knowledge in relation with the identification of the most significant variables and their definition (range, universe of discourse, number of linguistic terms, etc). Second, automatic generation of several fuzzy partitions from experimental data (uniform partitions, but also partitions fitted to data distribution by means of clustering algorithms like k-means and/or hierarchical fuzzy partitioning). Third, selecting the best partitions taking into account both expert knowledge and data distribution.

Figure 1. An example of SFP with five linguistic terms

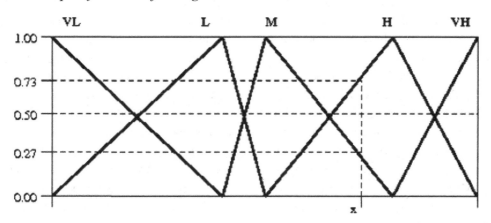

Once all involved linguistic variables (with all their related linguistic terms and attached fuzzy sets) have been properly defined, a global semantics is established. Then, linguistic rules of form "If Premise Then Conclusion", like rule R_k in Equation (2), can be set to describe the classifier behavior.

$$R_k: IF (V_1 is A_i) AND ... AND (V_{NI} is A_j) \quad THEN (Output is C_m) \qquad (2)$$

Both Premise and Conclusion are made up of linguistic propositions of form "V is A" where one of the previously defined linguistic terms, A, is assigned to one of the selected variables, V. For instance, "Age is Average" or "Prognosis is Short". Of course, this kind of expressions can be given by a physician or automatically extracted from data. HILK offers three different algorithms for rule induction: Wang & Mendel Algorithm, Fuzzy Decision Trees, and Fast Prototyping Algorithm. All of them produce rules sharing the global semantics previously defined; in this way rules can be compared directly at linguistic level and this favors interpretability.

The third main step in the HILK methodology corresponds to the knowledge base improvement stage. An iterative refinement process is applied both on partitions and rules. Such an activity can be performed by following a twofold strategy. On the one hand, this is the time for the physician to check the knowledge base, in order to apply his/her experience to confirm or modify the discovered data relationships. On the other hand, some kind of automatic procedures can be applied for the sake of model refinement. Of course, in this phase accuracy and interpretability of the classifier must be steadily inspected so as to implement the best trade-off between them. HILK offers automatic procedures for two kinds of improvement: linguistic simplification and partition optimization.

In the first case the aim is getting a more compact and general FRBC, keeping high accuracy while increasing comprehensibility. An iterative process starts looking for redundant elements (terms, variables, rules, etc.) that can be removed without altering the system accuracy (whose worsening should not exceed a predefined threshold). Then, it tries to merge elements always used together. Finally, it forces removing elements apparently needed but not contributing too much to the final accuracy. For each iteration, the process operates first on rules, then on partitions and stops when no more interpretability improvement is feasible without penalizing the accuracy of the model.

In the second case, partition optimization is devoted to increase the system accuracy while preserving the previously achieved interpretability. The process carries out a membership function tuning, constrained to keep the SFP property. Two search strategies are available: local search based on the proposal made by Solis & Wets; and global search Genetic-Tuning.

Finally, regarding the inference process, the designed FRBCs are endowed with the usual fuzzy classification structure based on the Max-Min inference scheme, and the winner rule fuzzy reasoning mechanism. Thus, given an NI-dimensional input vector $X=\{x_1,\ldots,x_i,\ldots,x_{NI}\}$, by applying the usual Max-Min fuzzy inference mechanism the FRBC provides an activation degree associated to each class C_m from a predefined set of NC classes. Of course, several classes can be activated at the same time with activation degree greater than zero. As a result, for each rule, the firing degree is computed as the minimum membership degree of x to all the attached A_i fuzzy sets, for all the NI inputs. Then, the output class is derived from the maximum firing degree of all rules yielding C_m as output class.

Please, notice that the interested reader is referred to (Alonso et al., 2008; Alonso & Magdalena, 2011c) for further details about HILK methodology and all involved algorithms related to knowledge induction. Moreover, the additional reading section includes some references which are likely to be informative.

Case Study: Prognosis of Immunoglobulin-A Nephropathy

To show the effectiveness of the proposed methodology, we describe its application on a real-world medical problem concerning the prognosis prediction in subjects affected by Immunoglobulin-A Nephropathy (IgAN).

IgAN is a renal disease and represents the most frequent primitive glomuronephritis in the world and one of the main causes of the terminal chronic renal failure (Beerman et al., 2007). Within about 20 years, 25-30% of subjects with IgAN diagnosis evolve in an end-stage renal disease (ESRD), thus requiring renal transplantation or dialysis

replacement. Such circumstances imply a number of issues negatively interfering with the patient's living standards; additionally, ESRD treatments produce a considerable cost for national health systems in the world. Therefore, prognosis of IgAN is crucial and its prediction is of greatest importance. As a consequence, several research efforts reported in literature have been addressed to the identification of features useful for predicting the decline of the renal function, thus providing information about the subsequent ESRD.

The need for a predictive model, capable of predicting the expected time for ESRD, is straightforward. Such model should rely both on clinical data and other specific measurements for evaluating the disease risk of a subject, so as to make a diagnosis and, more importantly, to propose a prognosis. Commonly, it is not easy to manage this kind of data, which is characterized by complex non-linear relations often only partially explainable by the available data features. Furthermore, the nature of some data features is not precise, as they are collected by interviews with the patients or approximate assessments.

In this context, useful predictive systems should be able to assist the physician by proposing an estimate of the prognosis and the reasons of the estimate. In this way the physician can integrate the estimate provided by the system with his/her knowledge for further considerations. This motivates the need of an interpretable predictive system which is also based on fuzzy logic for dealing with the inherent imprecision of the predictive problem. In perspective, this may represent a relevant achievement since the obtained information could enable the discovery of new patterns underlying data, useful to propose targeted therapies.

Description of Available Clinical Data

The dataset we analyzed has been provided by the Unit of Nephrology of "Policlinico di Bari" (Italy) and it is composed of 660 entries related to subjects affected by IgAN. For each subject, the

Table 1. The adopted set of features

Name	Type	Description
Gender	Categorical	Patient's gender (male/female)
Age at RB	Numerical	Patient's age at RB time (years)
Age at Onset	Numerical	Patient's age at the symptoms occurrence (years)
Onset type	Categorical	Type of symptom manifested (micro/macro hematuria)
Grade	Categorical	Histological grade assessed after RB (G1, G2, G3)[2]
RB sCr	Numerical	Urine Creatinine at RB (μmol/l)
RB uPr	Numerical	Urine Proteinuria at RB (g/day)
Hyp	Categorical	Hypertension (yes/no)
Prognosis	Categorical	Evolution time of ESRD (short/medium/long)

reported data refer to clinical information collected at different moments: partly during renal biopsy (RB), that is the moment when the pathology is verified, and others during one or more follow-ups (FU), corresponding to subsequent check-up visits.

The medical dataset has been subjected to a pre-processing phase in order to arrange the experimentation. Firstly, as the predictive model is supposed to provide for the evolution time to ESRD, only the subset of the dataset representing subjects who reached ESRD has been considered. Thus the dataset has been reduced to 98 records only. Pre-processing of data also affected the number of involved features. Studies on the progression of IgAN provide a significant feature subset. Accordingly, the initial total number of 43 features has been reduced. Furthermore, special attention has been paid on the RB/FU distinction. Data deriving from FU observations are surely relevant for refining ESRD prediction; however, in a preliminary stage, we are much more interested in deriving a predictive model which could prove to be useful during the first contacts with the patients, i.e. when only RB information has been collected. This may assist physicians in formulating a very first diagnosis (which could be later adjusted by monitoring the patients during the check-up visits). Additionally, inclusion of FU information in the experimentation would definitely increase the computational burden of

the model due to the well known "curse of dimensionality". Therefore, we resolved to exclude FU features from our analysis.

Some other interventions of ours concerned a better specification of the information reported in the dataset. In particular, we extracted a new feature – derived from existing ones – representing the numbers of years between the RB and the ESRD. Such a piece of information is very significant since it embodies the actual object of prediction. We call this new feature "Prognosis", representing the expected output of the predictive model. The set of features retained for experimentation is composed by nine elements: eight are intended as input features for the predictive problem to be tackled; one is intended as the single output feature to be predicted. All the features are briefly described in Table 1.

Since prediction problems can be translated into classification tasks (by partitioning the features to be predicted), the Prognosis feature has been processed in order to obtain temporal intervals (information granules). This choice is necessary to allow a rough indication of the prognosis severity; moreover, the prediction of an exact number of years to ESRD would be senseless because of the uncertainties of the variables at hand. Since preliminary discussions with experts showed that no meaningful subdivision of the Prognosis feature could be advised from a medi-

Figure 2. HILK methodology customized for the case study under consideration

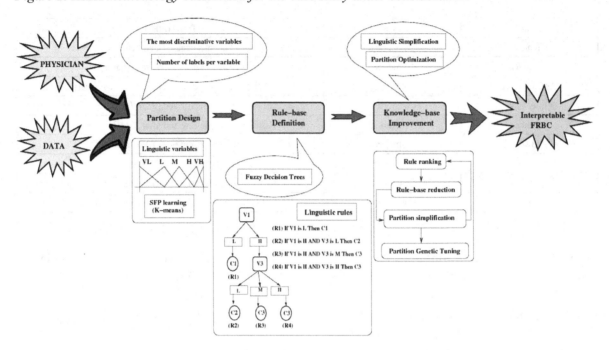

cal point of view, both the number of intervals and their amplitude have been automatically evaluated by a clustering process. The *K*-means clustering algorithm was adopted to identify three temporal clusters. For each of them, a linguistic label has been proposed: it represents the information underlying the granule and its semantic is strictly co-intensive with the physicians' knowledge. The resulting linguistic granules defined for the Prognosis feature are: short (identifying subjects whose renal survive is ranging between zero and about 5 years); medium (ranging between about 5 and 13 years); long (ranging between about 13 and 25 years).

Design of an Interpretable FRBC for IgAN Prognosis

To carry on the experimentation, we employed GUAJE (Alonso & Magdalena, 2011a; Alonso & Magdalena, 2011b), a free software tool which implements the HILK fuzzy modelling methodology previously presented. The whole modelling

process is made up of the three following main steps where we applied the options of HILK that are detailed in Figure 2:

1. **Partition Design:** As concerning our session of experiments, we resolved to generate partitions of the pre-processed data by means of centroids deriving from the well-known *K*-means algorithm (Hartigan & Wong, 1979). As reported in Table 1, the input features involved in the classification task are both numerical and categorical. The latter ones have been modeled by defining a fuzzy singleton for each category. The numerical features underwent the partitioning process: each numerical feature has been partitioned by five fuzzy sets obtained with the *K*-means algorithm. The number of fuzzy sets has been chosen as a trade-off between accuracy (the higher the number of fuzzy sets per input, the higher the accuracy) and interpretability (the lower the number of fuzzy sets per input, the higher the interpretability).

Both the fuzzy singletons and the fuzzy partitions have been labeled by linguistic terms whose semantic is strictly co-intensive with the experts knowledge, in order to maximize the interpretability of the resulting model.

2. **Rule-Base Definition**: Once obtained the fuzzy partitions, a fuzzy rule base has been automatically derived from data. Among the different methods for rule-based learning available in GUAJE, we adopted the Fuzzy Decision Tree (FDT) algorithm, which proved to produce the best results both in terms of interpretability and accuracy of the derived models. The applied FDT (Ichihashi et al., 1996) is a fuzzy version of the popular decision trees defined by Quinlan. It generates a neuro-fuzzy decision tree (directly from data) which is translated into quite general incomplete rules (only a subset of input variables is considered). In addition, input values are sorted according to their importance (minimizing the entropy).

3. **Knowledge-Base Improvement**: We have first run the linguistic simplification procedure provided by GUAJE and then, for partition optimization the Genetic Tuning strategy is selected with the aim of avoiding local minimum. It is an all-in-one optimization procedure based on a global search strategy which draws inspiration from the evolutionary processes that take place in nature (Cordón & Herrera, 1997).

The pseudocode of the simplification procedure is detailed below:

```
stop= false;
while (stop is false)
   RuleRanking();
   // Rank rules according to
   // increasing complexity

   // Rule base reduction
```

```
   SimplifyRB();
   // Remove redundancies and
   // solve contradictions
   MergeRB();
   // Merge rules that are
   // linguistically compatible
   ForceRR();
   // Trial and error process to
   // remove rules
   ForcePR();
   // Trial and error process to
   // remove premises

   // Partition simplification
   RemoveUV();
   // Remove variables that were
   // defined but are not used in
   // the rules
   RemoveUL();
   // Remove linguistic terms that
   // were defined but are not
   // used in the rules
   MergeLabels();
   // Merge linguistic terms (for
   // instance, L OR M)
   ForceVR();
   // Trial and error process to
   // remove variables

   // Checking stop condition
   if (FRBC has not been modified
       in the last cycle)
         stop= true;
end-while;
```

It consists of an iterative procedure where simplification affects both rules and partitions. It should be noticed that every modification in the knowledge base implies checking that accuracy is not reduced below a threshold established by the expert-physician. Otherwise, modifications are discarded. We opted by the most conservative strategy what means setting threshold equals

Table 2. Confusion matrix and unclassified cases

Observed	Inferred			Unclassified cases	*Total cases*
	Short	Medium	Long		
Short	**36.7%**	7.1%	1%	4.1%	*49%*
Medium	13.3%	**13.3%**	7.1%	4.1%	*37.8%*
Long	2.0%	7.1%	**4.1%**	0.0%	*13.2%*
Total	*52.0%*	*27.6%*	*12.2%*	*8.2%*	*100%*

Table 3. Excerpt from a sample rule base

Condition	Prognosis
Age at RB is very low and Grade is G2 and RB sCr is very low	Long
Grade is G3 and RB sCr is very low and RB uPr is very low or low	Medium
Age at RB is low or average and RB sCr is low and RB uPr is very low	Medium
Age on Onset is very high and RB sCr is low and RB uPr is low	Medium
Grade is G3 and RB sCr is very low and RB uPr is average or high	Short
Gender is male and Age at RB is low and Age at Onset is average and RB sCr is low and RB uPr is low	Short
Age at Onset is high and RB sCr is low and RB uPr is low	Short

to zero. This implies preserving initial accuracy during the simplification procedure.

Finally, the Genetic Tuning procedure was performed with a short number of generations (100) over a quite reduced population (only 10 individuals) due to the small size of the available experimental data. We consider binary tournament, BLX-α crossover (α=0.3, probability=0.6), uniform mutation (probability=0.1) and elitism. Further specific details can be found in (Alonso & Magdalena, 2011c).

Results and Discussion

The previously illustrated methodology has been applied to derive interpretable fuzzy classifiers starting from the analysis of data. The models have been tested through a leave-one-out cross-validation and the obtained results are reported in Table 2, in the form of a confusion matrix.

The obtained models may not be able to provide a class for each input instance. This happens whenever the classifier response lies on the bor-

derline of different classes (i.e. the fuzzy inference produces two outcomes whose numerical difference is below a certain threshold). Such a circumstance is reported in Table 2 ("Unclassified cases" column), amounting to 8.2% of cases. The overall value of classification accuracy is 54.1% (obtained by summing the bold values of the confusion matrix) and the values in the table show how the most critical situations are well managed by the classifiers. In fact, some particular cases, such as a kind of "false positive" (when a short prognosis value is predicted in front of a long observed value), and – most importantly – a kind of "false negative" (when a long prognosis value is predicted in front of a short observed value) are reported with the reduced percentage values of 2% and 1%, respectively.

Table 3 depicts the representation of a sample rule-base excerpt, derived from one of the rule-bases obtained during the cross-validation session. The reported rules, expressed by means of natural language terms, lend themselves to be read by physicians in order to assist their prog-

Table 4. Interpretability assessment (averaged)

Number of rules	Total rule length	Average fired rules	Logical View index
28.4	93.9	3.6	90%

Table 5. Comparative results

Model	Best Parameters	Accuracy
Multi-Layer Perceptron (MLP-Back Prop.)	Learning rate: 0.5	50.00%
Multi-Layer Perceptron (MLP-RPROP)	Max number of iterations: 5	52.04%
Support Vector Machine (SVM)	Kernel: Polynomial	57.1%
Fuzzy Inference System (RecBF-DDA)	T-norm: prod, Shrink function: rule-based	49.4%
Our model		54.1%

nosis formulation. In addition, more user-friendly representations could improve the accessibility of the knowledge base for deeper analysis.

In Table 4 some indexes are shown to provide information about the interpretability of the models. In particular, the reported values (averaged over all the models obtained during the cross-validation session) concern: the number of rules composing the knowledge bases, the total rule length (i.e. the total number of atoms composing all the rules inside a knowledge base), the averaged number of rules firing at each inference, the Logical View index. The latter represents an original non-structural parameter adopted to evaluate interpretability of a knowledge base by considering cointension with the semantics embedded into the fuzzy rules.

A comparative analysis has been carried out to verify how the model compares with other well-known adaptive models that acquire knowledge from data. We selected four models that are aimed at maximizing classification accuracy but are not designed for interpretability. The four models are:

- **Multi-Layer Perceptron (MLP):** With one hidden layer consisting of 28 neurons (this number has been chosen to equal the average number of rules obtained with our model). The nodes have the sigmoid transfer function and are trained through back-propagation with momentum;
- **MLP-RPROP:** The same configuration as above but trained with RProp algorithm;
- **Support Vector Machine (SVM):** Polynomial kernel and overlapping penalty set to 2.0;
- **Fuzzy Rule-Based Model:** Trained with RecBF-DDA algorithm.

The first model has been designed by the WEKA tool[3], while the last three models have been designed by the KNIME tool[4]. A number of trials have been run in order to determine the best values for the main parameters of each model. Leave-one-out strategy has been applied for fair comparison. Accuracy results are reported in Table 5. We notice that the proposed model shows comparable results in terms of classification accuracy, which remains noticeably low. At this stage we can reasonably assert that a significant amount of the classification error is inherent to the available data. However, in contrast with the comparing models, the proposed fuzzy model is completely transparent and accessible for end-users, who can explore the knowledge expressed as rules (possibly to revise and improve them according to his/her experience).

FUTURE RESEARCH DIRECTIONS

HILK is a general methodology for designing interpretable fuzzy models based on the combination of expert knowledge and knowledge automatically extracted from data, all along the design process. The basic building blocks (Partition design, rule-base definition, and knowledge base improvement) are general enough to let continuously incorporating the most recent enhancements in the field. Recent developments, still under consolidation, include multi-objective optimization and assessment of semantic cointension.

Multi-objective optimization is an approach to deal with the simultaneous optimization of different – and often conflicting – objectives of model design, like accuracy and interpretability. Current studies concern the most appropriate formalization of such goals for an effective optimization. Semantic cointension, on the other hand, is a new way for assessing interpretability by looking at the ability of the model in communicating semantic knowledge through its linguistic representation. This approach is relatively new, and initial studies are limited to the logical view of fuzzy rule-based classifiers. Nevertheless, this line of research is promising and is currently the subject of deeper insights for more general models as well as for devising new techniques of model design specifically aimed at maximizing semantic cointension.

In a broader point of view, although the relevance of interpretability for intelligent data analysis and data mining was pointed out long time ago, the interest in looking for formalizations and significant advances is growing more and more recently. As a consequence, studies on interpretable models, and especially fuzzy models, are currently very active. Future research trends mainly focus on the methodological level, where several research lines are explored. Interpretability assessment is one of these lines, where novel interpretability measures are proposed so as to be better tailored to application specific domains. Also, methods and workflows for automatic extraction of interpretable fuzzy knowledge are continuously refined. On a more theoretical level, the very subjective notion of interpretability is still under study. The main goal is to give machines the ability to reason and explain knowledge as humans do. This greatly impacts on the forms and methods of knowledge representation. Studies on structural vs. semantic interpretability constraints on knowledge representations go in this direction.

CONCLUSION

Medicine is one of the most challenging yet attractive application areas of intelligent data analysis. One of the greatest challenges is to provide for comprehensible explanations of acquired knowledge. Interpretability is a stringent requirement for physicians, who should be considered as end-users of a system that supports them in taking decisions on often complex problems. To this aim, a linguistic explanation of knowledge acquired through intelligent data analysis appears as a promising approach.

Linguistic fuzzy rule-based models are capable to provide for linguistic explanations in terms of fuzzy rules that can be given by an expert or designed through empirical learning methods. Nevertheless, their design is not straightforward. It must take into account the interpretability requirement since fuzzy set theory – on which fuzzy rules are built – is not enough to guarantee linguistic interpretability, i.e., fuzzy models are not interpretable *per se*, thus fuzzy modeling must be made carefully. Fortunately, we can trust on the HILK methodology, based on fuzzy set theory, that is capable of driving the designer in the production of explanatory fuzzy rule-based models that satisfy a number of interpretability constraints and, hence, linguistic interpretation. HILK is based on several steps, and directly involves the designer in several choices; this enables the integration of domain knowledge in the design phase, as well as an iterative control of the various steps. HILK can be considered as a methodological framework, where each step can be extended with new methods for designing interpretable fuzzy models as long as they are available.

An implementation of HILK is given in GUAJE, a free software tool for designing interpretable fuzzy rule-based models. As a proof of concept, we have presented the application of HILK to a real-world medical problem concerning the estimation of prognosis in patients affected by IgA Nephropathy, by using GUAJE. The application showed the diverse steps undertaken in the modeling phase, and an example of resulting rule base. Accuracy was comparable to other well-known black-box models, such as neural networks or support vector machines, but the resulting model has the added value of linguistic explanation. As a proof of concept, the presented model cannot be intended as definitive, and further refinements are possible, especially with a tight involvement of domain experts in the design process. This is the ultimate goal of our research: to provide a human-centric environment for intelligent data analysis.

ACKNOWLEDGMENT

This work has been partially funded by the Spanish government through the "Juan de la Cierva" program JCI-2011-09839

REFERENCES

Abbod, M. F., von Keyserlingk, D. G., Linkens, D. A., & Mahfouf, M. (2001). Survey of utilisation of fuzzy technology in medicine and healthcare. *Fuzzy Sets and Systems*, *120*, 331–349. doi:10.1016/S0165-0114(99)00148-7

Alonso, J. M., & Magdalena, L. (2011a). *GUAJE: Generating understandable and accurate fuzzy models in a Java environment*. Free software under GPL license. Retrieved September 15, 2011, from http://www.softcomputing.es/guaje

Alonso, J. M., & Magdalena, L. (2011b). Generating understandable and accurate fuzzy rule-based systems in a java environment. In A. M. Fanelli, W. Pedrycz, & A. Petrosino (Eds.), *Fuzzy Logic and Applications (9th International Workshop WILF2011), LNAI 6857* (pp. 212-219). Springer.

Alonso, J. M., & Magdalena, L. (2011c). HILK++: An interpretability-guided fuzzy modeling methodology for learning readable and comprehensible fuzzy rule-based classifiers. *Soft Computing*, *15*(10), 1959–1980. doi:10.1007/s00500-010-0628-5

Alonso, J. M., Magdalena, L., & Guillaume, S. (2008). HILK: A new methodology for designing highly interpretable linguistic knowledge bases using the fuzzy logic formalism. *International Journal of Intelligent Systems*, *23*(7), 761–794. doi:10.1002/int.20288

Beerman, I., Novak, J., Wyatt, R. J., Julian, B. A., & Gharavi, A. G. (2007). The genetics of IgA nephropathy. *Nature Clinical Practice. Nephrology*, *3*, 325–338. doi:10.1038/ncpneph0492

Berthold, M. R., & Hand, D. J. (2010). *Intelligent data analysis*. Berlin, Germany: Springer-Verlag.

Cordón, O., & Herrera, F. (1997). A three-stage evolutionary process for learning descriptive and approximate fuzzy-logic controller knowledge bases from examples. *International Journal of Approximate Reasoning*, *17*(4), 369–407. doi:10.1016/S0888-613X(96)00133-8

Gacto, M. J., Alcalá, R., & Herrera, F. (2011). Interpretability of linguistic fuzzy rule-based systems: An overview of interpretability measures. *Information Sciences*, *181*(20), 4340–4360. doi:10.1016/j.ins.2011.02.021

Hartigan, J. A., & Wong, M. (1979). A k-means clustering algorithm. *Applied Statistics*, *28*, 100–108. doi:10.2307/2346830

Ichihashi, H., Shirai, T., Nagasaka, K., & Miyoshi, T. (1996). Neuro-fuzzy ID3: A method of inducing fuzzy decision trees with linear programming for maximizing entropy and an algebraic method for incremental learning. *Fuzzy Sets and Systems*, *81*, 157–167. doi:10.1016/0165-0114(95)00247-2

Mencar, C., & Fanelli, A. M. (2008). Interpretability constraints for fuzzy information granulation. *Information Sciences, 178*, 4585–4618. doi:10.1016/j.ins.2008.08.015

Michalski, R. S. (1983). A theory and methodology of inductive learning. In Michalski, R. S., Carbonell, T. J., & Mitchell, T. M. (Eds.), *Machine learning: An artificial intelligence approach* (pp. 111–161). Palo Alto, CA: TIOGA Publishing Co. doi:10.1016/0004-3702(83)90016-4

Nauck, D., & Kruse, R. (1999). Obtaining interpretable fuzzy classification rules from medical data. *Artificial Intelligence in Medicine, 16*, 149–169. doi:10.1016/S0933-3657(98)00070-0

Zadeh, L. A. (1973). Outline of a new approach to the analysis of complex systems and decision processes. *IEEE Transactions on Systems, Man, and Cybernetics, 3*, 28–44. doi:10.1109/TSMC.1973.5408575

Zadeh, L. A. (1975). The concept of a linguistic variable and its application to approximate reasoning. *Information Sciences, Part I - 8*, 199–249, *Part II - 8*, 301-357. *Part III, 9*, 43–80.

ADDITIONAL READING

Alonso, J. M. (2007). *Interpretable fuzzy systems modelling with cooperation between expert and induced knowledge*. Unpublished doctoral dissertation, Technical University of Madrid, Spain.

Althoff, K.-D., Bergmann, R., Wess, S., Manago, M., Auriol, E., & Larichev, O. I. (1998). Case-based reasoning for medical decision support tasks: The Inreca approach. *Artificial Intelligence in Medicine, 12*(1), 25–41. doi:10.1016/S0933-3657(97)00038-9

Bargiela, A., & Pedrycz, W. (2003). *Granular computing: An introduction*. Boston, MA: Kluwer Academic Publishers.

Bartosik, L. P., Lajoie, G., Sugar, L., & Cattran, D. C. (2001). Predicting progression in IgA nephropathy. *American Journal of Kidney Diseases, 38*(4), 728–735. doi:10.1053/ajkd.2001.27689

Bezdek, J. C. (1981). *Pattern recognition with fuzzy objective function algorithms*. New York, NY: Plenum Press.

Boose, J. H., & Gaines, B. R. (1988). *Knowledge acquisition tools for expert systems*. New York, NY: Academic Press.

Breiman, L., Friedman, J. H., Olshen, R. A., & Stone, C. J. (1984). *Classification and regression trees*. Belmont, CA: Wadsworth International Group.

Casillas, J., Cordón, O., Herrera, M., & Magdalena, L. (Eds.). (2003). *Accuracy improvements in linguistic fuzzy modeling*. Heidelberg, Germany: Springer-Verlag.

Casillas, J., Cordón, O., Herrera, M., & Magdalena, L. (Eds.). (2003). *Interpretability issues in fuzzy modeling*. Heidelberg, Germany: Springer-Verlag.

Coppo, R., & D'Amico, G. (2005). Factors predicting progression of IgA nephropathies. *Journal of Nephrology, 18*(5), 503–512.

Dubois, D. (2005). Editorial: Forty years of fuzzy sets. *Fuzzy Sets and Systems, 156*(3), 331–333. doi:10.1016/j.fss.2005.05.027

Dybowski, R., & Gant, V. (2001). *Clinical applications of artificial neural networks*. Cambridge University Press. doi:10.1017/CBO9780511543494

Gabriel, T. R., & Berthold, M. R. (2004). Influence of fuzzy norms and other heuristics on mixed fuzzy rule formation. *International Journal of Approximate Reasoning, 35*, 195–202. doi:10.1016/j.ijar.2003.10.004

Guillaume, S. (2001). Designing fuzzy inference systems from data: An interpretability-oriented review. *IEEE Transactions on Fuzzy Systems*, *9*(3), 426–443. doi:10.1109/91.928739

Guillaume, S., & Magdalena, L. (2006). Expert guided integration of induced knowledge into a fuzzy knowledge base. *Soft Computing – A Fusion of Foundations. Methodologies and Applications*, *10*(9), 773–784.

Hand, D. J., & Yu, K. (2001). Idiot's Bayes – not so stupid after all? *International Statistical Review*, *69*(3), 385–399. doi:10.2307/1403452

Haykin, S. S. (2009). *Neural networks and learning machines* (3rd ed.). New Jersey: Pearson Prentice Hall.

Hjorth, J. S. U. (1994). *Computer intensive statistical methods validation, model selection, and bootstrap*. London, UK: Chapman & Hall.

Hüllermeier, E. (2005). Fuzzy methods in machine learning and data mining: Status and prospects. *Fuzzy Sets and Systems*, *156*, 387–406. doi:10.1016/j.fss.2005.05.036

Jang, J.-S. R., Sun, C.-T., & Mizutani, E. (1997). *Neuro-fuzzy and soft computing. A computational approach to learning and machine intelligence*. Prentice Hall.

Kuncheva, L. I. (2000). *Fuzzy classifier design*. Springer.

Kwiatkowska, M., & McMillan, L. (2010). A semiotic approach to data in medical decision making. In *IEEE International Conference on Fuzzy Systems* (pp. 436-442).

Lin, C.-T., & Lee, C. S. G. (1996). *Neural fuzzy systems. A neuro-fuzzy synergism to intelligent systems*. Prentice Hall.

Manno, C., Strippoli, G. F. M., D'Altri, C., Torres, D., Rossini, M., & Schena, F. P. (2007). A novel simpler histological classification for renal survival in IgA nephropathy: A retrospective study. *American Journal of Kidney Diseases*, *49*(6), 763–775. doi:10.1053/j.ajkd.2007.03.013

Mencar, C. (2004). *Theory of fuzzy information granulation: Contributions to interpretability issues*. Unpublished doctoral dissertation, University of Bari, Italy.

Mencar, C., Castiello, C., Cannone, R., & Fanelli, A. M. (2011). Interpretability assessment of fuzzy knowledge bases: A cointension based approach. *International Journal of Approximate Reasoning*, *52*(4), 501–518. doi:10.1016/j.ijar.2010.11.007

Miller, G. A. (1956). The magical number seven, plus or minus two: Some limits on our capacity for processing information. *Psychological Review*, *63*(2), 81–97. doi:10.1037/h0043158

Pedrycz, W. (1993). *Fuzzy control and fuzzy systems*. Tauton, UK: Research Studies Press Ltd.

Plutowski, M., Sakata, S., & White, H. (1994). Cross-validation estimates IMSE. In Cowan, J. D., Tesauro, G., & Alspector, J. (Eds.), *Advances in Neural information processing systems* (pp. 391–398). San Mateo, CA: Morgan Kaufman.

Quinlan, J. R. (1986). Induction of decision trees. *Machine Learning*, *1*, 81–106. doi:10.1007/BF00116251

Quinlan, J. R. (1993). *C4.5: Programs for machine learning*. San Mateo, CA: Morgan Kaufmann Publishers.

Riedmiller, M., & Braun, H. (1993). A direct adaptive method for faster backpropagation learning: The RPROP algorithm. In *Proceedings of the IEEE International Conference on Neural Networks (ICNN): Vol. 16* (pp. 586-591). Piscataway, NJ: IEEE

Ruspini, E. H. (1969). A new approach to clustering. *Information and Control, 15*(1), 22–32. doi:10.1016/S0019-9958(69)90591-9

Sadegh-Zadeh, K. (2000). Fundamentals of clinical methodology: 4- Diagnosis. *Artificial Intelligence in Medicine, 20*(3), 227–241. doi:10.1016/S0933-3657(00)00066-X

Sadegh-Zadeh, K. (2000). Fuzzy health, illness, and disease. *The Journal of Medicine and Philosophy, 25*, 605–638. doi:10.1076/0360-5310(200010)25:5;1-W;FT605

Seising, R. (2006). From vagueness in medical thought to the foundations of fuzzy reasoning in medical diagnosis. *Artificial Intelligence in Medicine, 38*, 237–256. doi:10.1016/j.artmed.2006.06.004

Ster, B., & Dobnikar, A. (1996). Neural networks in medical diagnosis: Comparison with other methods. In A. Bulsari (Ed.), *European Conference on Artificial Neural Networks* (pp. 427-430).

Valente de Oliveira, J. (1999). Semantic constraints for membership function optimization. *IEEE Transactions on Systems, Man, and Cybernetics. Part A, Systems and Humans, 29*(1), 128–138. doi:10.1109/3468.736369

Wang, L.-X., & Mendel, J. M. (1992). Generating fuzzy rules by learning from examples. *IEEE Transactions on Systems, Man, and Cybernetics, 22*(6), 1414–1427. doi:10.1109/21.199466

Zadeh, L. A. (1965). Fuzzy sets. *Information and Control, 8*, 338–353. doi:10.1016/S0019-9958(65)90241-X

Zadeh, L. A. (2008). Is there a need for fuzzy logic? *Information Sciences, 178*, 2751–2779. doi:10.1016/j.ins.2008.02.012

KEY TERMS AND DEFINITIONS

ESRD: End-stage Renal Disease.

FRBC: Fuzzy Rule-Based Classifier. A fuzzy model designed for classification tasks, i.e., for assigning a class (from a predefined set of classes) to every element of a given input set.

Fuzzy Logic: A special kind of formal logic able to tackle with uncertainty and imprecision. It constitutes the mathematical apparatus under fuzzy set theory to deal with approximate reasoning.

GUAJE: A free software tool which implements the HILK methodology with the aim of generating understandable and accurate fuzzy models in a Java environment.

HILK: Highly Interpretable Linguistic Knowledge. Fuzzy modeling methodology aimed to yield interpretable FRBC through integration of knowledge provided by an expert or automatically derived from experimental data.

IgAN: Immunoglobin A Nephropathy is a disease which affects the kidney and has become one of the main causes of chronic renal failures.

Interpretability: Ability (skill or talent) to conceive the significance of something. It should be considered as an umbrella covering several issues (sometimes taken as synonyms in a wrong and confusing way) like understandability, comprehensibility, intelligibility, readability, transparency, etc.

Interpretable Fuzzy Model: A mathematical model based on fuzzy logic which fulfills enough interpretability constraints in order to become capable of being understood, explicated or accounted for.

ENDNOTES

[1] http://www.nlm.nih.gov/medlineplus/medlineplus.html
[2] See Manno et al., 2007
[3] http://www.cs.waikato.ac.nz/ml/weka/
[4] http://www.knime.org

Chapter 18
Extraction of Medical Pathways from Electronic Patient Records

Dario Antonelli
Politecnico di Torino, Italy

Elena Baralis
Politecnico di Torino, Italy

Giulia Bruno
Politecnico di Torino, Italy

Silvia Chiusano
Politecnico di Torino, Italy

Naeem A. Mahoto
Politecnico di Torino, Italy

Caterina Petrigni
Politecnico di Torino, Italy

ABSTRACT

With the introduction of electronic medical records, a large amount of patients' medical data has been available. An actual problem in this domain is to perform reverse engineering of the medical treatment process to highlight medical pathways typically adopted for specific health conditions. This chapter addresses the ability of sequential data mining techniques to reconstruct the actual medical pathways followed by patients. Detected medical pathways are in the form of sets of exams frequently done together, sequences of exam sets frequently followed by patients and frequent correlations between exam sets. The analysis shows that the majority of the extracted pathways are consistent with the medical guidelines, but also reveals some unexpected results, which can be useful both to enrich existing guidelines and to improve the public sanitary service.

DOI: 10.4018/978-1-4666-1803-9.ch018

INTRODUCTION

A huge amount of medical data storing the medical history of patients has made available in recent years by the introduction of electronic medical records. Data mining techniques can be profitably exploited to support healthcare decision making, by extracting a variety of information from these large medical data collections. For example, it is possible to analyze the relationships between medical treatment and final patient condition, or the medical pathways frequently followed by patients with a given disease.

An actual problem in this domain is to perform reverse engineering of the medical treatment process to highlight medical pathways typically adopted for specific health conditions, as well as discovering deviations with respect to predefined care guidelines. This information can support healthcare organizations in improving the current treatment process or assessing new guidelines.

Care guidelines represent standard medical pathways that have been defined for a variety of clinical conditions. They specify the sequence and timing of actions necessary to provide treatments to patients with optimal effectiveness and efficiency. Sometimes care guidelines include suggestions to treat a particular health state but the real application depend on specific cases and there is not a unique right guideline. Also in this scenario it is important to extract the frequent medical pathways to analyze the most frequent patients' behavior and thus measure the patients' accessibility to the sanitary system.

The approach proposed in this chapter relies on sequential pattern mining to analyze a collection of patients' medical data and extract from it the medical pathways. The analysis is performed on the patients' medical treatments of a group of pregnant women provided by a Healthcare Territorial Agency in the Piedmont region of Italy. Sequential pattern mining is used to reconstruct

the actual diagnostic services accessed with high frequency by patients and even their temporal relationships. To this aim, raw medical logs are collected, cleaned, and integrated into a sequence data structure on which the mining process takes place.

Detected medical pathways include the sets of exams frequently done together, the sequences of exam sets frequently followed by patients and the frequent correlations between exam sets. Our analysis show that the majority of the extracted pathways are consistent with the medical guidelines, but also revealed some unexpected results. For example, some important exams occur with a lower frequency than expected, while some exams not included in the guidelines frequently appear in the considered medical data. These results are useful both to enrich guidelines by considering the exams actually done by patients and to improve the public sanitary service by investigating causes that lead patients to do exams privately.

BACKGROUND

The use of data mining techniques in healthcare institutes has taken great attention due to the large amount of generated data (Hardin, 2007). A lot of research has been carried out for enhancing and improving medical practices, disease management and resource utilization.

The medical treatment relationships and condition of a patient for a given disease can be extracted by means of data mining techniques (Cerrito, 2007). The decision support tools for clinical healthcare based on data mining techniques are addressed in Siddiq (2009), Kazemazadeh (2006) and Palniappan (2008). However, these works do not exploit real datasets for experiments. In Stoblba (2007), data warehousing and data mining techniques are emphasized essential to provide evidence-based guidelines for clinicians. Health care resources optimal utilization is focused in Dart (2003) and Rossille (2008).

Chen (2007) presents possible side effects of using multiple drugs during pregnancy period with the use of association rule mining approach. The SmartRule technique is used to mine association rules from a saved tabular pregnancy data and finds Maximum Frequent Itemsets (MFI) based on user specified minimum support threshold. The subset of MFIs is selected with targeted attributes by users to derive association rules for a given support and confidence level. The author tries to highlight and warn the drugs that may cause harm to unborn babies.

Gosain (2009) addresses decision tree and association rule mining techniques for finding human immune-deficiency virus (HIV) in order to get insight impacts in management strategies against HIV. This work analyses a real world dataset and investigates its association with data stored through the antiretoviral therapy system, which is a software developed for medical organizations. Decision tree technique identified patterns of higher support and confidence based on several attributes such as age, gender and education qualification. Further association rule mining technique is applied for predicting frequent correlations in the patterns of the dataset with patient's history in the system.

Cerrito (2006) explores electronic records using SAS Enterprise Miner and SAS Text Miner to optimize clinical decision-making. The 6-months records of patients, having complained of shortness-of-breath, were examined to find the differences in physician decision-makings using above said tools. Based on differences, optimal protocols and enhanced treatment procedures can be applied to improve patient care and reduce cost.

A preliminary application of the frequent sequence extraction to exam log data was proposed by Baralis (2010) to analyze the medical pathways of diabetic patients.

EXTRACTION AND EVALUATION OF PREGNANCY MEDICAL PATHWAYS

This section describes the guidelines available for the considered pregnancy case study and the proposed approach to extract and analyses medical pathways actually performed by patients.

Pregnancy Case Study and Medical Guidelines

Prenatal diagnostic testing involves testing the fetus before birth to determine whether the fetus has certain abnormalities, including certain hereditary or spontaneous genetic disorders. Some of these tests, such as Ultrasonography and certain blood tests, are often part of routine prenatal care (DOH, 2010; NICE, 2003).

In Italy, for the ministerial decree of the 1998, pregnant women are entitled to a set of examinations free of charge in order to monitor the physiological pregnancy. Pregnancy examinations are differently distributed week by week. Particularly, within the thirteen weeks usually the following exams are done: Hemochrome or Complete Blood Count (CBC), Rubella Virus Antibodies, Toxoplasmosis antibody, Virus Immune Deficiency Antibodies (HIV), concentration of Glucose in the blood, Urine microscopic exam (Urinalysis), Obstetric Ultrasound (Ultrasonography), Anti-erythrocyte antibody detection (or Indirect Coombs Test). Between the nineteenth and the twenty-third week the Urinalysis and the Ultrasonography are repeated. Then, between the twenty-fourth and the twenty-seventh week the concentration of Glucose in the blood and the Urinalysis are repeated, and between the twenty-eighth and the thirty-second week the CBC, the Urinalysis and the Ultrasonography are repeated. Then, between the thirty-third and the thirty-seventh week the Hepatitis B antibody test (HBV) and the Hepatitis C antibody test (HCV) are

Table 1. Guidelines for pregnancy exams

Exam code	Exam name (abbreviation)	Week
90.62.2	Complete Blood Count (CBC)	1-13
90.09.2	Aspartate Aminotransferase (AST)	1-13
90.04.5	Alanine Aminotransferase (ALT)	1-13
91.26.4	Rubella Virus Antibody	1-13
91.09.4	Toxoplasma Antibodies	1-13
91.22.4	Virus Immune Deficiency Antibodies (HIV)	1-13
90.27.1	Glucose	1-13
90.44.3	Urine Microscopic (Urinalysis)	1-13
88.78	Obstetric Ultrasound (Ultrasonography)	1-13
90.49.3	Anti-Erythrocutes	1-13
90.44.3	Urine Microscopic (Urinalysis)	14-18
90.44.3	Urine Microscopic (Urinalysis)	19-23
88.78	Obstetric Ultrasound (Ultrasonography)	19-23
90.27.1	Glucose	24-27
90.44.3	Urine Microscopic (Urinalysis)	24-27
90.62.2	Complete Blood Count (CBC)	28-32
90.22.3	Ferritin	28-32
90.44.3	Urine Microscopic (Urinalysis)	28-32
88.78	Obstetric Ultrasound (Ultrasonography)	28-32
91.18.5	Hepatitis B Virus (HBV)	33-37
91.19.5	Hepatitis C Virus (HCV)	33-37
90.62.2	Complete Blood Count (CBC)	33-37
90.44.3	Urine Microscopic (Urinalysis)	33-37
91.22.4	Virus Immune Deficiency Antibodies (HIV)	33-37
90.44.3	Urine Microscopic (Urinalysis)	38-40
88.78	Obstetric Ultrasound (Ultrasonography)	>=41
75.34.1	Cardiotocography (CTG)	>=41
90.94.2	Culture Urine Test (Uration)	>=41

done, and the CBC, the Urinanalysis and the HIV are repeated. Finally, between the thirty-eighth and the fortieth week the Urinanalysis is repeated, and as of the forty-first week the Ultrasonography and the Cardiotocography are done (NICE, 2003).

In Table 1 the timing of each exam is reported. The exam codes refer to the International Classification of Diseases - Clinical Modification (ICD IX-CM, 2011), which is used in assigning codes to diagnosis and surgical procedures.

Pathway Extraction and Evaluation

The proposed approach to detect the diagnostic pathways actually followed by patients is organized in three main phases, as shown in Figure 1. First, in the Data Collection and Segmentation phase, patients' exam log data are organized in a sequence database and segmented to separately analyze groups of patients with similar characteristics. Then, in the Pathway Mining phase, each

Figure 1. Phases of the proposed approach for pathway extraction and evaluation

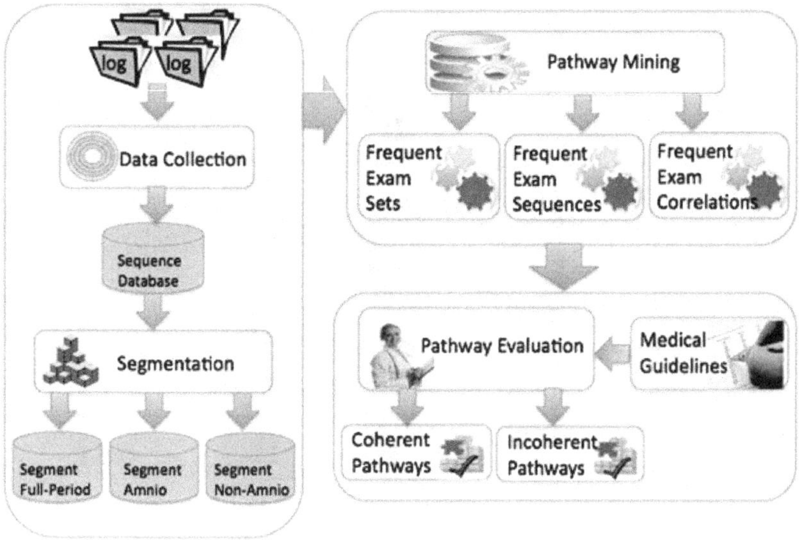

segment is analyzed by means of data mining techniques to extract the emerging diagnostic pathways actually followed by patients. Finally, in the Pathway Evaluation phase, the extracted pathways are evaluated based on available medical guidelines. The three phases are detailed in the following sections.

Data Collection and Segmentation

The exam log data analyzed in this chapter were provided by the Local Sanitary Agency of the Asti province (Italy). They include 29,679 records logging all the exams performed by the 905 women that gave birth to a child between July and December 2007. The histogram of the ages of the considered women is reported in Figure 2. Such women have been identified by searching the DRG (Diagnosis Related Group) codes corresponding to a delivery on the Hospital Discharge Records. Using DRG codes, patients are classified by diagnosis, average length of hospital stay, and

therapy received. For all the identified women the supplied services in terms of executed exams are selected.

The exam log data were transformed into a database of 905 sequences, where each sequence corresponds to the temporal list of exams done by a patient. The number of distinct exams appearing in the dataset is 327. The maximum, minimum and average number of exam done by patients are 172, 1, and 32 respectively.

The sequence database is partitioned into three segments, i.e., groups of patients with similar characteristic. The first segment includes patients with almost the full pregnancy period. In fact, the 9-months history is not available for all patients, probably because some of them had exams in a predicate structure. To analyze the complete medical pathways, we include in this segment, named $Segment_{Full-Period}$, only those patients who covered a period of at least 190 days (i.e., 6 months). This segment contains 455 patients.

Figure 2. Histogram of women age

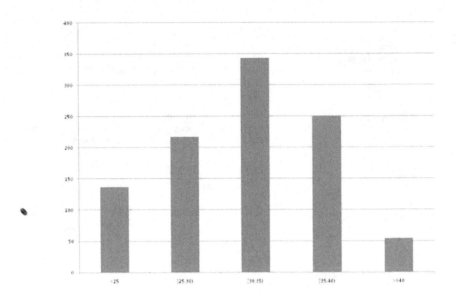

Another segmentation has been done to group patients that did particular exams, which can reveal abnormal conditions. One of the crucial exams in pregnancy is Amniocentesis. Amniocentesis is an invasive exam used to determine genetic disorders about the baby and diagnose uterine infection. It examines the amniotic fluid that surrounds the baby in the womb and it is usually done within the second trimester of pregnancy for women older than 35 years (NICE, 2003). To analyze pathways specific for women in more critical conditions, we divided patients in two segments, one including women that did the Amniocentesis (a total of 73 patients) and the other including women that did not the Amniocentesis (832 patients), named $Segment_{Amnio}$ and $Segment_{Non-Amnio}$ respectively. We extracted pathways from both segments and compared the results.

Pathway Mining

In the Pathway Mining phase, data mining techniques are exploited to extract the medical pathways actually done by patients. Medical pathways are in the form of (i) frequent exam sets,

(ii) frequent exam sequences, and (iii) frequent exam correlations.

Frequent Exam Sets

Exam sets represent the exams done by each patient without considering the time intervals among them neither the exams' repetitions. To extract the frequent exam sets, the sequence database is represented as a set database reporting the set of different exams done by each patient. Then, the frequent exam sets are extracted from the set database. Currently, the BIDE algorithm (Wang 2004) is exploited for frequent sets extraction. BIDE is an effective state-of-the art extraction algorithm, which adopts the BI-Directional Extension closure checking scheme to prune the search space. The Java implementation of the BIDE algorithm has been kindly provided by Fournier-Vigier (2010).

In our approach, to avoid the generation of redundant information and compactly represent the solution set, only the subset of closed exam sets are extracted. An exam set is closed when it is not included in other exam sets with the same frequency (Bastide, 2000). For example, let E1 be an exam and {E2, E3} an exam set including exams E2 and E3. If all patients that did {E2,E3} also did exam E1, it can be said that set {E2,E3} is redundant because it is included in the set {E1,E2, E3}. Set {E1,E2, E3} is instead a closed set. For simplicity, we omit the term "closed" in the following.

Frequent Exam Sequences

The analysis of frequent exam sequences done by patients allows highlighting the temporal relationships among exams, i.e., which exams frequently precede or follow other exams. A sequence is a temporal relationship among set of exams. For example, the sequence <{E1}{E2,E3}> means that exam E1 is done before the exam set {E2,E3}. The extraction of the frequent exam sequences is done directly from the sequence database produced in the Data Collection and Segmentation phase. As for the exam sets, also the exam sequence are extracted by means of the BIDE algorithm (Wang 2004). Also in this case, to avoid the generation of redundant information and compactly represent the solution set, only the subset of closed exam sequences is extracted, i.e., the sequences which are not included in other sequences with the same frequency (Wang 2004).

For example, being included in sequence <{E1}{E2,E3}>, sequences <{E1}>, <{E2}>, <{E3}>, <{E2,E3}>, <{E1}{E2}>, <{E1}{E3}> that have the same frequency of <{E1}{E2,E3}>, are redundant and can be discarded. Sequence <{E1}{E2,E3}> is instead a closed sequence. For simplicity, we omit also for exam sequences the term "closed" in the following.

Frequent Exam Correlations

Association rule learning is a popular method for discovering interesting relations between variables in databases (Agrawal, 1995). The problem of association rule mining is defined as following. Let I={E1, E2, E3,..} be a set of items (corresponding to patients' exams in our case), and

D={T_1,T_2,T_3,...} a set of transactions. An association rule is defined as an implication between two sets of items (called itemsets) in the form X → Y, where X,Y ⊆ I and X ∩ Y= Ø, e.g., {E1} → {E2,E3}. X is called the antecedent of the rule and Y the consequent. To select interesting rules from the set of all possible rules, constraints on various measures of significance and interest can be used. The best-known constraints are minimum thresholds on support and confidence. The support sup(X) of an itemset X is defined as the percentage of transactions in the dataset which contain X. The confidence of a rule conf(X → Y) is defined as sup(X∪Y)/sup(X). The confidence is the conditional probability of finding Y having found X (i.e., P(Y|X)). An association rule is called frequent if its support and confidence values are greater or equal to minimum threshold values. A closed association rule is a comprehensive representation of a set of association rules and it is extracted only from frequent closed itemsets instead from all the itemsets (Szathmary, 2006). Also in this case, we omit also for exam sequences the term "closed" in the following for simplicity.

Pathway Evaluation

In this section we analyze the exam sets, exam sequences, and exam correlations frequently occurring in the three segments. The majority of the extracted pathways are consistent with the guidelines reported in Table 1, but they also reveals some unexpected results, such as a frequency lower than expected for some important exams and a frequency higher than expected for exams that are not in the guidelines.

Pathways in Segment$_{Full-Period}$

Since guidelines are usually analyzed for trimesters, we divided the time period of each patient in three trimesters. Then, we analyzed the frequent exam sets, sequences and correlation in each trimester, and in all the period.

Frequent Exam Sets

Table 2 shows the extracted frequent exam sets in each trimester and in all the period. The majority of the extracted pathways are consistent with the guidelines reported in Table 1. The exams that occur with higher frequency in the 1st trimester (e.g., Ultrasonography, Glucose, Toxoplasma, ALT, AST, HIV) are those suggested by the guidelines in the first weeks of pregnancy. The exams that are more frequent in the 3rd trimester (e.g., HBV, HCV, Echocardiography, Cardiotocography, Uration, Total Biluribine) are those that, according to guidelines, should be done in the last weeks of pregnancy. The only exam occurring with higher frequency in the 2nd trimester is Amniocentesis. This results is coherent with guidelines, which prescribe the Amniocentesis exam between the 15th and the 20th week. The remaining exams have similar frequency in the three trimesters, being check up exams routinely repeated (e.g. CBC and Urinanalysis).

The analysis of the sets of exams usually performed together show results that are coherent with the guidelines. The ALT and AST exams are usually done together, as well as CBC, Urinanalysis, and Glucose.

Our analysis also reveals some unexpected results, as listed in the following.

- *For some exams, the actual frequency is lower than expected* (e.g., Ultrasonography, Cardiotocography, Rubella Virus Antibody). A possible explanation of this behavior is that some exams, such as Ultrasonography, can be comfortably and quickly done in private studies. This aspect can highlight some limitations in accessing services provided by the public sanitary agency, for example due to a long waiting time for exam booking.

A different situation is represented by exams such as the Rubella Virus Antibody exam. This exam is very critical, because if the mother is infected, the child may born with congenital rubella syndrome, which entails a range of serious incurable illnesses. This exam has been done by a limited percentage of patient, about 45%. The reason of this behavior can be that people already know if they did Rubella and thus know if they already have the antibodies.

- *Some exams occur with a high frequency even if they are not available in the guidelines.* This aspect is due to the fact that the ministerial decree of 1998, still valid in 2007, report medical guidelines that can be obsolete or at least incomplete with respect the actual medical knowledge. Since pregnancy is a complex process that strongly depends on the woman condition, doctors currently varies the prescribed exams based on the actual condition of the patient. More recent documents of other Italian regions include additional recommended exams. Prothrombin Time, Creatinine, Echocardiography, and Antithrombin III are example of exams that are not available in the guidelines, but occur with a high frequency in the analyzed exam logs (i.e., 50%, 48%, 47% and 44% respectively). Another example is given by the ALT, AST, and Glucose exams. Guidelines prescribe these exams only once in the whole pregnancy period, but they occur with a higher frequency both in the 1st and in the 3rd trimester in the considered exam logs. These variations are documented in a variety of websites which describe the importance of doing these additional exams during pregnancy (Monti, 2011).

Frequent Exam Sequences

We first analyzed the frequent exam sequences in each trimester. We observed that these sequences are characterized by a quite low frequency. This

Table 2. Frequent exam sets in each trimester and in all period in Segment$_{Full-Period}$

Exam sets	1st Trimester	2nd Trimester	3rd Trimester	All
{Ultrasonography}	**89%**	59%	65%	89%
{Glucose}	**60%**	35%	50%	79%
{Toxoplasma}	**57%**	49%	47%	77%
{ALT}	**57%**	27%	50%	78%
{AST}	**56%**	27%	50%	77%
{ALT, AST}	**56%**	27%	50%	77%
{CBC, Urinalysis, Glucose}	**52%**	25%	37%	76%
{HIV}	**45%**	11%	31%	62%
{Rubella Virus Antibody}	**41%**	6%	3%	45%
{CBC, Urinalysis, HIV}	**40%**	8%	27%	59%
{Anti-Erythrocutes}	**35%**	11%	13%	45%
{Amniocentesis}	5%	**6%**	--	10%
{CBC}	66%	62%	**76%**	92%
{Urinalysis}	66%	72%	**73%**	91%
{HBV}	36%	13%	**49%**	67%
{Cardiotocography}	9%	8%	**45%**	47%
{Prothrombin time}	18%	12%	**45%**	50%
{Echocardiography}	8%	8%	**44%**	47%
{Partial thromboplastin time}	18%	12%	**44%**	50%
{Antithrombin III}	14%	14%	**40%**	44%
{HCV}	29%	11%	**39%**	55%
{Creatinine}	31%	16%	**34%**	48%
{Uration}	22%	14%	**34%**	42%
{Total Bilirubin}	25%	15%	**31%**	41%
{Ferritin}	13%	11%	**24%**	33%

aspect show that there aren't exam sequences usually done by the majority of patients. This result is coherent with the guidelines, which do not include repetition of exams in a single trimester, except from the Urinalysis.

In the 1st trimester, the most frequent sequences concern the repetition of CBC and Urinanalysis exams, i.e., sequences <{CBC}{CBC}> and <{Urinalysis}{Urinalysis}> (in 24% and 21% of patients, respectively). Both sequences occur also in the 2nd trimester (23% and 32%), and in the 3rd semester with higher frequency (38% and 33%). Sequence <{Ultrasonography}{Ul-

trasonography}> is found both in the 2nd and in the 3rd semester, with frequency 27% and 20%, respectively. In the 3rd trimester, other frequent sequences occur, involving the repetition of the Cardiotocography exam. Sequence <{Cardiotocography}{Cardiotocography}> has frequency 31%, while sequence <{Cardiotocography}{Cardiotocography}{Cardiotocography}> has frequency 20%.

We then analyzed exam sequences across trimesters (i.e., each exam sets is extracted from a different semester). Analogously to above, also this analysis show that there isn't a behavior

Table 3. Frequent exam sequences of the three trimesters in Segment$_{Full-Period}$

Exam Sequences	Frequency
<{Ultrasonography}{Urinalysis}>	73%
<{Ultrasonography}{CBC}>	73%
<{Urinalysis}{Urinalysis}>	64%
<{Ultrasonography}{Ultrasonography}>	64%
<{CBC}{CBC}>	60%
<{HIV}{Urinalysis}>	38%
<{Glucose}{Glucose}>	37%
<{Ultrasonography}{Urinalysis}{CBC}>	44%
<{Ultrasonography}{Urinalysis}{ Urinalysis }>	43%
<{Ultrasonography}{Urinalysis}{Urinalysis, CBC}>	40%
<{Ultrasonography}{Ultrasonography}{CBC}>	38%
<{Ultrasonography}{Ultrasonography}{ Urinalysis}>	37%
<{Ultrasonography}{CBC}{CBC}>	36%
<{Ultrasonography}{Urinalysis}{Ultrasonography}>	36%
<{Ultrasonography}{Ultrasonography}{Ultrasonography}>	35%
<{Ultrasonography}{Toxoplasma}{Urinalysis }>	31%
<{Urinalysis}{Urinalysis}{Urinalysis}>	27%
<{Ultrasonography}{Urinalysis}{Echocardiography}>	26%
<{CBC}{CBC}{CBC}>	24%
<{Ultrasonography}{Urinalysis}{Cardiotocography}>	23%
<{Ulrasonography, HIV}{Urinalysis}{CBC}>	21%
<{Toxoplasma, AST, ALT}{Urinalysis}{CBC, Urinalysis}>	20%

followed by most of the patients. The extracted sequences are reported in the Table 3. For example, sequence <{Ultrasonography}{Urinalysis}> has a frequency of 73%, showing that 73% of patients performed the Ultrasonography exam in a trimester and the Urinalysis exam in a following trimester. The low frequency of the extracted sequences is not coherent with the guidelines, which specify the sequence of exams to do in the trimesters, and can be due to the fact that patients did some exams in private structures.

The most frequent sequence including one exam set for each trimester is <{Ultrasonography}{Urinalysis}{CBC}>, with a frequency of 44%. This sequence show that only 44% of patients did the Ultrasonography exam in the first trimester,

Urinalysis in the second one, and CBC in the third one. All other exam sequences are characterized by a lower frequency.

Frequent Exam Correlation

Table 4 reports the frequent correlations extracted from Segment$_{Full-Period}$. We observe that the majority of the correlations contain the CBC exam, being the most frequent exam in the segment. In addition, many extracted rules have a confidence of 100%, showing that there is a strong dependency between the exam sets in the rule antecedent and the rule consequent.

For example, rule {AST, ALT} → {CBC} has support 77% and confidence 100%. The support value shows that 77% of patients did exams

Table 4. Frequent correlations in the Segment$_{Full\text{-}Period}$

Frequent Correlations	Support	Confidence
{Ultrasonography} → {Urinalysis}	81%	91%
{Glucose} → {CBC}	79%	99%
{CBC, AST} → {ALT}	77%	100%
{AST, ALT} → {CBC}	77%	100%
{Toxoplasma} → {CBC}	75%	98%
{Toxoplasma} → {Ultrasonography}	69%	90%
{Ultrasonography, Glucose} → {Urinalysis}	68%	97%
{HBV} → {CBC}	67%	100%
{Urinalysis, HBV} → {CBC}	66%	100%
{HBV} → {CBC, Urinalysis}	66%	99%
{Toxoplasma, Glucose} → {Urinalysis}	65%	99%
{Glucose, HIV} → {CBC}	58%	100%
{Urinalysis, HCV} → {CBC}	54%	100%
{CBC, Partial thromboplastin time} → {Prothrombin time}	49%	99%
{ Prothrombin time, Partial thromboplastin time} → {CBC}	49%	100%
{ Prothrombin time, Partial thromboplastin time, Urinalysis} → {CBC}	48%	100%
{ Prothrombin time, Partial thromboplastin time, Glucose} → {CBC}	47%	100%
{CBC, Prothrombin time, AST} → {ALT}	47%	100%
{CTG} → {Ultrasonography}	42%	91%
{CBC, Glucose, Rubella Virus Antibody} → {Urinalysis}	42%	100%
{Rubella virus antibody, HIV} → {CBC, Urinalysis}	41%	100%
{Antithrombin III, ALT, AST} → {CBC}	41%	100%
{Antithrombin III, Glucose, Urinalysis} → {CBC}	41%	100%
{ALT, Total Bilirubin} → {CBC}	40%	100%
{Antithrombin III, Ultrasonography} → {CBC}	40%	100%

AST, ALT, and CBC. The confidence value shows that all patients who did the ALT and AST exams, also performed the CBC exam. This results is reasonable because the three exams are part of the blood exams.

Some rules don't have a confidence of 100% even if they should have. For example, rule {Glucose} → {CBC} has a confidence of only 99% and {Toxoplasma} → {CBC} of 98%. These exceptions probably refer to specific suspicious cases in which the doctor prescribed Toxoplasma or Glucose additionally to the routine CBC.

Pathways in Segment$_{Amnio}$ and Segment$_{Non\text{-}Amnio}$

We analyzed the frequent exam sets, sequences and correlation in segments Segment$_{Amnio}$ and Segment$_{Non\text{-}Amnio}$.

Frequent Exam Sets and Exam Sequences

Table 5 reports the frequent exam sets and exam sequences in segments Segment$_{Amnio}$ and Segment$_{Non\text{-}Amnio}$. Results from Segment$_{Amnio}$ are generally characterized by a higher frequency than in Seg-

Table 5. Frequent exam sets and exam sequences in Segment$_{Amnio}$ and Segment$_{Non-Amnio}$

Exam sets	Segment$_{Amnio}$	Segment$_{No-Amnio}$	Diff
{Ultrasonography}	100%	76%	24%
{CBC}	88%	77%	21%
{HBV}	68%	52%	16%
{CBC, Urinalysis, HBV}	63%	49%	14%
{HIV, Urinalysis, CBC}	56%	43%	13%
{HIV}	56%	45%	11%
{HBV, HCB}	53%	42%	11%
{HCV}	53%	43%	10%
{Urinalysis, Glucose, CBC}	68%	59%	9%
{Glucose}	73%	64%	9%
{Urinalysis}	85%	77%	8%
{CBC, ALT, AST}	67%	60%	7%
{ALT}	68%	61%	7%
{AST}	67%	61%	6%
{ALT, AST}	67%	61%	6%
{Toxoplasma}	63%	61%	2%
Exam sequences			
<{AST, ALT}{AST, ALT}>	45%	--	45%
<{Ultrasonography}{Ultrasonography}>	82%	48%	34%
<{CBC, Urinalysis} {CBC, Urinalysis}>	73%	44%	29%
<{CBC}{CBC}>	78%	52%	26%
<{CBC, Glucose}{CBC, Glucose}>	51%	26%	25%
<{Urinalysis}{Urinalysis}>	78%	54%	24%
<{Ultrasonography}{Ultrasonography} {Ultrasonography}>	62%	29%	33%
<{CBC}{CBC}{CBC}>	59%	33%	26%
<{Urinalysis}{Urinalysis}{Urinalysis}>	51%	36%	15%
<{Urinalysis}{Urinalysis}{Urinalysis}{Urinalysis}>	--	22%	22%

ment$_{Non-Amnio}$. For example, the Ultrasonography exam is done by 100% of patients in Segment$_{Amnio}$, but only by 76% of patients in Segment$_{Non-Amnio}$. The HBV, HCV and HIV exams are always at least 10% more frequent in Segment$_{Amnio}$ with respect to Segment$_{Non-Amnio}$. Some exams, such as ALT, AST and Toxoplasma, have a similar frequency in the two segments. Also most of the sequences have a frequency higher in Segment$_{Amnio}$ than in Segment$_{Non-Amnio}$. The different behavior observed in the two segments is due to the characteristics of the corresponding patients. Segment$_{Amnio}$ includes patients who did the Amniocentesis exam. This exam is usually prescribed in case of a more critical patient condition. It follows that these patients require more frequent and complete pregnancy exams. Furthermore, the Amniocentesis exam is usually done in women older than 35 years, that are potentially more careful in following the medical prescriptions.

Table 6. Frequent correlations in the Segment$_{No-Amnio}$

Frequent Correlations	Support	Confidence
{Glucose} → {CBC}	62%	97%
{AST} → {ALT}	61%	100%
{Toxoplasma} → {CBC}	59%	96%
{HBV} → {CBC}	51%	99%
{ALT} → {CBC}	51%	97%
{HBV} → {Urinalysis}	50%	96%
{Urinalysis, HBV} → {CBC}	49%	99%
{Urinalysis, HIV} → {CBC}	43%	99%
{HCV} → {HBV}	42%	97%
{HBV, HCV} → {CBC}	41%	99%
{Urinalysis, HCV} → {CBC}	40%	99%
{CBC, AST, HIV} → {ALT}	40%	100%
{Partial thromboplastin time} → {Prothrombin time}	39%	99%
{CBC, CTG} → {Urinalysis}	30%	97%
{Antithrombin III, Partial thromboplastin time} → {Prothrombin time}	30%	100%

Frequent Exam Correlations

Table 6 reports the most frequent association rules extracted from Segment$_{Non-Amnio}$. Most rules correspond to the rules extracted from segment Segment$_{Full-Period}$, but their support and confidence values are usually lower than in Segment$_{Ful-Period}$. For example, the support and confidence values for rule {Glucose} → {CBC} are 79% and 99% in Segment$_{Full Period}$, and 62% and 97% in Segment$_{Non-Amnio}$. Probably the correlations are lower because patients in Segment$_{Non-Amnio}$ did many exams in private structures.

Analogously to Segment$_{Full-Period}$, also in Segment$_{Non-Amnio}$ some rules have a confidence value lower than expected. For example, rule {Partial thromboplastin time} → {Prothrombin time} has confidence 99%, meaning that in 1% of cases the Partial thromboplastin time exam has been done without the Prothrombin time exam. The expected correct confidence value is instead 100%, because the two exams are usually done together to measure the extrinsic and intrinsic coagulation pathways.

The association rules found in Segment$_{Amnio}$ are similar to the ones found in Segment$_{Non-Amnio}$, but they are characterized by support and confidence values usually higher than in Segment$_{Non-Amnio}$ and in Segment$_{Full-Period}$. Thus, the presence of the Amniocentesis exam does not introduce new exam correlations, but increases the strength of these correlations. This result shows that patients in this segment are all characterized by a similar behavior.

FUTURE RESEARCH DIRECTIONS

The management of a complex healthcare system like the one governed by HTA is based on the possibility of accessing accurate and complete information on the performances of the system. By exploiting electronic medical records, a large number of information can be extracted from data. If some additional a-priori knowledge would be available, it can be exploited to focus the analysis on specific pregnancy conditions, for example by applying a different data segmentation. Future research directions will investigate the management of additional information, such as patients' age, to further drive the analysis and extract medical pathways related to particular conditions. Furthermore, following researches will investigate the extraction of closed sequences and rules from other datasets to monitor the evolution of actual pathways over years.

CONCLUSION

The chapter discusses an approach to analyze patients' exam log data to detect frequent medical pathways followed by patients. It aims at describing a method to evaluate the actual application of medical guidelines in the healthcare system by means of sequential data mining techniques. It shows how to extract the diagnostic pathways followed more frequently, and reports examples of extracted pathways. Obtained results can be exploited both to enrich guidelines by considering the exams actually done by patients and to improve the public sanitary service by investigating causes that lead patients to do exams privately. Thus, the aim of the chapter is on one side to demonstrate that it is possible to evaluate the actual application of diagnostic guidelines in the healthcare system, and on the other side to show how to extract the diagnostic pathways followed more frequently in order to improve the existing guidelines taking into account the actual practice.

REFERENCES

Agrawal, R., & Srikant, R. (1995). Mining sequential patterns. *11th International Conference on Data Engineering (ICDE'95),* Taipei, Taiwan, (pp. 3-14).

Baralis, E., Bruno, G., Chiusano, S., Domenici, V. C., Mahoto, N. A., & Petrigni, C. (2010). Analysis of medical pathways by means of frequent closed sequences. *International Conference on Knowledge-Based and Intelligent Information & Engineering Systems,* Cardiff, Wales, (pp. 418-425).

Cerrito, P. B. (2007). Mining the electronic medical record to examine. *Physician Decisions Studies in Computational Intelligence, 48,* 113–126. doi:10.1007/978-3-540-47527-9_5

Cerrito, P. B., & Cerrito, J. C. (2006). Data and text mining the electronic medical record to improve care and to lower costs. *Proceedings of the Thirty-first Annual SAS®Users Group International Conference.* Cary, NC: SAS Institute Inc., paper077-31.

Chen, Y., Pedersen, L. H., Chu, W. W., & Olsen, J. (2007). Drug exposure side effects from mining pregnancy data. *ACM SIGKDD Explorations Newsletter -Special issue on data mining for health informatics, 9*(1).

Dart, T., Cui, Y., Chatellier, G., & Degoulet, P. (2003). Analysis of hospitalized patient flows using data mining. *Studies in Health Technology and Informatics, 95,* 263–268.

DOH. (2010). New York State Medicaid update. *The Official Newsletter of the New York Medicaid Program, Prenatal Care Special Edition, 26*(2).

Fournier-Vigier, P. (2010). *A sequential pattern mining framework.* Retrieved March 10, 2011, from http://www.philippe-fournier-viger.com/spmf/

Gosain, A., & Kumar, A. (2009). Analysis of health care data using different data mining techniques. *International Conference on Intelligent Agent & Multi-Agent Systems, 2009 (IAMA 2009),* (pp. 1-6).

Hardin, J. M., & Chieng, C. (2007). Data mining and clinical decision support systems. *Clinical Decision Support Systems. Healthcare Informatics, 1*, 44–63. doi:10.1007/978-0-387-38319-4_3

ICD IX-CM. (2011). *Free online searchable 2009 ICD-9-CM.* Retrieved April 3, 2011 from http://icd9cm.chrisendres.com

Kazemzadeh, R. S., & Sartipi, K. (2006). Incorporating data mining applications into clinical guidelines. *Proceedings of the 19th IEEE Symposium on Computer-Based Medical Systems (CBMS'06).*

Monti, M. (2011). *Ostetricia e Ginecologia on line.* Retrieved April 5, 2011, from http://www.ginecolink.net/percorso_non_medici/EsamiGrav.htm

NICE. (2003). *Antenatal care, routine care for the healthy pregnant woman.* National Collaborating Centre for Women's and Children's Health by NICE, Clinical Guidelines. RCOG Press, 2003.

Nyblom, H., Berggren, U., Balldin, J., & Olsson, R. (2004). High AST/ALT Ratio may indicate advanced alcoholic liver disease rather than heavy drinking. *Alcohol and Alcoholism (Oxford, Oxfordshire), 39*(4), 336–339. doi:10.1093/alcalc/agh074

Palniappan, S., & Ling, C. S. (2008). Clinical decision support using OLAP with data mining. *International Journal of Computer Science and Network Security, 8*(9).

Rossille, D., Cuggia, M., Arnault, A., Bouget, J., & Le Beux, P. (2008). Managing an emergency department by analysing HIS medical data: A focus on elderly patient clinical pathways. *Health Care Management Science, 11*, 139–146. doi:10.1007/s10729-008-9059-6

Siddiq, J., Akhgar, B., Gruzdz, A., Zaefarian, G., & Ihnatowicz, A. (2009). *Automated diagnosis system to support colon cancer treatment: MATCH.* Fifth International Conference on Information Technology: New Generations.

Stolba, N., & Tjoa, A. M. (2007). The relevance of data warehousing and data mining in the field of evidence based medicine to support healthcare decision-making. *International Journal of Computer Systems Science and Engineering, 3*(3), 143–149.

Szathmary, L. (2006). *Symbolic data mining methods with the Coron Platform.* University Henri Poincaré, Nancy 1, laboratory of LORIA - INRIA Lorraine, France.

ADDITIONAL READING

Abdullah, U., Ahmad, J., & Ahmed, A. (2008). Analysis of effectiveness of Apriori algorithm in medical billing data mining. *4th International Conference on Emerging Technologies IEEE-ICET 2008,* (pp. 327 – 331). FUIEMS, Found. Univ., Islamabad.

Afridi, M. J., & Farooq, M. (2011). OG-Miner: An intelligent health tool for achieving millennium development goals (MDGs) in m-health environments. *Proceedings of the 44th Hawaii International Conference on System Sciences (HICSS 2011),* (pp. 1-10).

Brossette, S. E., Sprague, A. P., Hardin, J. M., Waites, K. B., Jones, W. T., & Moser, S. A. (1998). Association rules and data mining in hospital infection control and public health surveillance. *Journal of the American Medical Informatics Association, 5*(4), 373–378. doi:10.1136/jamia.1998.0050373

Chen, J., He, H., Li, J., Jin, H., McAullay, D., & Williams, G. … Kelman, C. (2005). Representing association classification rules mined from health data. *Proceedings of 9th International Conference on Knowledge-Based Intelligent Information and Engineering Systems (KES 2005).*

Choi, K., Chung, S., Rhee, H., & Suh, Y. (2010). Classification and sequential pattern analysis for improving managerial efficiency and providing better medical service in public healthcare centers. *Journal of Korean Society of Medical Informatics*, *16*(2), 67–76.

Cios, K. J., & Moore, W. (2002). Uniqueness of medical data mining. *Artificial Intelligence in Medicine*, *26*(1-2), 1–24. doi:10.1016/S0933-3657(02)00049-0

Concaro, S., Sacchi, L., Fratino, P., & Bellazzi, R. (2009). Mining healthcare data with temporal association rules: Improvements and assessment for a practical use. *Artificial Intelligence in Medicine*, *5651*, 16–25. doi:10.1007/978-3-642-02976-9_3

Delen, D., Fuller, C., Mccann, C., & Ray, D. (2009). Analysis of healthcare coverage: A data mining approach. *Expert Systems with Applications*, *36*(2), 995–1003. doi:10.1016/j.eswa.2007.10.041

Fayyad, U., Piatetsky-Shapiro, G., & Padhraic, S. (1996). From data mining to knowledge discovery in databases. *AI Magazine*, *17*(3).

Gorthi, A., Firtion, C., & Vepa, J. (2009). Automated risk assessment tool for pregnancy care. *31st Annual International Conference of the IEEE Engineering in Medicine and Biology Society EMBC'09*, (pp. 6222 – 6225).

Gosain, A., & Kumar, A. (2009). Analysis of health care data using different data mining techniques. *International Conference on Intelligent Agent & Multi-Agent Systems, 2009 (IAMA 2009)*, (pp. 1-6).

Kaur, H., & Wasan, S. K. (2006). Empirical study on applications of data mining techniques in healthcare. *Journal of Computer Science*, *2*(2), 194–200. doi:10.3844/jcssp.2006.194.200

Kurgan, L. A., Cios, K. J., Tadeusiewicz, R., Ogiela, M., & Goodenday, L. S. (2001). Knowledge discovery approach to automated cardiac SPECT diagnosis. *Artificial Intelligence in Medicine*, *23*(2), 149–169. doi:10.1016/S0933-3657(01)00082-3

Lin, F., Chou, S., Pan, S., & Chen, Y. (2001). Mining time dependency patterns in clinical pathways. *International Journal of Medical Informatics*, *62*, 11–25. doi:10.1016/S1386-5056(01)00126-5

Lucas, P. (2004). Bayesian analysis, pattern analysis, and data mining in health care. *Current Opinion in Critical Care*, *10*(5), 399–403. doi:10.1097/01.ccx.0000141546.74590.d6

Mohammed, N., Fung, B. C. M., Hung, P. C. K., & Lee, C. (2009). Anonymizing healthcare data: A case study on the blood transfusion service. *Proceedings of the 15th ACM SIGKDD international conference on Knowledge discovery and data mining*, June 28-July 01, 2009, Paris, France.

Ordonez, C., Ezquerra, N. F., & Santana, C. A. (2006). Constraining and summarizing association rules in medical data. *Knowledge and Information Systems*, *9*(3), 259–283. doi:10.1007/s10115-005-0226-5

Patil, B. M., Joshi, R. C., & Toshniwal, D. (2010). Association rule for classification of type-2 diabetic patients. *Second International Conference on Machine Learning and Computing (ICMLC) 2010*, Bangalore, India, (pp. 330-334).

Prather, J. C., Lobach, D. F., Goodwin, L. K., Hales, J. W., Hage, M. L., & Hammond, W. E. (1997). Medical data mining: Knowledge discovery in a clinical data warehouse. *Proceedings of the AMIA Annual Fall Symposium, 1997*, 106–110.

Quinn, A., Jelinek, H. F., Stranieri, A., & Year-wood, J. (2008). AWSum - Applying data mining in a health care scenario. *International Conference on Intelligent Sensors, Sensor Networks and Information Processing, (ISSNIP 2008)*, (pp. 291-296).

Ramaraj, E., & Venkatesan, N. (2005). An efficient pattern mining analysis in healthcare database. *International Conference for Intelligent System*, University Technology PETRONAS, Malaysia, (pp. 549-555).

Siau, K. (2003). Health care informatics. *IEEE Transactions on Information Technology in Biomedicine, 7*(1), 1–7. doi:10.1109/TITB.2002.805449

Silver, M., Sakata, T., Su, H. C., Herman, C., Dolins, S. B., & O'Shea, M. J. (2001). Case study: how to apply data mining techniques in a healthcare data warehouse. *Journal of Healthcare Information Management, 15*(2).

Viveros, M. S., Nearhos, J. P., & Rothman, M. J. (1996). Applying data mining techniques to a health insurance information system. *Proceedings of the 22th International Conference on Very Large Data Bases (VLDB '96)*, Mombai, India, (pp. 286-294).

Zhuang, Z., Churilov, L., Burstein, F., & Sikaris, K. (2009). Combining data mining and case-based reasoning for intelligent decision support for pathology ordering by general practitioners. *European Journal of Operational Research, 195*(3), 662–675. doi:10.1016/j.ejor.2007.11.003

KEY TERMS AND DEFINITIONS

Association Rule: An implication between two sets of elements (antecedent and consequent) which measures by means of the support and confidence values, how much the antecedent and the consequent are dependent.

Closed Sequence: A sequence that is not contained in another sequence with same frequency.

Data Mining: The process of extracting hidden information from datasets, which include algorithms for classification, clustering, association rules and sequence extraction.

Exam Log Data: Data recording electronic patients' exam records with time stamps.

Medical Pathway: The treatment course followed by patients for a given disease.

Segmentation: The activity of partitioning data into segments by exploiting specific criteria to group data.

Sequence Extraction: A data mining technique that involves finding existing sequences of elements in the data.

Chapter 19
Building a Lazy Domain Theory for Characterizing Malignant Melanoma

Eva Armengol
Artificial Intelligence Research Institute (IIIA-CSIC), Spain

Susana Puig
Hospital Clínic i Provincial de Barcelona, Spain

ABSTRACT

In this chapter, the authors propose an approach for building a model characterizing malignant melanomas. A common way to build a domain model is using an inductive learning method. Such resulting model is a generalization of the known examples. However, in some domains where there is not a clear difference among the classes, the inductive model could be too general. The approach taken in this chapter consists of using lazy learning methods for building what the authors call a lazy domain theory. The main difference between both inductive and lazy theories is that the former is complete whereas the latter is not. This means that the lazy domain theory may not cover all the space of known examples. The authors' experiments have shown that, despite of this, the lazy domain theory has better performance than the inductive theory.

INTRODUCTION

Malignant melanoma (MM) is the most dangerous type of skin cancer. The MM is the second most frequent kind of cancer among people between 15 and 34 years old. In the last thirty years the incidence of MM has been increased more rapidly than other kinds of cancer. Many studies show that an early detection of MM increases the survival rate since when tumors are thin the lesion can be excised and the survival is around the 95% after 5 years. However, when the tumor has spreading to the nodes the risk of metastases increases and, thus the survival rate decreases. The early diagnosis of melanoma is a difficult task that dermatologist face every day. When a lesion is suspicious of being a

DOI: 10.4018/978-1-4666-1803-9.ch019

melanoma it is removed and the final diagnosis is performed based on histopathology criteria.

The clinical diagnosis of MM is based on the ABCD rule that takes into account the *Asymmetry, Border irregularity, Color* and *Diameter* of the lesion. Although the ABCD rule has been proved to be effective for an early diagnosis, there are necessary more accurate methods to correctly diagnose lesions that do not present clear malignant characteristics. It is important that a dermatologist can detect suspicious skin lesions during a clinical session, therefore it should be very useful to have a clear and easy characterization of MM in early stages. *Dermoscopy* is a non-invasive technique introduced by dermatologists two decades ago. This technique provides a more accurate evaluation of skin lesions, and can therefore, avoid the excision of lesions that are benign. Therefore, dermatologists need to achieve a good dermatoscopic classification of lesions prior to extraction (Puig et al., 2007). Hofmann-Wellenhof et al. (2002) suggested a classification of benign melanocytic lesions. Argenziano et al. (2007) hypothesized that dermoscopic classification may be better than the classical clinico pathological classification of benign melanocytic lesions (*nevi*). Dermoscopy improves accuracy for the diagnosis of melanoma in nearly 25%. However, some benign lesions may mimic melanoma and some melanomas may be similar to benign lesions, consequently many unnecessary extractions are produced. It is assessed that one of 30 lesions excised by non-expert dermatologists only one of them is MM. When dermatologists have high expertise, the ratio decreases to one MM for each 4 excisions. For this reason, the benign/malignant ratio of excised lesions is 1 malignant for 30 benign for non-expert dermatologists, whereas this ratio is 1 MM to 4 benignant when the dermatologist has high expertise. The *reflectance confocal microscopy* is a new non-invasive diagnostic technique that allows the visualization of skin cells in vivo. This technique also increase the accuracy of the experts diagnosis but even in the hands of experts

and in combination with dermoscopy information, accuracy never reaches 100%.

Thus, we are especially interested on characterizing skin lesions in the frontier of both malignant and benign lesions. In our experiments we used descriptions of skins lesions that have already been excised, i.e., they are lesions that dermatologists considered that could be malignant melanomas. However some of them, after a histopathology analysis resulted to be benign. This means that they provide a good set of suspicious lesions from which to generate a domain model able to discriminate between both malignant and benignant lesions with similar characteristics. We propose to take descriptions of known skin lesions and to use a lazy learning method to obtain a domain theory. Skin lesions are described using two sets of features, dermatoscopic and confocal, and our goal is to find a subset of features characterizing malignant lesions.

What we propose is to use lazy learning methods for building a domain theory useful for the classification of skin lesions. We experimented with two lazy learning methods: *k* nearest neighbor and *Lazy Induction of Descriptions* (LID). The *k* nearest neighbor (*k*-NN in short) method is based on the idea that similar objects have similar classification. Once an unseen object has been classified, we propose to build an explanation of the classification based on the anti-unification concept, i.e., the explanation is formed by the attributes shared by all the objects assessed as the most similar to the unseen object. The LID method is a lazy learning method useful for classification tasks. In addition of classifying a new domain object, LID also gives a symbolic description that can be interpreted in several ways. One of these interpretations is as a partial description of a class.

When the lazy learning method is used during a training phase (i.e., we know in advance the correct classification of the domain objects) the explanation of the classification can be interpreted as a rule of a domain theory in the same sense that the rules produced by inductive learning methods.

Thus, when all these rules are stored we obtain a domain theory. However such domain theory is *lazy* since it has been obtained during the process of classification of a concrete domain object. We used this procedure on a database containing descriptions of skin lesions and we compared the results with those produced by a decision tree (i.e., from an inductive learning method). Our experiments show that the lazy learning methods build a domain model having, in terms of both sensitivity and specificity, better performance than the produced by the decision tree.

BACKGROUND

Frawley et at (1992) defined *knowledge discovery* as "the non-trivial extraction of implicit, unknown and potentially useful information from data". The goal of a knowledge discovery (KD) process is to explore a set of known data in order to find patterns. Most of the techniques used for KD are based on inductive learning methods (Mitchell, 1997) that generalize the input data to generate a model (or domain theory) that can be useful in the future for classify unseen data. This means that, because of objects of a domain can be divided in several classes, the domain theory has to include discriminatory descriptions for each one of these classes. Mitchell (1997) pointed out that this is a global approximation to concepts since all the known examples are used to generate a domain theory, i.e., the induced theory is complete with respect to the set of known examples. In our approach we want to support domain experts in building a domain theory, producing descriptions of classes that can be easily understood and giving them the opportunity to systematically analyze the classes proposed.

A different approach for classifying unseen examples is to use some lazy learning method (instance-based, case-based reasoning, etc.). Thus, a new problem is classified as belonging to a class by assessing its similarity with a set of known examples. However, lazy learning methods do not produce explicit generalizations and, therefore, they do not generate domain theories. Our point is that if we could generate some explicit generalization of the classification process from a lazy learning method, we could generate a domain theory. These generalizations could be seen as local approximations since they describe an area around the problem that has been solved. In a previous work (Armengol, 2008) we proposed to generate domain theories using the explanations of the classifications produced by a lazy learning method. Notice that the domain theory formed by local approximations is not complete with respect to the set of known examples, since it only describes areas of the problem space around the new problems. We call the theory generated from local approximations a *lazy domain theory*. This is the same idea of *explanation-based learning (EBL)* methods (Mitchell et al., 1986; Dejong & Mooney, 1986) that generate domain rules from one example. Methods of this family solve a problem and then analyzes the problem solving trace in order to generalize it. The generalized trace is an *explanation* that is used as a new domain rule for solving new problems more efficiently. This explanation is represented using the same formalism as the one used for describing problems, therefore it is perfectly understandable and usable by the system. Examples of systems using EBL are EBG (Dejong & Mooney, 1986), PRODIGY (Carbonell et al., 1995) and SOAR (Laird et al., 1987) among others.

EBL methods are capable of building new domain rules (explanations) by generalizing the problem solving trace of a particular problem. Lazy learning methods do not explicitly generalize the examples but they always use the complete set of examples. Thus, an unseen problem is classified according to its similitude to a subset of known examples. In this sense, both EBL and lazy learning methods build *local approximations* of concepts (Mitchell, 1997) since the similar examples define an area around the new example and the explanation of the similarity can be taken as a general description of that area. Case-based reasoning (CBR) methods (Kolodner, 1993) predict the classification of a problem based on its similarity to already solved cases. Several approaches on CBR generate some kind of structure that can be interpreted as an explanation. An example of such system is CHEF (Hammond, 1989) whose goal is to produce a cooking recipe from a set of ingredients. The process followed by CHEF is to retrieve a similar recipe and to adapt it by replacing some ingredients. Another approach is that proposed by Leake (Leake, 1996) that use the experience acquired by a CBR system to improve its performance. The knowledge structures he proposes and what he defines as *experience* or *introspection* can be seen as explanations of different parts of the problem solving process.

In the context of CBR for solving classification problems, we want to use generalizations for explaining the result to the domain expert, and on the other hand, we want that the system can take benefit of these explanations when solving new problems. In (Armengol & Plaza, 2006) we proposed an explanation scheme that is independent of the CBR method used for solving the problem. This explanation scheme is based on the notion of the *anti-unification* concept (Armengol & Plaza, 2000). The anti-unification of a set of objects is a description (AU) that contains attributes shared by the set of objects and each attribute takes as value the most specific of all the values holding in the original set. Our approach is that the anti-unification is an explanation of why the cases in *C* have been considered as the more similar to *p*, since it is a description of all that is shared among the retrieved cases and the new problem. This explanation scheme supports the user in understanding the classification of an unseen problem. Two applications of this explanation scheme, one on toxicology domain and the other on telecommunications domain, can be found in (Armengol & Plaza, 2006; Corral et al., 2009) respectively.

Our claim is that in some domains the inductive learning methods are not appropriated because they produce overgeneralization. This means that, although the model fits the known data, it fails in the classification of unseen objects. An example of this kind of domains is *Predictive Toxicology,* where the goal is to find a model for carcinogenesis. The difficulty in that domain is that there are chemical compounds with a very similar chemical structure with different carcinogenic activity. For this reason the construction of a carcinogenic model from inductive learning methods is not actually useful without the support of other domain knowledge that is not included in the description of the chemical compounds. For instance, the existence of a bromide atom is indicative of carcinogenesis, but this information cannot be extracted in a inductive way, it has to be supplied by the expert and added to the model. A similar situation occurs in the characterization of skin lesions since early malignant melanoma can share many characteristics with benignant lesions and, therefore a dermatologist can easily confuse them.

There are several tools that automatically diagnose malignant melanoma. For instance, MELAFIND (http://medgadget.com/archives/2005/08/melafind_system.html) is a device designed to determine whether skin moles and lesions are malignant. It uses a database of around 6000 already biopsied lesions to find similarities with a new potentially malignant skin lesion. In (Vestergaard & Menzies, 2008) there is an interesting comparison of the performance of several automatic instruments with human experts. The main conclusion of this comparison is that there is not automatic method clearly outperforming human experts. All these automatic instruments have been built with a different goal than our approach since they want to take the role of dermatologists and analyze and interpret an image of an skin lesion in order to diagnose it. The goal of our approach is not to diagnose from an image but from the interpretation of an image given by a dermatologist. In fact we do not want to take the dematologist's role but support them in diagnosing skin lesions.

What we propose is to use, as it is done in (Armengol, 2008), a lazy learning method for building a domain theory able to characterize the malignancy of skin lesions. However, because we also want to obtain a domain model characterizing skin lesions, we propose a method to explain the result of the classification. Such method, allows the construction of a domain theory from local approximations to concepts. An example of a lazy construction of a domain model is the method called *Lazy Decision Trees* (LDT) proposed by (Friedman et al., 1996). Differently from pure inductive techniques, LDT builds a decision tree in a lazy way, i.e., each time that a new problem has to be classified, the system reuses, if possible, the existing tree. Otherwise, a new branch classifying the new problem is added to the tree. Notice that, in fact, the decision tree represents a general model of a domain and LDT builds it in a lazy way.

LAZY DOMAIN THEORIES

The most common learning techniques for knowledge discovery are those based on inductive algorithms. The domain model resulting from the application of these algorithms is a complete domain theory, in the sense that it covers all the space of known examples. However, in some domains where there is not a clear difference among the classes, the inductive model could be too general. In other words, the area on the frontier of two classes could be described by descriptions that, although they are correct on the known examples, they are actually non-discriminant on unseen examples belonging to this area. The classification of skin lesions presents two interesting characteristics. On one hand, the frontier among benign skin lesions and malignant melanomas is not clear (i.e., there are benignant lesions with

many characteristics of malignant melanomas and vice versa). On the other hand, there is not a model for classifying skin lesions widely agree. In this paper we show that using a lazy learning method, instead of an inductive one, it is possible the improvement of the classification performance and, in addition, it also produces a domain model as accurate as the one build by inductive learning methods.

What we propose is the use of lazy learning methods for classifying a given problem and to generate a domain model from the explanation of the classification. Each one of the explanations can be seen as a local description of a class; therefore, it can be stored for future use. The set of explanations constitutes a *lazy domain theory*. Explanations are understood here as generalizations and, as such, we interpret them as domain rules in the same sense that inductive learning methods do. Differently than domain theories generated by inductive learning methods, theories generated from explanations are partial. In our approach we discuss the feasibility of "global" in front of "partial" domain theories from experimental results.

In the next sections we first explain the general process we propose for building a lazy domain theory. Then we briefly explain two lazy learning methods, k-NN and LID and how to generate a domain theory from each one of them.

Generating a Domain Theory with a Lazy Learning Method

In this section we explain how to generate a lazy domain theory from the explanations build during the classification process using a lazy learning method. Let S be the training set containing domain objects with known and correct classification, and T the domain theory, initially empty. The procedure we propose is the following (see Figure 1): to use a lazy learning method (LLM) with leave-one-out to classify each object in S. Then, for each object o_i belonging to S to proceed as follows:

Figure 1. Scheme of the procedure generating a domain theory using a learning method

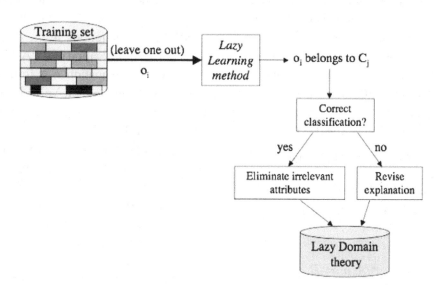

If LLM proposed the correct classification, then

1. Generate the explanation E_i of the classification
2. Simplify E_i by eliminating irrelevant attributes (if necessary)
3. Include the (simplified) explanation in T

If LMM cannot uniquely classify o_i, i.e., it proposes at least two classes, then for each class c_i

1. Generate one explanation E_{ci} of the membership of o_i to each class
2. Simplify each E_{ci} by eliminating irrelevant attributes (if necessary)
3. Include the (simplified explanations) in T; otherwise, T is not modified

Notice that T is composed of discriminant descriptions since the explanations of one class are simplified whereas they are not satisfied by examples of other classes. Otherwise they are not included in the theory.

We conducted experiments using two lazy learning methods: k-NN and LID. In the next

sections we briefly explain both methods and how to generate a lazy domain theory with each one of them.

Explaining the *k*-NN Classification

A common method for classification is the k-NN. This method is based on the idea that similar objects have similar classification. Given a training set S and a problem p to classify, the k-NN algorithm is composed of the following steps:

1. To assess the similarity between p and each one of the elements of S,
2. To take the subset S_k of S composed of the k elements of S having the highest similarity to p,
3. To classify p as belonging to the class of the majority of elements in S_k.

The key point of this algorithm is the particular similarity measure used to compare the objects. Commonly the similarity ranges from 0 to 1, therefore it can be seen as the dual of a distance measure (i.e., $similarity = 1 - distance$). There are several distances commonly used (for instance, Euclidean, Minkowski, or Mahalanobis) and the user has to evaluate the most appropriate for the domain at hand. Let us suppose that domain objects are described as tuples of n attributes a_1 ... a_n. When the values of these attributes are symbolic, the usual way to assess the distance between two domain objects A and B is

$$D(A, B) = \sum_{i=1}^{n} d(A.a_i, B.a_i), \text{ where } A.a_i \text{ and}$$

$B.a_i$ are the values that the attribute a_i takes in A and B respectively, and $d(A.a_i, B.a_i)$ is defined as follows:

$$d(A. a_i, B. b_i) = \begin{cases} 1, & A, a_i = B. a_i \\ 0, & \text{otherwise} \end{cases}$$

The explanation of the k-NN is a classification for the problem p, however sometimes this result is too poor for the expert. Some automatic systems are not accepted for common use because of the lack of understandability of its outcome. In other words, the system has to be able to explain its result in order to convince experts that the result has not been obtained by chance. Experts and no experts need to understand the reasoning process in achieving the classification. In particular, the explanation of the k-NN should be the resulting similarity value and the explanation of the formula used to reach it, but it is difficult to understand. Often an alternative explanation of the k-NN method is to show the k cases assessed as the most similar to the new problem. Nevertheless, when the cases have a complex structure, simply showing the most similar cases to the user may not be enough. We use the explanation scheme introduced in (Armengol & Plaza, 2006) based on the *anti-unification concept* (Armengol & Plaza, 2000). The anti-unification of a set of objects is a description (AU) defined as the most specific generalization of these objects. The AU is formed by the attributes common to the set of objects assessed as the most similar to the problem p. Each attribute in AU takes as value the most specific of all the values holding in the original set. We consider a simplification of the AU in the following way: an explanation E is formed by all the attributes taking the same value in both p and all the elements in S_k. For instance, we can explain the similarity of the objects *m-85* and *m-102* shown in Figure 2 by means of the explanation shown in the right part of the same figure. Notice that:

1. The attributes as morphology and typical-basal are only present in one of the objects, therefore they are not in the explanation,
2. The attributes as colors, n-struct and junctional-nests-features are common to both objects but with different values, therefore they are not in the explanation,
3. All attributes in the explanation are present with the same value in both objects.

In order to eliminate irrelevant attributes of E we propose the following procedure:

1. To sort the attributes with some relevance criteria,
2. To take the first attribute a_i,
3. To eliminate a_i from E,
4. If E -$\{a_i\}$ is satisfied by examples of only one class then take $E' = E$ - $\{a_i\}$ and return to step 2 with E'; otherwise a_i cannot be eliminated so take the next attribute a_{i+1} and return to step 3.

In our experiments we used as relevance criteria the López de Mántaras (LM) distance (López de Mántaras, 1991) that measures the distance among the correct partition (that classifies correctly the known examples) with the partition induced by an attribute. Let us recall its definition: Let X be a finite set of objects; $\mathcal{P} = \{P_1, \dots, P_n\}$ be a partition of X in n sets; and $\mathcal{Q} = \{Q_1, \dots, Q_m\}$

Figure 2. The right description is formed by the common attributes and values of objects m-85 and m-102. It is an adaptation of the anti-unification concept.

```
(define (Object :id m-85)          (define (Object :id m-102)         (define (Object :id EXPLANATION)
  (asymmetry twoaxes)               (asymmetry twoaxes)                 (asymmetry twoaxes)
  (colors 2)                        (colors 3)                          (nt yes)
  (n-estruct 3)                     (n-estruct 2)                       (projections 0)
  (nt yes)                          (nt yes)                            (structureless-areas 0)
  (projections 0)                   (projections 0)                     (glob yes)
  (structureless-areas 0)           (structureless-areas 0)             (regression yes)
  (glob yes)                        (glob yes)                          (glob-perif 0)
  (regression yes)                  (regression yes)                    (Cobblestone no)
  (glob-perif 0)                    (glob-perif 0)                      (disarranged 0)
  (HC typical)                      (HC atypical)                       (Corneal 0)
  (Cobblestone no)                  (Cobblestone no)                    (pagetoid-infiltration yes)
  (disarranged 0)                   (disarranged 0)                     (PG_form dendritic)
  (Corneal 0)                       (Corneal 0)                         (PG_global pleomorphic)
  (pagetoid-infiltration yes)       (pagetoid-infiltration yes)         (cerebriform-struct 0)
  (grade 1)                         (grade 3)                           (Dermal-papilla yes)
  (PG_form dendritic)               (PG_form dendritic)                 (DP_localization localized)
  (PG_global pleomorphic)           (PG_global pleomorphic)             (DP_irregular 1)
  (cerebriform-struct 0)            (cerebriform-struct 0)              (junsheetlike-cells no)
  (Dermal-papilla yes)              (Dermal-papilla yes)                (spindled 0)
  (DP_localization localized)       (DP_localization localized)         (cerebriform-clusters 0)
  (DP_irregular 1)                  (DP_irregular 1)                    (Dermal-cells no)
  (DP_papilla edged nonedged)       (DP_papilla edged)                  (bright-or-spots no)
  (Junctional-nests-features clusters)  (Junctional-nests-features no)  (C_vessels no)
  (typical-basal mild)              (junsheetlike-cells no)             (collagen no)
  (junsheetlike-cells no)           (spindled 0)                      )
  (morphology juncpleomorph)        (Dermal-nests no)
  (spindled 0)                      (cerebriform-clusters 0)
  (Dermal-nests yes)                (Dermal-cells no)
  (dense-clusters regular)          (bright-or-spots no)
  (cerebriform-clusters 0)          (C_vessels no)
  (Dermal-cells no)                 (collagen no)
  (bright-or-spots no)            )
  (C_vessels no)
  (collagen no)
)
```

be a partition of X in m sets. The LM distance between them is computed as follows:

$$LM(P,Q) = 2 - \frac{I(P) + I(Q)}{I(P \cap Q)} \text{ ,where}$$

$$I(P) = -\sum_{i=1}^{n} p_i \log_2 p_i; \ p_i = \frac{|P_i|}{|X|} \ ;$$

$$I(Q) = -\sum_{j=1}^{m} p_j \log_2 p_j; \ p_j = \frac{|Q_j|}{|X|} \ ;$$

$$I(P \cap Q) = -\sum_{i=1}^{n}\sum_{j=1}^{m} p_{ij} \log_2 p_{ij}; \ p_{ij} = \frac{|P_i \cap Q_j|}{|X|} \ .$$

For each attribute describing a domain object, we computed its LM distance to the correct partition and then we ordered the attributes from highest to lowest distance. This order reflects that an attribute inducing a partition with high distance to the correct partition is irrelevant, therefore it can be eliminated. With this elimination procedure, the explanation shown in Figure 2 becomes in the one shown in Figure 3.

The Lazy Induction of Descriptions Method

Lazy Induction of Descriptions (LID) (Armengol & Plaza, 2001) is a lazy learning method for classification tasks that determines the most relevant attributes of a problem and searches in a case base for cases sharing these relevant attributes.

Figure 3. Simplification of the explanation shown in Figure 2

```
(define (Object :id SIMPLIFIED-EXPLANATION)
    (asymmetry twoaxes)
    (nt yes)
    (projections 0)
    (structureless-areas 0)
    (glob yes)
    (regression yes)
    (glob-perif 0)
    (pagetoid-infiltration yes)
    (PG_form dendritic)
    (PG_global pleomorphic)
    (DP_localization localized)
    (DP_irregular 1)
)
```

The problem p is classified when LID finds a set of relevant attributes whose values are shared by a subset of cases all belonging to the same solution class C_i. Then LID classifies the problem as belonging to C_i. We call *similitude term* the description formed by these relevant attributes and *discriminatory set* the set of cases satisfying a similitude term. In fact, a similitude term is a generalization of both p and the cases in the discriminatory set.

Given a problem for solving p, the LID algorithm (Figure 4) initializes D_0 as a description with no attributes, the discriminatory set S_{D_0} as the set of cases satisfying D_0, i.e., all the available cases, and C as the set of solution classes into which the known cases are classified. Let D_i be the current similitude term and S_{D_i} be the set of all the cases satisfying D_i. When the stopping condition of LID is not satisfied, the next step is to select an attribute for specializing D_i. The specialization of D_i is achieved by adding attributes to it. Given a set F of attributes candidate to specialize D_i, the next step of the algorithm is the selection of an attribute $f \in F$. Selecting the

most discriminatory attribute in F is heuristically done using a distance measure. Such distance is used to compare each partition P_f induced by an attribute f with the correct partition P_c. The correct partition has as many sets as solution classes. Each attribute $f \in F$ induces in the discriminatory set a partition P_f with as many sets as the number of different values that f satisfies in the cases. Given a distance measure " and two attributes f and g inducing respectively partitions P_f and P_g, we say that f is *more discriminatory than g* if and only if " $(P_f, P_c) <$ " (P_g, P_c). This means that the partition P_f is closer to the correct partition than the partition P_g. The selection of the most discriminatory attribute is heuristically done using the LM distance over the candidate attributes. Let f_d be the most discriminatory attribute in F; the specialization of D_i defines a new similitude term $D_{i+1} = D_i \bigcup f_d$ that is satisfied by a subset of cases $S_{D_{i+1}} \subseteq S_{D_i}$. Next, LID is recursively called with $S_{D_{i+1}}$ and D_{i+1}. The recursive call of LID has $S_{D_{i+1}}$ instead of S_{D_i} because the cases that are not satisfied by D_{i+1} will not satisfy any further specialization.

Figure 4. The LID algorithm: p is the problem to be solved, D_i is the similitude term, S_{D_i} is the discriminatory set associated with D_i, C is the set of solution classes, class(S_{D_i}) is the class C_i in C to which all the elements in S_{D_i} belong.

LID has two stopping situations: 1) all the cases in the discriminatory set S_{D_j} belong to the same solution class C_i, or 2) there is no attribute allowing the specialization of the similitude term. When the stopping condition 1) is satisfied p is classified as belonging to C_i. When the stopping condition 2) is satisfied, S_{D_j} contains cases from several classes.

The last similitude term produced by LID can be interpreted in several ways. One of them is that it can be seen as a partial discriminant description of C_i since all the cases satisfying the similitude term belong to C_i (according to one of the stopping conditions of LID). Therefore, the similitude term can be used as a generalization of knowledge in the sense of either PROTOS (Bareiss et al., 1988) EBL (Mitchell et al., 1986; Dejong & Mooney, 1986) or inductive learning methods (Quinlan, 1986). Since the similitude term contains the important attributes used to classify a problem, it can also be interpreted as a justification or explanation of the problem classification. Notice that in any of the interpretations above, LID explanations can be taken by the system as domain rules since they contain the relevant attributes for classifying a problem.

EXPERIMENTS

We carried out experiments with a database containing descriptions of 192 skin lesions, 50 of them are malignant melanomas (MM) and 142 are benignant. These lesions are described by 11 dermatoscopic attributes and 22 confocal attributes. All attributes take symbolic values although it is possible the existence of unknown values. We conducted 70 experiments consisting on the random generation of two disjoint sets: the training set, from which lazy domain theory is generated; and the test set whose elements will be classified using the generated theory. We prefer this kind of evaluation instead of using 10-fold cross-validation because we also want to analyze the lazy theories generated from training sets of different size.

To classify a problem p of the test set, our procedure exhaustively checks all the rules of the theory (either the one generated using k-NN or the one generated using LID) and gives as classification the class (or classes) having some description satisfied by p. A description d of a class C_i is satisfied by p when every attribute-value pair in d is also present in p. The result of this classification may be the following: 1) one class (benign or MM); 2) a multiple solution (i.e., both classes) meaning that the lesion is suspicious since it satisfies descriptions of both classes; and 3) no answer (NA) meaning that the lesion does not satisfy any class description.

Concerning the k-NN method, we experimented with several values of k: 3, 5 and 7. From some preliminary experiments we have seen that the coverage of the domain theory generated on the training set produced the best results taking $k = 3$.

We evaluated the results of the experiments from two aspects: 1) the comprehensibility and feasibility of the lazy domain theory; and 2) the predictivity of the theory. In order to better appreciate the feasibility of the lazy domain theory, we also performed the same kind of experiments with a domain theory generated using a decision tree. We used the J48 algorithm for constructing decision trees given in the Weka platform (Hall et al., 2009). We do not performed an analysis of the computational cost of both generating the domain theory and classifying the objects of the test set. However even in the case of training sets over 120 objects the whole process (theory generation and classification of all the test set objects) does not take more than few seconds.

Analysis of the Lazy Domain Theory

From the experiments it can be shown that lazy theories from both k-NN and LID are very similar. Both have a high number of discriminant descriptions for the class *benign* and only a few for the class MM. These descriptions involve a similar subset of attributes. Also, that independently on the size of the training sets, there are subsets of class descriptions that, with little differences, appear in all the experiments. Experts known that the confocal attribute pagetoid-infiltration (see an image of such attribute in Figure 5) with value *yes* is a clear characteristic of MM, although some benignant lesions can also present pagetoid infiltration (there are suspicious lesions that are commonly excised and, after biopsy, they are classified as benignant). For this reason, we specially analyzed the descriptions of the lazy theories for the benignant class with some of the attributes related having pagetoid infiltration. Descriptions shown in Figure 6 have been generated with *k*-NN and they correspond to benignant lesions having pagetoid infiltration. These descriptions, with some variations due to the objects contained in the training set, have been generated in all the experiments. We represented them in a tree form, however there is not any kind of neither order nor preference between attributes, it only represents attributes that are common to several rules. In other words, (pagetoid-infiltration = *yes*) and (dermal-cells = no) are common to the three rules, whereas junctional-nests-features = *no*, C-vessels = *no*, junsheetlikecells = *no*, and dermal-nests = *no* are present in only two of them.

The lazy theory generated using LID has overfitting because there are a lot of class descriptions satisfied by only one object of the training set. However, concerning benignant lesions with some attribute related with having pagetoid infiltration, the descriptions are similar to those generated using *k*-NN.

Figure 7 shows two decision trees: one of them involves the attribute pagetoid-infiltration and it is according with the dermatologist's knowledge since most of lesions with an irregular dermal papilla (DP_irregular = *1*) having pagetoid infiltration are MM. The other decision tree involves only the attribute junsheetlike-cells that represents the presence or absence of atypical cells arranged in sheet-like structures visualized in superficial papillary dermis. This kind of cells is an indicative of MM. Due to the pruning process of the algorithm J48 (Quinlan, 1993) for constructing decisions trees, class descriptions are not discriminatory, however as we will analyze in the next section, the predictivity of the theory is around 75% and it never classifies a lesion as suspicious. Instead, using the lazy domain theories, a lesion may be classified as suspicious or even it may not be

Figure 5. Reflectance confocal microscopy image of a skin lesion with pagetoid infiltration

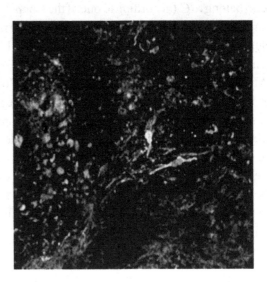

classified. In the next section we will analyze the predictivity in more detail in terms of sensitivity and specificity.

Concerning the size of the training sets, we see that both theories (the one generated using LID and the one generated using *k*-NN) are stable in the sense that there is a set of descriptions that, with minor differences, have been generated in all the experiments indepently on the size of the training sets. However, this does not happens when the domain theory is generated using decision trees. A possible explanation is that decision trees take into account all the attributes present in all the available examples whereas lazy learning methods only take into account the attributes describing the problem to be classified. Notice that this different behaviour between decision trees and the lazy learning methods is a consequence of having, respectively, global and local approximations to concepts.

There are several conclusions concerning the expert's opinions about the domain theories. Firstly, we see that the domain theory generated by a decision tree sometimes take into account

Figure 6. Three rules for the benign class generated using k-NN. Authors represented them in a tree form, however there is not any kind of neither order nor preference between the attributes. Numbers between parentheses are the support of the rules.

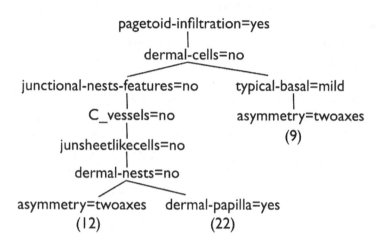

Figure 7. Two decision trees generated using the J48 algorithm

pagetoid-infiltration = yes
| DP_irregular = 0: benign (5.94/1.77)
| DP_irregular = 1: mm (9.46/1.23)
pagetoid-infiltration = no: benign (23.61/3.0)

junsheetlike-cells = 0: benign (66.34/16.74)
junsheetlike-cells = 1: mm (4.66/0.39)

attributes that, although they correctly classify according to the training set at hand, they are considered as secondary by the experts. However, as we show in Figure 7, sometimes decision trees generated very interesting domain theories according to the expert's knowledge. Secondly, theories generated by both lazy methods always take into account a subset of attributes considered as relevant by the experts. Again, we explain this fact due to the difference between the global and local approximations of concepts. Descriptions obtained by means of local approximations take into account the attributes describing the problem to be classified, therefore most of these descriptions focus on the most important characteristics of the problem that are also those considered as

important by the experts when they describe a skin lesion. Thus, local descriptions focus on the same attributes than experts do. Therefore, the main conclusion is that lazy domain theories are coherent with the expert's knowledge. Also, these theories give some rules than, even they are not confirmed by the expert's experience, they are reasonable enough to be analized in more detail.

Analysis of the Predictivity of the Lazy Domain Theory

In this section we compare the predictivity of the theories using the *Receiver Operating Characteristic* (ROC) curves. A ROC graph (Fawcett, 2006) is a technique for visualizing, organizing and selecting classifiers based on their performance. This kind of representation is useful specially when error costs are not the same in all the classes. For instance, in our domain is clearly worst to consider as benign a malignant lesion that the inverse situation. The ROC curves take into account the *true positive rate* (TPR) and the *false positive rate* (FPR) for the comparison of methods. These measures are calculated from the *sensitivity* (SE) and the *specificity* (SP), being

$$SE = \frac{TP}{TP + FN} \qquad\qquad SP = \frac{TN}{TN + FP}$$

where TP stands for true positive; TN for true negative; FP for false positive; and FN for false negative. The TPR is the sensitivity and the FPR is $1 - SP$.

One point (FPR, TPR) in the ROC space is better than another if it is in the northwest part of the graphic, i.e., if its TPR is higher, its FPR rate is lower, or both. A classifier represented by a point in the diagonal means that it has a random behavior. Points upper to the diagonal means that the classifier exploits some information from the data. Points down to the diagonal means that the classifier performs worse than a random classifier. Thus, a point is better than another if TPR is higher and FPR is lower. Moreover, given two points (FPR_1 , TPR_1) and (FPR_2 , TPR_2) such that $FPR_1 < FPR_2$ and $TPR_1 < TPR_2$, the performance of the two methods is incomparable and the cost of false positives has to be taken into account in order to choose between them.

The ROC curves are used to compare the performance of methods. A common way to do this comparison is by means of the calculation of the *area under the ROC curve* (AUC). The range of AUC is the interval [0, 1], however, because the area corresponding to a random classifier is 0.5, i.e., the area under the diagonal, the AUC of a classifier should to be upper to 0.5. The AUC of a classifier is equivalent to the probability that

the classifier will rank a randomly chosen positive instance higher than a randomly chosen negative instance. See (Fawcett, 2006) for an excellent tutorial on ROC curves.

For each one of the experiments (70 for each method) we calculated the TPR and the FPR. Because of it is possible that a lesion either cannot be classified or it is classified as suspicious, in the evaluation of the results we do not take into account neither no answers nor multiple answers. In other words, the sensitivity and specificity have been calculated taking into account only the classifications in one (correct or incorrect) class. The *k*-NN lazy theory produces around a 21% of no classifications and around a 3% of suspicious lesions; and the LID lazy theory produces around a 20% of no classifications and around a 12% of suspicious lesions. The predictivity of the lazy theories is around 63% and 55% for *k*-NN and LID respectively.

Figure 8 shows the ROC curves generated using the average of sensitivity and specificity of the 70 random experiments we performed with each method. From this graphic we seen that the theory generated with *k*-NN has lower rate of false positives than both the theory generated with LID and the one generated with the decision tree. However, LID produces a higher rate of true positives than the others. The AUC of the methods is 0.6160, 0.609 and 0,677 for decision trees (DT), for the domain theory generated by k-NN (T-*k*-NN) and the domain theory generated by LID (T-LID) respectively. Thus, the AUC shows that, although the mean predictivity of the lazy theories is lower than the produced by the decision tree, they have better performance when analyzing TPR and FPR . In particular, T-LID despite of having overfitting, produces highest number of true positives than the other theories and T-kNN has lowest FPR.

An explanation of the better performance of the lazy theories should be its over fitting. The decision tree tries to reduce it and consequently,

Figure 8. ROC curves representing the average of 70 random experiments with the three methods: decision trees (DT), the lazy theory generated with k-NN (T-kNN), and the lazy theory generated with LID (T-LID)

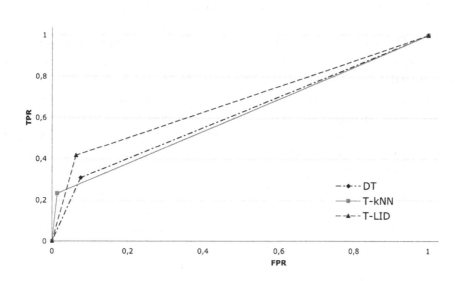

it offers compact class descriptions satisfying the known objects. However, that theory can fail in recognizing some unseen suspicious lesions. Instead, due to the over fitting, lazy domain theories have class descriptions that are more specific than those of the produced by the decision tree. This means that there will be unseen object that will not be classified because they belong to areas of the domain for which there is no characterization. Nevertheless, there are other areas that are better characterized due to this specificity of the descriptions.

In fact, in (Armengol, 2008) we compared lazy domain theories formed by sets of explanations from LID with the eager theory built by the ID3 method (Quinlan, 1986). In our experiments we showed that, for some domains, eager and lazy theories have similar predictive ability. The difference is that because the explanations that make up the lazy domain theory are more specific than inductive rules, there is a high percentage of unseen problems that the lazy theory cannot classify although the classification, when it is proposed,

is usually correct. The result obtained with the current experimentation in MM seems to confirm that previous result.

FUTURE RESEARCH DIRECTIONS

A future research direction is to combine the lazy domain theories generated using k-NN and LID into an ensemble of classifiers. An *ensemble* consists of a set of individually trained classifiers whose predictions are combined for classifying unseen domain objects (Opitz & Maclin, 1999). Because the results of the experiments show that both lazy domain theories seem to be complementary, we think that an ensemble could improve the perfomance in classifying MM. Our intuition is that an ensemble formed by a classifier using T-kNN and another classifier using T-LID, will produce low FPR and high TPR. For this reason a future research line could be to experiment with ensembles combining both theories.

When the available examples are unbalanced with respect to the solution classes, there are some methods, such as (Ha & Bunke, 1997) or SMOTE (Chawla et al., 2002), allowing the automatic generation of new examples in order to balance the classes. This kind of techniques is also used on emsembles of classifiers. Although the examples we have available in our data base are unbalanced, it could be interesting to analyze in depth whether or not these techniques are appropriated for our domain. Nevertheless, our main concern is that experts have not a clear model about the relevant characteristics differentiating early malignant melanomas from benign lesions, thus it could be possible that a random generation of examples will produce misclassifications.

Another interesting line of research should be the use of meta-learning techniques (Vilalta et al., 2010). The goal of these techniques is to learn the appropriate method for learning. In other words, a classification problem can be solved using several independent classifiers (for instance, T-kNN and T-LID) and we know that these classifiers have different properties (for instance, T-kNN produces less FPR than T-LID) and, as a consequence, they are good in different areas of the problem space. Meta-learning techniques automatically analyze the performance of both classifiers and characterize the situations in which can be used each one of them. We think that this kind of techniques could improve the detection of early MM.

Finally we also plan to use fuzzy techniques to describe the classes. Because early malignant melanomas are very similar to some benignant lesions, we think that fuzzy descriptions of classes could improve the predictivity ratio of the theories.

CONCLUSION

In the approach presented here, we exploit the concept of lazy domain theory for knowledge discovery. Although lazy domain theories are formed by approximations of concepts (i.e., spe-cific rules), this information is very valuable to experts to obtain a picture of some parts of the domain. The lesions used in the experiments are suspicious lesions removed because they have some characteristics of melanoma, although most of them are benignant. Thus, the available set of lesions represents conflictive areas of the domain. The results generated in the present study demonstrate the difficulties in the discrimination between melanoma and benign lesions in the early stages of the malignant process. Interestingly, lazy domain theories offer new definitions of classes that are useful in the recognition of a subgroup of melanomas or benign lesions to improve the accuracy of experts. The lazy domain theories discover the main traits associated to malignant melanoma as the presence of either pagetoid infiltration in confocal microscopy or asymmetry in two axes in dermoscopy.

REFERENCES

Argenziano, G., Zalaudek, I., Ferrara, G., Hofmann-Wellenhof, R., & Soyer, H. P. (2007). Proposal of a new classication system for melanocytic naevi. *The British Journal of Dermatology, 157*(2), 217–227. doi:10.1111/j.1365-2133.2007.07972.x

Armengol, E. (2008). Building partial domain theories from explanations. *Knowledge Intelligence, 2*(8), 19–24.

Armengol, E., & Plaza, E. (2000). Bottom-up induction of feature terms. *Machine Learning, 41*(3), 259–294. doi:10.1023/A:1007677713969

Armengol, E., & Plaza, E. (2001). Lazy induction of descriptions for relational case-based learning. In L. De Reaedt & P. Flach, (Eds.), *European Conference on Machine Learning: Vol 2167 Lecture Notes in Articial Intelligence,* (pp. 13–24). Springer.

Armengol, E., & Plaza, E. (2006). Symbolic explanation of similarities in case-based reasoning. *Computing and Informatics, 25*(2-3), 153–171.

Bareiss, E. R., Porter, B. W., & Wier, C. C. (1988). PROTOS: An examplar-based learning apprentice. *International Journal of Man-Machine Studies, 29*(5), 549–561. doi:10.1016/S0020-7373(88)80012-9

Carbonell, J., Etzioni, O., Gil, Y., Joseph, R., Knoblock, C., Minton, S., & Veloso, M. (1995). Planning and learning in PRODIGY: Overview of an integrated architecture. In Ramand, A., & Leake, D. B. (Eds.), *Goal-driven learning*. MIT Press.

Chawla, N. V., Bowyer, K. W., Hall, L. O., & Kegelmeyer, W. P. (2002). SMOTE: Synthetic minority over-sampling technique. *Journal of Artificial Intelligence Research, 16*, 321–357.

Corral, G., Armengol, E., Fornells, A., & Golobardes, E. (2009). Explanations of unsupervised clustering applied to data security analysis. *Neurocomputing, 72*, 2754–2762. doi:10.1016/j.neucom.2008.09.021

Dejong, G., & Mooney, R. (1986). Explanation-based learning: An alternative view. *Machine Learning*, 145–176. doi:10.1007/BF00114116

Fawcett, T. (2006). An introduction to ROC analysis. *Pattern Recognition Letters, 27*, 861–874. doi:10.1016/j.patrec.2005.10.010

Frawley, W. J., Piatetsky-Shapiro, G., & Matheus, C. J. (1992). Knowledge discovery in databases: An overview. *AI Magazine, 13*, 57–70.

Friedman, J. H., Kohavi, R., & Yun, Y. (1996). Lazy decision trees. In *Proceedings of the Thirteenth National Conference on Artificial Intelligence*, Vol. 1, (pp. 717–724).

Ha, T. M., & Bunke, H. (1997). Off-line, handwritten numeral recognition by perturbation method. *Pattern Analysis and Machine Intelligence, 19*(5), 535–539. doi:10.1109/34.589216

Hall, M., Frank, E., Holmes, G., Pfahringer, B., Reutemann, P., & Witten, I. H. (2009). The WEKA data mining software: An update. *SIGKDD Explorations, 11*(1). doi:10.1145/1656274.1656278

Hammond, K. J. (1989). *Case-base planning. Viewing planning as a memory task. Perspectives in Artificial Intelligence, 1*. Academic Press, Inc.

Hofmann-Wellenhof, R., Blum, A., Wolf, I. H., Zalaudek, I., Piccolo, D., & Kerl, H. (2002). Dermoscopic classification of clark's nevi (atypical melanocytic nevi). *Clinics in Dermatology, 20*(3), 255–258. doi:10.1016/S0738-081X(02)00217-1

Kolodner, J. (1993). *Case-based reasoning*. Morgan Kaufmann.

Laird, J. E., Newell, A., & Rosenbloom, P. S. (1987). Soar: An architecture for general intelligence. *Artificial. Intelligence, 33*, 1–64.

Leake, D. B. (1996). Experience, introspection and expertise: Learning to refine the case-based reasoning process. *Journal of Experimental & Theoretical Artificial Intelligence, 8*(3-4), 319–339. doi:10.1080/095281396147357

López de Mántaras, R. (1991). A distance-based attribute selection measure for decision tree induction. *Machine Learning, 6*, 81–92. doi:10.1023/A:1022694001379

Mitchell, T. M. (1997). *Machine learning. McGraw-Hill* (International Editions). Computer Science Series.

Mitchell, T. M., Keller, R. M., & Kedar-Cabelli, S. T. (1986). Explanation-based learning: A unifying view. *Machine Learning, 1*(1), 47–80. doi:10.1007/BF00116250

Opitz, D. W., & Maclin, R. (1999). Popular ensemble methods: An empirical study. *Journal of Artificial Intelligence Research, 11*, 169–198.

Puig, S., Argenziano, G., Zalaudek, I., Ferrara, G., Palou, J., & Massi, D. (2007). Melanomas that failed dermoscopic detection: A combined clinico-dermoscopic approach for not missing melanoma. *Dermatologic Surgery, 33*(10), 1262–1273. doi:10.1111/j.1524-4725.2007.33264.x

Quinlan, R. (1986). Induction of decision trees. *Machine Learning, 1*(1), 81–106. doi:10.1007/BF00116251

Quinlan, R. (1993). *C4.5: Programs for machine learning*. San Mateo, CA: Morgan Kaufmann Publishers.

Vestergaard, M. E., & Menzies, S. W. (2008). Automated diagnostic instruments for cutaneous melanoma. *Seminars in Cutaneous Medicine and Surgery, 27*(1), 32–36. doi:10.1016/j.sder.2008.01.001

Vilalta, R., Giraud-Carrier, C., & Brazdil, P. (2010). Meta-learning: Concepts and techniques. In Maimon, O., & Rokach, L. (Eds.), *The data mining and knowledge discovery handbook* (pp. 717–731). Springer.

ADDITIONAL READING

Allen, A. C., & Spitz, S. (2006). Malignant melanoma. A clinicopathological analysis of the criteria for diagnosis and prognosis. *Cancer, 6*(1), 1–45. doi:10.1002/1097-0142(195301)6:1<1::AID-CNCR2820060102>3.0.CO;2-C

Brazdil, P., Giraud-Carrier, C., Soares, C., & Vilalta, R. (2009). *Metalearning: Applications to data mining*. Cognitive Technologies. Springer, 2009.

Clancey, W. J. (1984). Classification problem solving. In. *Proceedings of AAAI, 1984*, 49–55.

Gamberger, D., & Lavrac, N. (2011). *Expert-guided subgroup discovery: Methodology and application*. Computing Research Repository (CoRR) abs/1106.4576. Ithaca, NY: Cornell University. Retrieved from http://arxiv.org/abs/1106.4576

Gibert, K., García-Rudolph, A., García-Molina, A., Roig-Rovira, T., Bernabeu, M., & Tormos, J. M. (2008). Knowledge discovery on the response to neurorehabilitation treatment of patients. In T. Alsinet, J. Puyol-Gruart, & C. Torras (Eds.), *Artificial Intelligence Research and Development, 184*, 170-177. IOS Press.

Gibert, K., Rodríguez-Silva, G., & Rodríguez-Roda, I. (2010). Knowledge discovery with clustering based on rules by states: A water treatment application. *Environmental Modelling & Software, 25*(6), 712–723. doi:10.1016/j.envsoft.2009.11.004

Goldstein, B. G., & Goldstein, A. O. (2001). Diagnosis and management of malignant melanoma. *American Family Physician, 63*(7), 1359–1369.

Grin, C. M., Kopf, A. W., Welkovich, B., Bart, R. S., & Levenstein, M. J. (1990). Accuracy in the clinical diagnosis of malignant melanoma. *Archives of Dermatology, 126*(6), 763–766. doi:10.1001/archderm.1990.01670300063008

Helma, C., King, R. D., Kramer, S., & Srinivasan, A. (2001). The predictive toxicology challenge 2000-2001. *Bioinformatics (Oxford, England), 17*(1), 107–108. doi:10.1093/bioinformatics/17.1.107

Huang, K., Yang, H., & King, I. (2008). *Machine learning: Modeling data locally and globally*. Springer.

Jain, A. K., Murty, M. N., & Flynn, P. J. (1999). Data clustering: A review. *ACM Computing Surveys, 31*(3), 264–323. doi:10.1145/331499.331504

Leake, D., & Mcsherry, D. (2005). Introduction to the special issue on explanation in case-based reasoning. *Artificial Intelligence Review, 24*(2), 103–108. doi:10.1007/s10462-005-4606-8

Leake, D. B. (1995). Adaptive similarity assessment for case-based explanation. International. *Journal of Expert Systems, 8*(2), 165–194.

Maimon, O., & Rokach, L. (Eds.). (2010). *Data mining and knowledge discovery handbook* (2nd ed.). Springer. doi:10.1007/978-0-387-09823-4

Malvehy, J., Braun, R., & Puig, S. (2006). *Handbook of dermoscopy*. Taylor & Francis Group.

Michalski, R. S., & Tecuci, G. (1994). *Machine learning: A multistrategy approach*. Morgan Kaufmann.

Roth-Berghofer, T. (2004). Explanations and case-based reasoning: Foundational issues. In *Advances in Case-based Reasoning (Vol. 3155, pp. 389–403*). Lecture Notes in Computer Science Springer. doi:10.1007/978-3-540-28631-8_29

Schank, R. C. (1986). The process of explanation: Explanation patterns. In *Explanation patterns: Understanding mechanically and creatively*. Routledge.

Schank, R. C., Kass, A., & Riesbek, C. K. (1994). *Inside case-based explanation*. Routledge.

Steiner, A., Pehamberger, H., & Wolff, K. (1987). In vivo epiluminescence microscopy of pigmented skin lesions, II: Diagnosis of small pigmented skin lesions and early detection of malignant melanoma. *Journal of the American Academy of Dermatology, 17*(4), 584–591. doi:10.1016/S0190-9622(87)70240-0

Tadepalli, P. (1989). Lazy explanation-based learning: A solution to the intractable theory problem. In *Proceedings International Joint Conference on Artificial Intelligence-89* (pp. 694-700). Detroit, MI.

Toivonen, H., Srinivasan, A., King, R. D., Kramer, S., & Helma, C. (2003). Statistical evaluation of the predictive toxicology challenge 2000-2001. *Bioinformatics (Oxford, England), 19*(10), 1183–1193. doi:10.1093/bioinformatics/btg130

Witten, I. H., Frank, E., & Hall, M. A. (2011). *Data mining: Practical machine learning tools and techniques* (3rd ed.). Morgan Kaufmann.

Xu, R., & Wunch, D. C. (2009). *Clustering*. Wiley-IEEE Press.

KEY TERMS AND DEFINITIONS

Classification Problems: Families of domains where the data can be put in different classes (namely the solution classes). For instance, cars can be classified according their trademark.

Dermatology: Is the branch of medicine dealing with the skin and its diseases.

Domain Theory: Set of general knowledge about a domain. A very frequently representation of domain theories is by means of rules, however other representations are possible.

Domain: Area of knowledge (i.e., medicine, biology, chemistry, law, etc).

Inductive Learning Methods: Family of machine learning methods that build domain theories by generalizing the input data.

Knowledge Discovery: Extraction of regular patterns from a set of data. These patterns form a domain theory that can be partially unknown from domain experts.

Lazy Learning Methods: Family of machine methods that solve new problems based on similarities. Differently than inductive learning methods, most of them do not perform explicit generalization of input data, i.e., they do not construct explicit domain theories.

Machine Learning: Branch of artificial intelligence concerned with the development of algorithms that allow problem solvers to take advantage of the experience acquired solving previous problems to improve its performance in solving future problems.

Medical Diagnosis: Process of attempting to determine and/or identify a possible disease or disorder. Notice that medical diagnosis can be seen as a classification problem.

Melanoma: Melanoma is a malignant tumor of melanocytes. Melanocytes are cells that produce the dark pigment, melanin, which is responsible for the color of skin. They predominantly occur in skin, but are also found in other parts of the body, including the bowel and the eye. Melanoma can occur in any part of the body that contains melanocytes.

Compilation of References

Abbod, M. F., von Keyserlingk, D. G., Linkens, D. A., & Mahfouf, M. (2001). Survey of utilisation of fuzzy technology in medicine and healthcare. *Fuzzy Sets and Systems*, *120*, 331–349. doi:10.1016/S0165-0114(99)00148-7

Adomavicius, G., & Tuzhilin, A. (2005). Toward the next generation of recommender systems: A survey of the state-of-the-art and possible extensions. *IEEE Transactions on Knowledge and Data Engineering*, *17*(6), 734–749. doi:10.1109/TKDE.2005.99

Afonso, V.X., Tompkins, W., Nguyen, T., Trautmann, S., & Luo, S. (1995). Filter bank-based processing of the stress ECG. In *IEEE 17th Annual Conference of the Engineering in Medicine and Biology Society*, (Vol. 2, pp. 887–888).

Afonso, V.X., Tompkins, W., Nguyen, T., & Luo, S. (1999). ECG beat detection using filter banks. *IEEE Transactions on Bio-Medical Engineering*, *46*(2), 192–202. doi:10.1109/10.740882

Ageberg, E. (2002). Consequences of a ligament injury on neuromuscular function and relevance to rehabilitation using the anterior cruciate ligament-injured knee as model. *Journal of Electromyography and Kinesiology*, *12*(3), 205–212. doi:10.1016/S1050-6411(02)00022-6

Agoris, P. D., Meijer, S., Gulski, E., & Smit, J. J. (2004) Threshold selection for wavelet denoising of partial discharge data. In *Conference Record of the 2004 IEEE International Symposium on Electrical Insulation*, (pp. 62-65). IEEE.

Agrawal, R., & Srikant, R. (1994). *Fast algorithms for mining association rules*.

Agrawal, R., & Srikant, R. (1995). Mining sequential patterns. *11th International Conference on Data Engineering (ICDE'95)*, Taipei, Taiwan, (pp. 3-14).

Agrawal, R., Imieli ski, T., & Swami, A. (1993). Mining association rules between sets of items in large databases. *SIGMOD Record*, *22*(2), 207–216. doi:10.1145/170036.170072

Ahlbom, A., Green, A., Kheifets, L., Savitz, D., & Swerdlow, A. (2004). Epidemiology of health effects of radiofrequency exposure. *Environmental Health Perspectives*, *112*(17), 1741–1754. doi:10.1289/ehp.7306

Ajaal, T. T., & Smith, R. W. (2009). Employing the Taguchi method in optimizing the scaffold production process for artificial bone grafts. *Journal of Materials Processing Technology*, *209*, 1521–1532. doi:10.1016/j.jmatprotec.2008.04.001

Akbani, R., Kwek, S., & Japkowitz, N. (2004). Applying support vector machines to imbalanced datasets. In Boulicaut, J. F., Esposito, F., Giannotti, F., & Pedreschi, D. (Eds.), *Machine Learning: ECML 2004* (*Vol. 3201*, pp. 39–50). Lecture Notes in Computer Science Berlin, Germany: Springer-Verlag. doi:10.1007/978-3-540-30115-8_7

Allison, J. S., Heo, J., & Iskandrian, A. E. (2005). Artificial neural network modeling of stress single-photon emission computed tomographic imaging for detecting extensive coronary artery disease. *The American Journal of Cardiology*, *95*(2), 178–181. doi:10.1016/j.amjcard.2004.09.003

Alonso, J. M., & Magdalena, L. (2011a). *GUAJE: Generating understandable and accurate fuzzy models in a Java environment.* Free software under GPL license. Retrieved September 15, 2011, from http://www.soft-computing.es/guaje

Alonso, J. M., & Magdalena, L. (2011b). Generating understandable and accurate fuzzy rule-based systems in a java environment. In A. M. Fanelli, W. Pedrycz, & A. Petrosino (Eds.), *Fuzzy Logic and Applications (9ᵗʰ International Workshop WILF2011), LNAI 6857* (pp. 212-219). Springer.

Alonso, J. M., & Magdalena, L. (2011c). HILK++: An interpretability-guided fuzzy modeling methodology for learning readable and comprehensible fuzzy rule-based classifiers. *Soft Computing, 15*(10), 1959–1980. doi:10.1007/s00500-010-0628-5

Alonso, J. M., Magdalena, L., & Guillaume, S. (2008). HILK: A new methodology for designing highly interpretable linguistic knowledge bases using the fuzzy logic formalism. *International Journal of Intelligent Systems, 23*(7), 761–794. doi:10.1002/int.20288

Ambert, K. H., & Cohen, A. M. (2009). A system for classifying disease comorbidity status from medical discharge summaries using automated hotspot and negated concept detection. *Journal of the American Medical Informatics Association, 16*(4), 447–458. doi:10.1197/jamia.M3095

Andras, P. (2002). Kernel-Kohonen networks. *International Journal of Neural Systems, 12*, 117–135. doi:10.1016/S0129-0657(02)00108-4

Andreasen, S., Woldbye, M., Falck, B., & Andersen, S. K. (1987). *MUNIN: A causal probabilistic network for interpretation of electomyographic findings.* Paper presented at the 10th International Joint Conference on Artificial Intelligence, Los Altos, CA.

Andreassen, S., Riekehr, C., Kristensen, B., Schonheyder, H. C., & Leibovici, L. (1999). Using probabilistic and decision-theoretic methods in treatment and prognosis modeling. *Artificial Intelligence in Medicine, 15*(2), 121–134. doi:10.1016/S0933-3657(98)00048-7

Andreassi, J. (2000). *Psychophysiology: Human behavior and physiological response.* Lawrence Erlabaum Associates, Inc.

Angus, D. C., Linde-Zwirble, W. T., Lidicker, J., Clermont, G., Carcillo, J., & Pinsky, M. R. (2001). Epidemiology of severe sepsis in the United States: Analysis of incidence, outcome and associated costs of care. *Critical Care Medicine, 29*, 1303–1310. doi:10.1097/00003246-200107000-00002

Anom. (2010). Introduction to investigating an outbreak. Excellence in Curriculum Innovation through Teaching Epidemiology and the Science of Public Health. Retrieved from http://www.cdc.gov/excite/classroom/outbreak/objectives.htm

Antal, P., Fannes, G., De Smet, F., Vandewalle, J., & De Moor, B. (2001). *Ovarian cancer classification with rejection by Bayesian belief networks.* Paper presented at the European Conference on Artificial Intelligence in Medicine.

Antal, P., Fannes, G., Timmerman, D., Moreau, Y., & De Moor, B. (2004). Using literature and data to learn Bayesian networks as clinical models of ovarian tumors. *Artificial Intelligence in Medicine, 30*(3), 257–281. doi:10.1016/j.artmed.2003.11.007

Aphinyanaphongs, Y., & Aliferis, C. (2005). Text categorization models for retrieval of high quality articles. *Journal of the American Medical Informatics Association, 12*(2), 207–216. doi:10.1197/jamia.M1641

Arbib, M. (2002). *The handbook of brain theory and neural networks.* MIT Press.

Argenziano, G., Zalaudek, I., Ferrara, G., Hofmann-Wellenhof, R., & Soyer, H. P. (2007). Proposal of a new classification system for melanocytic naevi. *The British Journal of Dermatology, 157*(2), 217–227. doi:10.1111/j.1365-2133.2007.07972.x

Arizmendi, C., Hernández-Tamames, J., Romero, E., Vellido, A., & del Pozo, F. (2010). Diagnosis of brain tumours from magnetic resonance spectroscopy using wavelets and Neural Networks. In *Proceedings of the Engineering in Medicine and Biology Society (EMBC), Annual International Conference of the IEEE,* (pp. 6074-6077).

Armengol, E., & Plaza, E. (2001). Lazy induction of descriptions for relational case-based learning. In L. De Reaedt & P. Flach, (Eds.), *European Conference on Machine Learning: Vol 2167 Lecture Notes in Artificial Intelligence,* (pp. 13–24). Springer.

Armengol, E. (2008). Building partial domain theories from explanations. *Knowledge Intelligence*, *2*(8), 19–24.

Armengol, E., & Plaza, E. (2000). Bottom-up induction of feature terms. *Machine Learning*, *41*(3), 259–294. doi:10.1023/A:1007677713969

Armengol, E., & Plaza, E. (2006). Symbolic explanation of similarities in case-based reasoning. *Computing and Informatics*, *25*(2-3), 153–171.

Arulampalam, M., Maskell, S., Gordon, N., & Clapp, T. (2002). A tutorial on particle filters of online nonlinear/non-Gaussian Bayesian tracking. *IEEE Transactions on Signal Processing*, *50*(2), 174–188. doi:10.1109/78.978374

Baker, R., Laurenson, L., Winter, M., & Pritchard, A. (2004). The impact of information technology on haemophilia care. *Haemophilia*, *10*(4), 41–46. doi:10.1111/j.1365-2516.2004.00995.x

Baldi, P., & Brunak, S. (2001). *Bioinformatics: The machine learning approach*. MIT Press.

Ball, M. J., Weaver, C. A., & Kiel, J. M. (2004). *Healthcare information management systems: Cases, strategies, and solutions* (3rd ed.). New York, NY: Springer.

Banan, H., Al-Sabti, A., Jimulia, T., & Hart, A. J. (2002). The treatment of unstable, extracapsular hip fractures with the AO/ASIF proximal femoral nail (PFN)—our first 60 cases. *Injury-International Journal of the Care of the Injured*, *33*, 401–405.

Baralis, E., Bruno, G., Chiusano, S., Domenici, V. C., Mahoto, N. A., & Petrigni, C. (2010). Analysis of medical pathways by means of frequent closed sequences. *International Conference on Knowledge-Based and Intelligent Information & Engineering Systems,* Cardiff, Wales, (pp. 418-425).

Baratto, L., Morasso, P. G., Re, C., & Spada, G. (2002). A new look at posturographic analysis in the clinical context: sway-density versus other parameterization techniques. *Motor Control*, *6*(3), 246–270.

Bareiss, E. R., Porter, B. W., & Wier, C. C. (1988). PROTOS: An examplar-based learning apprentice. *International Journal of Man-Machine Studies*, *29*(5), 549–561. doi:10.1016/S0020-7373(88)80012-9

Bar-Hillel, A., Hertz, T., Shental, N., & Weinshall, D. (2005). Learning a Mahalanobis metric from equivalence constraints. *Journal of Machine Learning Research*, *6*, 937–965.

Barro, S., Fernandez-Delgado, M., Vila-Sobrino, J. A., & Sanchez, E. (1998). Classifying multichannel ECG patterns with an adaptive neural network. *IEEE Engineering in Medicine and Biology*, *17*, 45–55. doi:10.1109/51.646221

Başar, E., Schürmann, M., Demiralp, T., Başar-Eroglu, C., & Ademoglu, A. (2001). Event-related oscillations are "real brain responses" – Wavelet analysis and new strategies. *International Journal of Psychophysiology*, *39*, 91–127. doi:10.1016/S0167-8760(00)00135-5

Beerman, I., Novak, J., Wyatt, R. J., Julian, B. A., & Gharavi, A. G. (2007). The genetics of IgA nephropathy. *Nature Clinical Practice. Nephrology*, *3*, 325–338. doi:10.1038/ncpneph0492

Bellabarba, C., Herscovici, D., Ricci, W. M., & Hudanich, R. (2003). Percutaneous treatment of peritrochanteric fractures using the gamma nail. *Journal of Orthopaedic Trauma*, *17*(8), S38–S50. doi:10.1097/00005131-200309001-00009

Ben-Gal, I. (2005). Outlier detection. In Maiman, O., & Rokach, L. (Eds.), *Data mining and knowledge discovery handbook: A complete guide for practitioners and researchers*. Kluwer Academic Publishers. doi:10.1007/0-387-25465-X_7

Bernard, A., & Hartemink, A. J. (2005). Informative structure priors: Joint learning of dynamic regulatory networks from multiple types of data. *Pacific Symposium on Biocomputing. Pacific Symposium on Biocomputing*, (pp. 459-470).

Berthold, M. R., & Hand, D. J. (2010). *Intelligent data analysis*. Berlin, Germany: Springer-Verlag.

Bevk, M., & Kononenko, I. (2006). Towards symbolic mining of images with association rules: Preliminary results on textures. *Intelligent Data Analysis*, *10*(4), 379–393.

Bilenko, M., Basu, S., & Mooney, R. J. (2004). Integrating constraints and metric learning in semi-supervised clustering. *Proceedings of the 21 International Conference on Machine Learning* (pp. 81-88). Banff, Canada.

Birbaumer, N., Flor, H., Ghanayim, N., Hinterberger, T., Iverson, I., & Taub, E. (1999). A brain-controlled spelling device for the completely paralyzed. *Nature, 398,* 297–298. doi:10.1038/18581

Bishop, C. M. (1996). *Neural networks for pattern recognition.* Clarendon Press.

Bishop, C. M. (2007). *Pattern recognition and machine learning.* Springer.

Bishop, C. M., Svensén, M., & Williams, C. K. I. (1998). GTM: The generative topographic mapping. *Neural Computation, 10*(1), 215–234. doi:10.1162/089976698300017953

Bishop, C. M., Svensén, M., & Williams, C. K. I. (1998b). Developments of the generative topographic mapping. *Neurocomputing, 21*(1-3), 203–224. doi:10.1016/S0925-2312(98)00043-5

Blanco, R., Larrañaga, P., Inza, I., & Sierra, B. (2001). *Selection of highly accurate genes for cancer classification by estimation of distribution algorithms.* Paper presented at the European Conference on Artificial Intelligence in Medicine, workshop on Bayesian Models in Medicine, Cascais, Portugal.

Blind, J., & Das, S. (2007). *Disease outbreak detection and tracking for biosurveillance: A data fusion approach.*

Blount, M., Batra, V. M., Capella, A. N., Ebling, M. R., Jerome, W. F., & Martin, S. M. (2007). Remote healthcare monitoring using personal care connect. *IBM Systems Journal, 46*(1), 95–113. doi:10.1147/sj.461.0095

Bodenheimer, T., Lorig, K., Holman, H., & Grumbach, K. (2002). Patient self-management of chronic disease in primary care. *Journal of the American Medical Association, 288*(19), 2469–2475. doi:10.1001/jama.288.19.2469

Bone, R. C., Balk, R. A., Cerra, F. B., Dellinger, R. P., Fein, A. M., & Knaus, W. A. (1992). Definitions of sepsis and organ failure and guidelines for the use of innovative therapies in sepsis. *Chest, 101*(6), 1644–1655. doi:10.1378/chest.101.6.1644

Bonhard, P., & Sasse, M. A. (2006). Knowing me, knowing you - Using profiles and social networking to improve recommender systems. *BT Technology Journal, 25*(3), 84–98. doi:10.1007/s10550-006-0080-3

Bosansky, B., & Lhotska, L. (2009). Agent-based process-critiquing decision support system. In *2nd International Symposium on Applied Sciences in Biomedical and Communication Technologies,* (pp. 1-6).

Bosnić, Z., & Kononenko, I. (2009). An overview of advances in reliability estimation of individual predictions in machine learning. *Intelligent Data Analysis, 13*(2), 385–401. doi:doi:10.3233/IDA-2009-0371

Braham, N., Le Beux, P., & Fontaine, D. (1987). An experimental knowledge-based system for simulation in hematology. *Proceedings of the third International Expert Systems Conference* (pp. 459-466).

Brawnwald, E., Fauci, A. S., Kasper, D. L., Hauser, S. L., Long, D. L., & Jameson, J. L. (2008). *Harrison's principles of internal medicine.* London, UK: McGraw-Hill Medical Publishing Division.

Brin, S., Motwani, R., Ullman, J. D., & Tsur, S. (1997). *Dynamic itemset counting and implication rules for market basket data.*

Brodatz, P. (1966). *Textures - A photographic album for artists and designers.* Reinhold.

Brown, A. M. (2001). A step-by-step guide to nonlinear regression analysis of experimental data using a Microsoft Excel spreadsheet. *Computer Methods and Programs in Biomedicine, 65,* 191–200. doi:10.1016/S0169-2607(00)00124-3

Brown, D., & Gray, G. A. (2005). *Implementation of a data fusion algorithm for RODS, a real-time outbreak and disease surveillance system. SAND2005-6007.* Sandia National Laboratories. doi:10.2172/876344

Bruijn, B., Cherry, C., Kiritchenko, S., Martin, J., & Zhu, X. (2010). *NRC at i2b2: One challenge, three practical tasks, nine statistical systems, hundreds of clinical records, millions of useful features.* Paper presented at the i2b2 Workshop on Challenges in Natural Language Processing for Clinical Data, Washington, DC.

Brun-Buisson, C., Doyan, F., Carlet, J., Dellamonica, P., Gouin, F., & Lepoutre, A. (1995). Incidence, risk Factors, and outcome of severe sepsis and septic shock in adults. *Journal of the American Medical Association, 274,* 968–974. doi:10.1001/jama.1995.03530120060042

Buchanan, B. G., Sutherland, G. L., & Feigenbaum, E. A. (1969). Heuristic Dendral: A program for generating explanatory hypotheses in organic chemistry. In Meltzer, B., & Michie, D. (Eds.), *Machine intelligence (Vol. 4)*. Edinburgh University Press.

Bucholz, R. W., Heckman, J. D., & Court-Brown, C. (2006). *Fractures in adult*. Philadelphia, PA: Lippincott Williams & Wilkins.

Buehler, J. W., Berkelman, R. L., Hartley, D. M., & Peters, C. J. (2003). Syndromic surveillance and bioterrorism-related epidemics. *Emerging Infectious Diseases, 9*(10), 1197–1204.

Buehler, J. W., Hopkins, R. S., Overhage, J. M., Sosin, D. M., & Tong, V. (2004a). Framework for evaluating public health surveillance systems for early detection of outbreaks. *Morbidity and Mortality Weekly Report Recommendations and Reports, 53*, 1–11.

Buehler, J. W., Hopkins, R. S., Overhage, J. M., Sosin, D. M., & Tong, V. (2004b). Framework for evaluating public health surveillance systems for early detection of outbreaks: Recommendations from the CDC Working Group. *Recommendations and Reports: Morbidity and Mortality Weekly Report, 53*(RR-5), 1.

Bunescu, R., & Mooney, R. (2005). A shortest path dependency kernel for relation extraction. In *Proceedings of the Conference on Human Language Technology and Empirical Methods in Natural Language Processing (HLT/EMNLP)* (pp. 724–731). Morristown, NJ: ACL.

Cacioppo, J., Tassinary, L. G., & Berntson, G. G. (Eds.). (2007). *Handbook of psychophysiology*. Cambridge University Press.

Carbonell, J., Etzioni, O., Gil, Y., Joseph, R., Knoblock, C., Minton, S., & Veloso, M. (1995). Planning and learning in PRODIGY: Overview of an integrated architecture. In Ramand, A., & Leake, D. B. (Eds.), *Goal-driven learning*. MIT Press.

Carme, B., Sobesky, M., Biard, M., Cotellon, P., Aznar, C., & Fontanella, J. (2003). Non-specific alert system for dengue epidemic outbreaks in areas of endemic malaria. A hospital-based evaluation in Cayenne (French Guiana). *Epidemiology and Infection, 130*(1), 93–100. doi:10.1017/S0950268802007641

Castro, R., Kneupner, K., Vega, J., De Arcas, G., López, J. M., & Purahoo, K. (2010). Real-time remote diagnostic monitoring test-bed in JET. *Fusion Engineering and Design, 85*(3-4), 598–602. doi:10.1016/j.fusengdes.2010.03.050

Ceglar, A., & Roddick, J. F. (2006). Association mining. *ACM Computing Surveys, 38*(2). doi:10.1145/1132956.1132958

Center for Disease Control. (1990). Increase in national hospital discharge survey rates for Septicemia: United States, 1979-1987. *Morbidity and Mortality Weekly Report, 39*, 31–34.

Centers for Disease Control and Prevention. (1993). Mortality patterns-United States, 1990. *Monthly Vital Statistics Report, 41*, 5.

Cerrito, P. B., & Cerrito, J. C. (2006). Data and text mining the electronic medical record to improve care and to lower costs. *Proceedings of the Thirty-first Annual SAS®Users Group International Conference*. Cary, NC: SAS Institute Inc., paper077-31.

Cerrito, P. B. (2007). Mining the electronic medical record to examine. *Physician Decisions Studies in Computational Intelligence, 48*, 113–126. doi:10.1007/978-3-540-47527-9_5

Chandola, V., Mithal, V., & Kumar, V. (2008). *A comparative evaluation of anomaly detection techniques for sequence data*.

Chandola, V., Banerjee, A., & Kumar, V. (2007). *Outlier detection: A survey*. USA: Technical Report. Univeristy of Minnesota.

Chandola, V., Banerjee, A., & Kumar, V. (2009). Anomaly detection: A survey. *ACM Computing Surveys, 41*(3), 15. doi:10.1145/1541880.1541882

Chao, C. K., Hsu, C. C., Wang, J. L., & Lin, J. (2007). Increasing bending strength of tibial locking screws: Mechanical tests and finite element analyses. *Clinical Biomechanics (Bristol, Avon), 22*, 59–66. doi:10.1016/j.clinbiomech.2006.07.007

Chao, C. K., Lin, J., Putra, S. T., & Hsu, C. C. (2010). A neurogenetic approach to a multiobjective design optimization of spinal pedicle screws. *Journal of Biomechanical Engineering-Transactions of the ASME, 132*(9), 091006–0910066. doi:10.1115/1.4001887

Chapman, W., Chu, D., & Dowling, J. N. (2007). Con-Text: An algorithm for identifying contextual features from clinical text. *In Proceedings of the Workshop on Biological, Translational, and Clinical Language Processing (BioNLP)* (pp. 81-88). Prague, Czech Republic.

Chapman, W. W., Fizman, M., Chapman, B. E., & Haug, P. J. (2001). A comparison of classification algorithms to automatically identify chest x-ray reports that support pneumonia. *Journal of Biomedical Informatics*, *34*(1), 4–14. doi:10.1006/jbin.2001.1000

Chawla, N. V., Japkowitz, N., & Koltz, A. (2004). Editorial: Special issue on learning from imbalanced data sets. *SIGKDD Explorations Newsletter – Special Issue on Learning from Imbalanced Datasets*, *6*(1), 1-6. doi: 10.1145/1007730.1007733

Chawla, N. V., Bowyer, K. W., Hall, L. O., & Kegelmeyer, W. P. (2002). SMOTE: Synthetic minority over-sampling technique. *Journal of Artificial Intelligence Research*, *16*(1), 321–357. Retrieved from http://www.jair.org/media/953/live-953-2037-jair.pdf

Chawla, N. V., Lazarevic, A., Hall, L. O., & Bowyer, K. W. (2003). SMOTEBoost: Improving prediction of the minority class in boosting. In Lavrac, N., Gamberger, D., Todorovski, L., & Blockeel, H. (Eds.), *Knowledge Discovery in Databases: PKDD 2003 (Vol. 2838*, pp. 107–119). Lecture Notes in Computer Science Berlin, Germany: Springer-Verlag. doi:10.1007/978-3-540-39804-2_12

Chen, Y., Pedersen, L. H., Chu, W. W., & Olsen, J. (2007). Drug exposure side effects from mining pregnancy data. *ACM SIGKDD Explorations Newsletter - Special issue on data mining for health informatics*, *9*(1).

Cheng, J.-L., Jeng, J.-R., & Chiang, Z.-W. (2006). Heart rate measurement in the presence of noises. In *Pervasive Health Conference and Workshops, 2006* (pp. 1-4).

Chen, X. W., Anantha, G., & Wang, X. (2006). An effective structure learning method for constructing gene networks. *Bioinformatics (Oxford, England)*, *22*(11), 1367–1374. doi:10.1093/bioinformatics/btl090

Chui, C. (1992). *An introduction to wavelets*. San Diego, CA: Academic Press.

Chun, C., Hurdle, W., & Unwin, A. (2008). *Handbook of data visualization*. Springer.

Clancey, W. J., & Shortliffe, E. H. (1984). *Readings in medical AI: The first decade*. Reading, MA: Addison-Wesley.

Claudio, G., Lavelli, A., & Romano, L. (2006). Exploiting shallow linguistic information for relation extraction from biomedical literature. *In Proceedings of the 11*[th] *Conference of the European Chapter of the Association for Computational Linguistics*. Trento, Italy.

Clyman, J. I., Black, H. R., & Miller, P. L. (1989). Assessing practice conformance for hypertension management using an expert system. *Computer Applications in Medical Care: Proceedings of the Thirteenth Annual Symposium*, Washington DC, USA, November 5-8.

Coast, A., Stern, R., Cano, G., & Briller, S. (1990). An approach to cardiac arrhythmia analysis using hidden Markov models. *IEEE Transactions on Bio-Medical Engineering*, *37*(9), 826–835. doi:10.1109/10.58593

Cobanoglu, M. C., Saygin, Y., & Sezerman, U. (2010). Classification of GPCRs using family specific motifs. *IEEE/ACM Transactions on Computational Biology and Bioinformatics*, *8*(6).

Cohen, A. M., Hersh, W. R., Peterson, K., & Yen, P. Y. (2006). Reducing workload in systematic review preparation using automated citation classification. *Journal of the American Medical Informatics Association*, *13*(2), 206–219. doi:10.1197/jamia.M1929

Cohen, G., Hilario, M., Sax, H., Hugonnet, S., & Geissbuhler, A. (2006). Learning from imbalanced data in surveillance of nosocomial infection. *Artificial Intelligence in Medicine*, *37*(1), 7–18. doi:10.1016/j.artmed.2005.03.002

Collins, P., Bolton-Maggs, P., Stephenson, D., Jenkins, B., Loran, C., & Winter, M. (2003). Pilot study of an Internet-based electronic patient treatment record and communication systems for haemophilia, Advoy.com. *Haemophilia*, *9*(3), 285–291. doi:10.1046/j.1365-2516.2003.00747.x

Cooley, M. (1987). Human centered systems: An urgent problem for systems designers. *AI & Society*, *1*(1), 21–43. doi:10.1007/BF01905888

Cooper, R., & Collins, C. (2008). *GWT in practice*. Manning Publications Co.

Cordón, O., & Herrera, F. (1997). A three-stage evolutionary process for learning descriptive and approximate fuzzy-logic controller knowledge bases from examples. *International Journal of Approximate Reasoning, 17*(4), 369–407. doi:10.1016/S0888-613X(96)00133-8

Corral, G., Armengol, E., Fornells, A., & Golobardes, E. (2009). Explanations of unsupervised clustering applied to data security analysis. *Neurocomputing, 72*, 2754–2762. doi:10.1016/j.neucom.2008.09.021

Cowell, R. G. (2001). Conditions under which conditional independence and scoring methods lead to identical selection of Bayesian network models. *Proceedings of the Seventeenth Conference on Uncertainty in Artificial Intelligence* (pp. 91-97). Morgan Kaufmann Publishers.

Cowell, R. G., Dawid, A. P., Lauritzen, S. L., & Spiegelhalter, D. J. (1999). *Probabilistic networks and expert systems*. Springer.

Cox, T. F., & Cox, M. A. A. (2001). *Multidimensional scaling* (2nd ed.). USA: Chapman & Hall/CRC.

Cristianini, N., Kandola, J., Elisseeff, J., & Shawe-Taylor, A. (2002). On the kernel target alignment. *Journal of Machine Learning Research, 1*, 1–31.

Cundick, R., Turner, C. W., Lincoln, M. J., Buchanan, J. P., Anderson, C., Homer, R., & Bouhaddou, O. (1989). ILIAD as a patient case simulator to teach medical problem solving. *Symposium on Computer Applications in Medical Care*, (pp. 902-906). Washington, DC: IEEE Computer Society.

Dart, T., Cui, Y., Chatellier, G., & Degoulet, P. (2003). Analysis of hospitalized patient flows using data mining. *Studies in Health Technology and Informatics, 95*, 263–268.

Deci, E. L., & Ryan, R. M. (1991). A motivational approach to self: Integration in personality. In R. Dienstbier (Ed.), *Nebraska Symposium on Motivation: Vol. 38, Perspectives on Motivation* (pp. 237-288). Lincoln, NE: University of Nebraska Press.

DeGroot, M. H. (1986). *Probability and statistics*. Addison-Wesley.

Dejong, G., & Mooney, R. (1986). Explanation-based learning: An alternative view. *Machine Learning*, (n.d), 145–176. doi:10.1007/BF00114116

Dellinger, R. P., Carlet, J. M., Masur, H., Gerlach, H., Calanda, T., & Cohen, J. (2004). Surviving sepsis campaign guidelines for management of severe sepsis and septic shock. *Intensive Care Medicine, 30*, 536–555. doi:10.1007/s00134-004-2210-z

DeMets, D. L., Furberg, C., & Friedman, L. (2006). *Data monitoring in clinical trials: A case studies approach*. Springer. doi:10.1007/0-387-30107-0

Dempster, A. P., Laird, N. M., & Rubin, D. B. (1977). Maximum likelihood from incomplete data via the EM algorithm. *Journal of the Royal Statistical Society. Series B. Methodological, 39*(1), 1–38.

Demšar, J., Zupan, B., & Leban, G. (2004). *Orange: From experimental machine learning to interactive data mining*. White paper. Retrieved August 16, 2009, from http://www.ailab.si/orange

Demšar, J. (2006). Statistical comparisons of classifiers over multiple data sets. *Journal of Machine Learning Research, 7*, 1–30.

DeShazo, J. P., & Turner, A. M. (2008). *Hands-on NLP: An interactive and user-centered system to classify discharge summaries for obesity and related co-morbidities*. Paper presented at the i2b2 Workshop on Challenges in Natural Language Processing for Clinical Data, Washington, DC.

Diamantini, C., & Potena, D. (2008). Borderline detection by Bayes vector quantizers. In *Proceedings of the 23rd Annual ACM Symposium on Applied Computing - Special Track on Data Mining*, Vol. 2, (pp. 904–908).

Diamantini, C., & Potena, D. (2009). Bayes vector quantizer for class-imbalance problem. *IEEE Transactions on Knowledge and Data Engineering, 21*(5), 638–651. doi:10.1109/TKDE.2008.187

Dickey, J. P., Pierrynowski, M. R., Bednar, D. A., & Yang, S. X. (2002). Relationship between pain and vertebral motion in chronic low-back pain subjects. *Clinical Biomechanics (Bristol, Avon), 17*, 345–352. doi:10.1016/S0268-0033(02)00032-3

DOH. (2010). New York State Medicaid update. *The Official Newsletter of the New York Medicaid Program, Prenatal Care Special Edition, 26*(2).

Dokur, Z., Olmez, T., Yazgan, E., & Ersoy, O. (1997). Detection of ECG waveforms by neural networks. *Medical Engineering & Physics*, *19*, 738–741. doi:10.1016/S1350-4533(97)00029-5

Donaldson, I. (2003). PreBIND and textomy: Mining the biomedical literature for protein-protein interactions using a support vector machine. *BMC Bioinformatics*, *4*, 11. doi:10.1186/1471-2105-4-11

Douglas, I. (2009). Global mapping of usability labs and centers. *Proceedings of Computer Human Interaction Conference, CHI 2009*, April 4 – 9, Boston, MA, USA, (pp. 4393-4398).

Douglas, I. W. (1986). *Medical expert systems: The problem of epilepsy*. M.Sc. Dissertation, University of Warwick.

Drews, J. (2000). Drug discovery: A historical perspective. *Science*, *287*, 1960. doi:10.1126/science.287.5460.1960

Durbin, R., Eddy, S. R., Krogh, A., & Mitchison, G. (2004). *Biological sequence analysis: Probabilistic models of proteins and nucleic acids*. Cambridge, UK: Cambridge University Press.

Du, Y. P., Liang, Y. Z., Jiang, J. H., Berry, R. J., & Ozaki, Y. (2004). Spectral regions selection to improve prediction ability of PLS models by changeable size moving window partial least squares and searching combination moving window partial least squares. *Analytica Chimica Acta*, *501*(2), 183–191. doi:10.1016/j.aca.2003.09.041

Estabrooks, A., & Japkowitz, N. (2001). A mixture-of-experts framework for learning from imbalanced data sets. In Hoffmann, F., Hand, D. J., Adams, N., Fisher, D., & Guimaraes, G. (Eds.), *Advances in Intelligent Data Analysis* (*Vol. 2189*, pp. 34–43). Lecture Notes in Computer Science Berlin, Germany: Springer-Verlag. doi:10.1007/3-540-44816-0_4

Evans, J. (2011). In medicine, iPad today means a Mac tomorrow. *Computerworld*, April. Retrieved July 20, 2011, from http://blogs.computerworld.com/18134/collected_in_medicine_ipad_today_means_a_mac_tomorrow

Fawcett, T. (2006). An introduction to ROC analysis. *Pattern Recognition Letters*, *27*, 861–874. doi:10.1016/j.patrec.2005.10.010

Fawcett, T., & Provost, F. (1997). Adaptive fraud detection. *Data Mining and Knowledge Discovery*, *1*(3), 291–316. doi:10.1023/A:1009700419189

Fayyad, U. M. (1993). Multi-interval discretization of continuous-valued attributes for classification learning. In R. Bajcsy (Ed.), *Proceedings of the International Joint Conferences on Artificial Intelligence*, (pp. 1022–1027). San Mateo, CA: Morgan Kaufmann.

Felgaer, P., Britos, P., & García-Martínes, R. (2006). Predition in health domain using Bayesian networks optimization based on induction learning techniques. *International Journal of Modern Physics C*, *17*(3), 447–455. doi:10.1142/S0129183106008558

Fiersen, G., Jannett, T., Jadallah, M., Yates, S., Quint, S., & Nagle, H. (1990). A comparison of the noise sensitivity of nine QRS detection algorithms. *IEEE Transactions on Bio-Medical Engineering*, *37*(1), 85–98. doi:10.1109/10.43620

Fingelkurts, A. A., Fingelkurts, A. A., & Kähkönen, S. (2005). Functional connectivity in the brain – Is it an elusive concept? *Neuroscience and Biobehavioral Reviews*, *28*, 827–836. doi:10.1016/j.neubiorev.2004.10.009

Fioretti, S., Scocco, M., Ladislao, L., Ghetti, G., & Rabini, R. A. (2010). Identification of peripheral neuropathy in type-2 diabetic subjects by static posturography and linear discriminant analysis. *Gait & Posture*, *32*(3), 317–320. doi:10.1016/j.gaitpost.2010.05.017

Fischer, E. A., Lo, J. Y., & Markey, M. K. (2004). *Bayesian networks of BI-RADS TM descriptors for breast lesion classification*. Paper presented at the 26th Annual International Conference of the IEEE EMBS.

Fischer, G., Lemke, A. C., & Mastaglio, T. (1990). Critics: An emerging approach to knowledge-based human-computer interaction. *Proceedings of Computer Human Interaction Conference, CHI 90*, April 1-5.

Fitzpatrick, J., & Sonka, M. (2000). *Handbook of medical imaging, medical image processing and analysis* (*Vol. 2*). Bellingham, WA: SPIE.

Foresee, F. D., & Hagan, M. T. (1997). Gauss-Newton approximation to Bayesian regularization. In *Proceedings of the International Joint Conference on Neural Networks, IJCNN 1997*, (pp. 1930-1935). Houston, Texas, USA.

Foster, D., McGregor, C., & El-Masri, S. (2006). A survey of agent-based intelligent decision support systems to support clinical management and research. In G. Armano, E. Merelli, J. Denzinger, A. Martin, S. Miles, H. Tianfield, & R. Unland (Eds.), *Proceedings of MAS BIOMED '05,* Utretch, Netherlands.

Fournier-Vigier, P. (2010). *A sequential pattern mining framework.* Retrieved March 10, 2011, from http://www. philippe-fournier-viger.com/spmf/

Fowlkes, W. Y., & Creveling, C. M. (1995). *Engineering methods for robust production design using Taguchi method in technology and product development.* Reading, MA: Addison Wesley.

Frank, I. H. W. E. (2005). *Data mining: Practical machine learning tools and techniques.* Morgan Kaufmann Publishers.

Frawley, W. J., Piatetsky-Shapiro, G., & Matheus, C. J. (1992). Knowledge discovery in databases: An overview. *AI Magazine, 13,* 57–70.

Friedman, J. H., Kohavi, R., & Yun, Y. (1996). Lazy decision trees. In *Proceedings of the Thirteenth National Conference on Artificial Intelligence,* Vol. 1, (pp. 717–724).

Friedman, N., Iftach, N., & Pe'er, D. (1999). Learning Bayesian network structure from massive datasets: The "sparse candidate" algorithm. *Proceedings of the Fifteenth Conference on Uncertainty in Artificial Intelligence.* Morgan Kaufmann Publishers.

Friedman, N. (2004). Inferring cellular networks using probabilistic graphical models. *Science, 303*(5659), 799–805. doi:10.1126/science.1094068

Friedman, N., Linial, M., Nachman, I., & Pe'er, D. (2000). Using Bayesian networks to analyze expression data. *Journal of Computational Biology, 7,* 601–620. doi:10.1089/106652700750050961

Frunza, O., & Inkpen, D. (2008). *Representation and classification techniques for clinical data focused on obesity and its co-morbidities.* Paper presented at the i2b2 Workshop on Challenges in Natural Language Processing for Clinical Data, Washington, DC.

Frunza, O., & Inkpen, D. (2011). Extracting relations between diseases, treatments, and tests from clinical data. In *Proceedings of the 24th Canadian Conference on Artificial Intelligence.* St. John's, Canada.

Frunza, O., Inkpen, D., Matwin, S., Klement, W., & O'Blenis, P. (2011). Exploiting the systematic review protocol for classification of medical abstracts. *Artificial Intelligence in Medicine, 51,* 17–25. doi:10.1016/j. artmed.2010.10.005

Frunza, O., Inkpen, D., & Tran, T. (2011). A machine learning approach for identifying disease-treatment relations in short texts. *IEEE Transactions on Knowledge and Data Engineering, 23*(6). doi:10.1109/TKDE.2010.152

Fukunaga, K. (1990). *Introduction to statistical pattern recognition* (2nd ed.). San Diego, CA: Academic Press Professional, Inc.

Gacto, M. J., Alcalá, R., & Herrera, F. (2011). Interpretability of linguistic fuzzy rule-based systems: An overview of interpretability measures. *Information Sciences, 181*(20), 4340–4360. doi:10.1016/j.ins.2011.02.021

Gamberger, D., Lavrac, N., & Krstacic, G. (2003). Active subgroup mining: A case study in coronary heart disease risk group detection. *Artificial Intelligence in Medicine, 28*(1), 27–57. doi:10.1016/S0933-3657(03)00034-4

Garcia, E. V., Cooke, C. D., Folks, R. D., Santana, C. A., Krawczynska, E. G., Braal, L. D., & Ezquerra, N. F. (2001). Diagnostic performance of an expert system for the interpretation of myocardial perfusion aspect studies. *Journal of Nuclear Medicine, 42*(8), 1185–1191.

García-Gómez, J. M., Luts, J., Juliá-Sapé, M., Krooshof, P., Tortajada, S., & Robledo, J. V. (2009). Multiproject–multicenter evaluation of automatic brain tumor classification by magnetic resonance spectroscopy. *Magnetic Resonance Materials in Physics. Biologie Medicale, 22*(1), 5–18.

Gatti, C. J., Doro, L. C., Langenderfer, J. E., Mell, A. G., Maratt, J. D., & Carpenter, J. E. (2008). Evaluation of three methods for determining EMG-muscle force parameter estimates for the shoulder muscles. *Clinical Biomechanics (Bristol, Avon), 23,* 166–174. doi:10.1016/j. clinbiomech.2007.08.026

Gehler, P. V., & Nowozin, S. (2008). Infinite kernel learning. *Proceedings of the NIPS 2008 Workshop on Kernel Learning: Automatic Selection of Optimal Kernels.*

General Electric. (2001). *ECToolbox protocol operators guide.*

German, R. R., Armstrong, G., Birkhead, G. S., Horan, J. M., & Herrera, G. (2001). Updated guidelines for evaluating public health surveillance systems. *MMWR. Recommendations and Reports*, *50*, 1–35.

Gilman, A. G. (1987). G proteins: Transducers of receptor-generated signals. *Annual Review of Biochemistry*, *56*, 615–649. doi:10.1146/annurev.bi.56.070187.003151

Giraldo, B., Garde, A., Arizmendi, C., Jane, R., Benito, S., Díaz, I., & Ballesteros, D. (2006) Support vector machine classification applied on weaning trials patients. In *Proceedings of the Engineering in Medicine and Biology Society, EMBS'06, 28th Annual International Conference of the IEEE*, (pp. 5587-5590). IEEE.

Gismondi, R. C., Almeida, R. M. V. R., & Infantosi, A. F. C. (2002). Artificial neural networks for infant mortality modelling. *Computer Methods and Programs in Biomedicine*, *69*, 237–247. doi:10.1016/S0169-2607(02)00006-8

González-Navarro, F. F., Belanche-Muñoz, L. A., Romero, E., Vellido, A., Julià-Sapé, M., & Arús, C. (2010). Feature and model selection with discriminatory visualization for diagnostic classification of brain tumors. *Neurocomputing*, *73*(4-6), 622–632. doi:10.1016/j.neucom.2009.07.018

Göransson, L., & Koski, T. (2002). *Using a dynamic Bayesian network to learn genetic interactions*. Stockholm, Sweden: Royal institute of Technology.

Gosain, A., & Kumar, A. (2009). Analysis of health care data using different data mining techniques. *International Conference on Intelligent Agent & Multi-Agent Systems, 2009 (IAMA 2009)*, (pp. 1-6).

Gotlin, R. S., & Huie, G. (2000). Anterior cruciate ligament injuries. Operative and rehabilitative options. *Physical Medicine and Rehabilitation Clinics of North America*, *11*(4), 895–928.

Gotts, N. M., Hunter, J. R. W., & Sinnhuber, R. K. (1984). *An intelligent model based system for diagnosis in cardiology- A research proposal. AIM-7 Research Report of the AI in Medicine Group.* University of Sussex.

Grigorescu, S., Petkov, N., & Kruizinga, P. (2002). Comparison of texture features based on gabor filters. *IEEE Transactions on Image Processing*, *11*(10), 1160–1167. doi:10.1109/TIP.2002.804262

Groopman, J. (2007). *How doctors think*. Boston, MA: Houghton Mifflin Company.

Groot, P., Hommersom, A., Lucas, P., Serban, R., ten Teije, A., & van Harmelen, F. (2007). The role of model checking in critiquing based on clinical guidelines. *Lecture Notes on Artificial Intelligence*, 411-420.

Groot, P., Hommersom, A., Lucas, P., Merk, R. J., ten Teije, A., van Harmelen, F., & Serban, R. (2008). Using model checking for critiquing based on clinical guidelines. *Artificial Intelligence in Medicine*, (n.d), 19–36.

Grouin, C., et al. (2010). *CARAMBA: Concept, assertion, and relation annotation using machine-learning based approaches.* Paper presented at the i2b2 Workshop on Challenges in Natural Language Processing for Clinical Data, Washington DC., DC.

Guthrie, G., Stacey, D. A., & Calvert, D. (2005). *Detection of disease outbreaks in pharmaceutical sales: Neural networks and threshold algorithms.*

Hagan, T. M., Demuth, H. B., & Beale, M. (1996). *Neural network design*. Boston, MA: PWS Publishing Company.

Hall, M., Frank, E., Holmes, G., Pfahringer, B., Reutemann, P., & Witten, I. H. (2009). The WEKA data mining software: An update. *SIGKDD Explorations*, *11*(1). doi:10.1145/1656274.1656278

Hamilton, P., & Tompkins, W. (1988). Adaptive matched filtering for QRS detection. In *IEEE 10th Annual International Conference Engineering in Medicine and Biology Society*, (pp. 147–148).

Hammond, K. J. (1989). *Case-base planning. Viewing planning as a memory task. Perspectives in Artificial Intelligence, 1*. Academic Press, Inc.

Hammond, P., Davenport, J. C., & Fitzpatrick, F. J. (1993). Logic-based integrity constraints and the design of dental prostheses. *Artificial Intelligence in Medicine*, *5*(5), 431–446. doi:10.1016/0933-3657(93)90035-2

Han, H., Wang, W. Y., & Mao, B. H. (2005). Borderline-SMOTE: A new over-sampling method in imbalanced data sets learning. *Advances in Intelligent Computing, 3644*, 878–887. doi:10.1007/11538059_91

Han, J., Cheng, H., Xin, D., & Yan, X. (2007). Frequent pattern mining: current status and future directions. *Data Mining and Knowledge Discovery, 15*(1), 55–86. doi:10.1007/s10618-006-0059-1

Han, J., & Kamber, M. (2001). *Data mining: Concepts and techniques*. Morgan Kaufmann.

Hardin, J. M., & Chieng, C. (2007). Data mining and clinical decision support systems. *Clinical Decision Support Systems. Healthcare Informatics, 1*, 44–63. doi:10.1007/978-0-387-38319-4_3

Hartford, J. M., Patel, A., & Powell, J. (2005). Intertrochanteric osteotomy using a dynamic hip screw for femoral neck nonunion. *Journal of Orthopaedic Trauma, 19*(5), 329–333.

Hartigan, J. A., & Wong, M. (1979). A k-means clustering algorithm. *Applied Statistics, 28*, 100–108. doi:10.2307/2346830

Hastie, T., Tibshirani, R., & Friedman, J. H. (2008). *The elements of statistical learning*. Springer.

Ha, T. M., & Bunke, H. (1997). Off-line, handwritten numeral recognition by perturbation method. *Pattern Analysis and Machine Intelligence, 19*(5), 535–539. doi:10.1109/34.589216

Haux, R. (2006). Health information systems - Past, present, future. *International Journal of Medical Informatics, 75*(3-4), 268–281. doi:10.1016/j.ijmedinf.2005.08.002

Haykin, S. (2008). *Neural networks and learning machines* (3rd ed.). Prentice Hall.

He, Z., Xu, X., Huang, Z., & Deng, S. (2005). FP-outlier: Frequent pattern based outlier detection. *Computer Science and Information Systems/ComSIS, 2*(1), 103-118.

Heckerman, D. E., Horvitz, E. J., & Nathwani, B. N. (1992). Toward normative expert systems: Part I. The Pathfinder project. *Methods of Information in Medicine, 31*(2), 90–105.

Heckerman, D. E., & Nathwani, B. N. (1992). Toward normative expert systems: Part II. Probability-based representations for efficient knowledge acquisition and inference. *Methods of Information in Medicine, 31*(2), 106–116.

Hernández, J. A. (2009). Optimum operating conditions for heat and mass transfer in foodstuffs drying by means of neural network inverse. *Food Control, 20*, 435–438. doi:10.1016/j.foodcont.2008.07.005

Hesse, B., & Gächter, A. (2004). Complications following the treatment of trochanteric fractures with the gamma nail. *Archives of Orthopaedic and Trauma Surgery, 124*, 692–698. doi:10.1007/s00402-004-0744-8

Hodge, V., & Austin, J. (2004). A survey of outlier detection methodologies. *Artificial Intelligence Review, 22*(2), 85–126. doi:10.1023/B:AIRE.0000045502.10941.a9

Hofmann-Wellenhof, R., Blum, A., Wolf, I. H., Zalaudek, I., Piccolo, D., & Kerl, H. (2002). Dermoscopic classi□cation of clark's nevi (atypical melanocytic nevi). *Clinics in Dermatology, 20*(3), 255–258. doi:10.1016/S0738-081X(02)00217-1

Horn, F., Weare, J., Beukers, M. W., Horsch, S., Bairoch, A., & Chen, W. (1998). GPCRDB: An information system for G protein-coupled receptors. *Nucleic Acids Research, 26*, 275–279. doi:10.1093/nar/26.1.275

Hsu, C. C., Chao, C. K., Wang, J. L., Hou, S. M., Tsai, Y. T., & Lin, J. (2005). Increase of pullout strength of spinal pedicle screws with conical core: Biomechanical tests and finite element analyses. *Journal of Orthopaedic Research, 23*(4), 788–794. doi:10.1016/j.orthres.2004.11.002

Hsu, C. C., Chao, C. K., Wang, J. L., & Lin, J. (2006). Multiobjective optimization of tibial locking screws design using a genetic algorithm: Evaluation of mechanical performance. *Journal of Orthopaedic Research, 24*, 908–916. doi:10.1002/jor.20088

Hsu, C. C., Lin, J., Amaritsakul, Y., Antonius, T., & Chao, C. K. (2009). Finite element analysis for the treatment of proximal femoral fracture. *CMC-Computers. Materials & Continua, 11*(1), 1–13.

Huang, D., & Pan, W. (2006). Incorporating biological knowledge into distance-based clustering analysis of microarray gene expression data. *Bioinformatics (Oxford, England)*, 22(10), 1259–1268. doi:10.1093/bioinformatics/btl065

Hubert, L., & Arabie, P. (1985). Comparing partitions. *Journal of Classification*, 2(1), 193–218. doi:10.1007/BF01908075

Hugin. (2011). *Hugin expert*. Retrieved from http://www.hugin.com

Hulsman, M., Reinders, M. J. T., & de Ridder, D. (2009). Evolutionary optimization of kernel weights improves protein complex comembership prediction. *IEEE/ACM Transactions on Computational Biology and Bioinformatics*, 6(3), 427–437. doi:10.1109/TCBB.2008.137

Hutwagner, L., Thompson, W., Seeman, G. M., & Treadwell, T. (2003). The bioterrorism preparedness and response early aberration reporting system (EARS). *Journal of Urban Health: Bulletin of the New York Academy of Medicine*, 80(Supplement 1), i89–i96.

Hwang, R. L., Lin, T. P., Liang, H. H., Yang, K. H., & Yeh, T. C. (2009). Additive model for thermal comfort generated by matrix experiment using orthogonal array. *Building and Environment*, 44, 1730–1739. doi:10.1016/j.buildenv.2008.11.009

Hyvärinen, A., Karhunen, J., & Oja, E. (2001). *Independent component analysis*. New York, NY: John Wiley & Sons, inc. doi:10.1002/0471221317

ICD IX-CM. (2011). *Free online searchable 2009 ICD-9-CM*. Retrieved April 3, 2011 from http://icd9cm.chrisendres.com

Ichihashi, H., Shirai, T., Nagasaka, K., & Miyoshi, T. (1996). Neuro-fuzzy ID3: A method of inducing fuzzy decision trees with linear programming for maximizing entropy and an algebraic method for incremental learning. *Fuzzy Sets and Systems*, 81, 157–167. doi:10.1016/0165-0114(95)00247-2

Imran, A., & O'Connor, J. J. (1998). Control of knee stability after ACL injury or repair: Interaction between hamstrings contraction and tibial translation. *Clinical Biomechanics (Bristol, Avon)*, 13(3), 153–162. doi:10.1016/S0268-0033(97)00030-2

Inbar, O., Lavie, T., & Meyer, J. (2009). Acceptable intrusiveness of online help in mobile devices. In *Proceedings of the 11th International Conference on Human-Computer Interaction with Mobile Devices and Services* (MobileHCI '09), (p. 26). New York, NY: ACM.

Ivanitsky, A. M., Nikolaev, A. R., & Ivanitsky, G. A. (2001). Cortical connectivity during word association search. *International Journal of Psychophysiology*, 42, 35–53. doi:10.1016/S0167-8760(01)00140-4

Jackson, J. E. (1991). *A user guide to principal components*. New York, NY: John Wiley & Sons, inc.

Japkowicz, N. (2000). The class imbalance problem: Significance and strategies. In *Proceedings of the International Conference on Artificial Intelligence (ICAI 2000)*, Vol. 1, (pp. 111-117).

Jeffery, I. B., Higgins, D. G., & Culhane, A. C. (2006). Comparison and evaluation methods for generating differentially expressed gene list from microarray data. *BMC Bioinformatics*, 7(359), 1–16.

Jelonek, J., & Stefanowski, J. (1997). Feature subset selection for classification of histological images. *Artificial Intelligence in Medicine*, 9(3), 227–239. doi:10.1016/S0933-3657(96)00375-2

Jensen, F. V. (2001). *Bayesian networks and decision graphs*. Springer. Jordan, M. I. (Ed.). (1998). *Learning in graphical models*. The MIT Press.

Jensen, O. (2001). Information transfer between rythmically coupled networks: Reading the hippocampal phase code. *Neural Computation*, 13, 2743–2761. doi:10.1162/089976601317098510

Jenssen, T. K., Laegreid, A., Komorowski, J., & Hovig, E. (2001). A literature network of human genes for high-throughput analysis of gene expression. *Nature Genetics*, 28(1), 21–28. doi:10.1038/ng0501-21

Jiang, J. H., Berry, R. J., Siesler, H. W., & Ozaki, Y. (2002). Wavelength interval selection in multicomponent spectral analysis by moving window partial least-squares regression with applications to mid-infrared and near-infrared spectroscopic data. *Analytical Chemistry*, 74(14), 3555–3565. doi:10.1021/ac011177u

Jolliffe, I. (2002). *Principal component analysis*. New York, NY: Springer.

Julià-Sapé, M., Acosta, D., Mier, M., Arús, C., & Watson, D. (2006). A multi-centre, web-accessible and quality control-checked database of in vivo MR spectra of brain tumour patients. *Magnetic Resonance Materials in Physics, Biology and Medicine. Magma (New York, N.Y.)*, *19*(1), 22–33. doi:10.1007/s10334-005-0023-x

Kahn, S. D. (2011). On the future of genomic data. *Science*, *331*(6018), 728–729. doi:10.1126/science.1197891

Katsis, C.D., Goletsis, Y., Likas, A., Fotiadis, D., & Sarmas, I. (2006). A novel method for automated EMG decomposition and MUAP classification. *Artificial Intelligence in Medicine*, *37*(1), 55–64. doi:10.1016/j.artmed.2005.09.002

Kazemzadeh, R. S., & Sartipi, K. (2006). Incorporating data mining applications into clinical guidelines. *Proceedings of the 19th IEEE Symposium on Computer-Based Medical Systems (CBMS'06)*.

Keyak, J. H., & Skinner, H. B. (1992). Three-dimensional finite element modeling of bone: Effects of element size. *Journal of Biomechanical Engineering-Transactions of the ASME*, *14*, 483–489.

Kira, K., & Rendell, L. (1992). A practical approach to feature selection. In D. Sleeman & P. Edwards, (Eds.), *Proceedings of the International Conference on Machine Learning*, (pp. 249–256). Aberdeen, UK: Morgan Kaufmann.

Kleihues, P., & Cavenee, W.K. (2000). *Pathology and genetics of tumours of the nervous system*. World Health Organization Classification of Tumours. Lyon, France: IARCPress.

Knaus, W. A., Draper, E. A., Wagner, D. P., & Zimmerman, J. E. (1985). APACHE II: A severity of disease classification system. *Critical Care Medicine*, *13*, 818–829. doi:10.1097/00003246-198510000-00009

Kohler, B., Hennig, C., & Orglmeister, R. (2002). The principles of software QRS detection. *IEEE Engineering in Medicine and Biology Magazine*, *21*(1), 42–57. doi:10.1109/51.993193

Kohonen, T. (2000). *Self-organizing maps*. Springer.

Kohonen, T. (2001). *Self-organizing maps* (3rd ed.). Berlin, Germany: Springer-Verlag.

Koller, D., & Friedman, N. (2009). *Probabilistic graphical models: Principles and techniques*. The MIT Press.

Kolodner, J. (1993). *Case-based reasoning*. Morgan Kaufmann.

Kononenko, I. (1993). Inductive and Bayesian learning in medical diagnosis. *Applied Artificial Intelligence*, *7*, 317–337. doi:10.1080/08839519308949993

Kononenko, I. (2001). Machine learning for medical diagnosis: History, state of the art and perspective. *Artificial Intelligence in Medicine*, *3*, 89–109. doi:10.1016/S0933-3657(01)00077-X

Kononenko, I., & Kukar, M. (2007). *Machine learning and data mining: Introduction to principles and algorithms*. Chichester, UK: Horwood Publishing.

Kosko, B. (1994). Fuzzy systems as universal approximators. *IEEE Transactions on Computers*, *43*(11), 1329–1333. doi:10.1109/12.324566

Koufakou, A., Ortiz, E., Georgiopoulos, M., Anagnostopoulos, G., & Reynolds, K. (2007). *A scalable and efficient outlier detection strategy for categorical data*.

Kouvidis, G. K., Sommers, M. B., Giannoudis, P. V., Katonis, P. G., & Bottlang, M. (2009). Comparison of migration behavior between single and dual lag screw implants for intertrochanteric fracture fixation. *Journal of Orthopaedic Surgery and Research*, *4*(16), 1–9.

Kroch, E., Vaughn, T., Koepke, M., Roman, S., Foster, D., & Sinha, S. (2006). Hospital boards and quality dashboards. *Journal of Patient Safety*, *2*(1), 10–19.

Kubat, M., Holte, R., & Matwin, S. (1998). Machine learning for the detection of oil spills in satellite radar images. *Machine Learning*, *30*(2-3), 195–215. doi:10.1023/A:1007452223027

Kubiak, E. N., Bong, M., Park, S. S., Kummer, F., Egol, K., & Koval, K. J. (2004). Intramedullary fixation of unstable intertrochanteric hip fractures. *Journal of Orthopaedic Trauma*, *18*(1), 12–17. doi:10.1097/00005131-200401000-00003

Kukar, M. (2001). *Estimating classifications' reliability and cost-sensitive combination of machine learning methods*. Doctoral dissertation, University of Ljubljana.

Kukar, M., & Grošelj, C. (1999). Machine learning in stepwise diagnostic process. In W. Horn, Y. Shahar, G. Lindberg, S. Andreassen & J. Wyatt (Eds.), *Proceedings of the Joint European Conference on Artificial Intelligence in Medicine and Medical Decision Making*, (pp. 315–325). Aalborg, Denmark: Springer.

Kukar, M., & Šajn, L. (2009). Improving probabilistic interpretation of medical diagnoses with multi-resolution image parameterization: A case study. In C. Combi, Y. Shahar & A. Abu-Hanna (Eds.), *12th Conference on Artificial Intelligence in Medicine*, (pp. 136–145). Springer.

Kukar, M., Grošelj, C., Kononenko, I., & Fettich, J. (1997). An application of machine learning in the diagnosis of ischaemic heart disease. In *Proceedings of the Sixth European Conference of AI in Medicine Europe AIME97*, Grenoble, France, (pp. 461–464).

Kukar, M., & Kononenko, I. (2002). Reliable classifications with machine learning. In Elomaa, T., Mannila, H., & Toivonen, H. (Eds.), *Machine Learning: ECML 2002* (*Vol. 2430*, pp. 1–8). Lecture Notes in Computer Science Berlin, Germany: Springer-Verlag. doi:10.1007/3-540-36755-1_19

Kukar, M., Kononenko, I., Grošelj, C., Kralj, K., & Fettich, J. (1999). Analysing and improving the diagnosis of ischaemic heart disease with machine learning. *Artificial Intelligence in Medicine*, *16*(1), 25–50. doi:10.1016/S0933-3657(98)00063-3

Kukar, M., Šajn, L., Grošelj, C., & Grošelj, J. (2007). Multi-resolution image parametrization in sequential diagnostics of coronary artery disease. In Bellazzi, R., Abu-Hanna, A., & Hunter, J. (Eds.), *Artificial intelligence in medicine* (pp. 119–129). Berlin, Germany: Springer. doi:10.1007/978-3-540-73599-1_13

Kurgan, L. A., Cios, K. J., & Tadeusiewicz, R. (2001). Knowledge discovery approach to automated cardiac spect diagnosis. *Artificial Intelligence in Medicine*, *23*(2), 149–169. doi:10.1016/S0933-3657(01)00082-3

Kurt, I., Ture, M., & Turhan Kurum, A. (2008). Comparing performances of logistic regression classification and regression tree, and neural networks for predicting coronary arterial disease. *Expert Systems with Applications*, *34*(1), 366–374. doi:10.1016/j.eswa.2006.09.004

Kuzmanovski, I., & Aleksovska, S. (2003). Optimization of artificial neural networks for prediction of the unit cell parameters in orthorhombic perovskites. Comparison with multiple linear regression. *Chemometrics and Intelligent Laboratory Systems*, *67*, 167–174. doi:10.1016/S0169-7439(03)00092-3

Kwok, J. T., & Tsang, I. W. (2003). Learning with idealized kernels. *Proceedings of the Twentieth International Conference on Machine Learning*, (pp. 400-407). Washington, DC.

Ladroue, C., Howe, F. A., Griffiths, J. R., & Tate, A. R. (2003). Independent component analysis for automated decomposition of in vivo magnetic resonance spectra. *Magnetic Resonance in Medicine*, *50*(4), 697–703. doi:10.1002/mrm.10595

Lai, P., & Kwong, K. (2010). Spatial analysis of the 2008 influenza outbreak of Hong Kong. *Computational Science and Its Applications–ICCSA*, *2010*, 374–388.

Laird, J. E., Newell, A., & Rosenbloom, P. S. (1987). Soar: An architecture for general intelligence. *Artificial. Intelligence*, *33*, 1–64.

Lanckriet, G. R. G., De Bie, T., Cristianini, N., Jordan, M. I., & Stafford Noble, W. (2004b). A statistical framework for genomic data fusion. *Bioinformatics (Oxford, England)*, *20*(16), 2626–2635. doi:10.1093/bioinformatics/bth294

Lanckriet, G., Cristianini, N., Barlett, P., El Ghaoui, L., & Jordan, M. (2004). Learning the kernel matrix with semidefinite programming. *Journal of Machine Learning Research*, *3*, 27–72.

Langlotz, C. P., & Shortliffe, E. H. (1983). Adapting a consultation system to critique user plans. *International Journal of Man-Machine Studies*, *19*, 479–496. doi:10.1016/S0020-7373(83)80067-4

Lantos, P. L., Vandenberg, S. R., & Kleihues, P. (1996). Tumours of the nervous system. In Graham, D. I., & Lantos, P. L. (Eds.), *Greenfield's neuropathology* (pp. 583–879). London, UK: Arnold.

Laws, K. I. (1980). *Textured image segmentation*. PhD thesis, Dept. Electrical Engineering, University of Southern California, Los Angeles, California, USA.

Leake, D. B. (1996). Experience, introspection and expertise: Learning to refine the case-based reasoning process. *Journal of Experimental & Theoretical Artificial Intelligence*, 8(3-4), 319–339. doi:10.1080/095281396147357

Lee, D. C., & Lee, J. I. (2004). Structural optimization design for large mirror. *Optics and Lasers in Engineering*, 42, 109–117. doi:10.1016/S0143-8166(03)00079-4

Lee, D. D., & Seung, S. (1999). Learning the parts of objects by non-negative matrix Factorization. *Nature*, 6755(401), 788–791.

Leroy, G., Chen, H. C., & Martinez, J. D. (2003). A shallow parser based on closed-class words to capture relations in biomedical text. *Journal of Biomedical Informatics*, 36(3), 145–158. doi:10.1016/S1532-0464(03)00039-X

Levy, M. M., Fink, M. P., Marshall, J. C., Abraham, E., Angus, D., & Cook, D. … Ramsay, G. (2003). *2001 SSCM/ESICM/ACCP/SIS International Sepsis Definitions Conference* (pp. 530-538).

Lindahl, D., Palmer, J., Pettersson, J., White, T., Lundin, A., & Edenbrandt, L. (1998). Scintigraphic diagnosis of coronary artery disease: Myocardial bulls-eye images contain the important information. *Clinical Physiology (Oxford, England)*, 6(18).

Lin, J. (2006). Encouraging results of treating femoral trochanteric fractures with specially designed double screw nails. *The Journal of Trauma Injury Infection and Critical Care*, 63(4), 866–874. doi:10.1097/TA.0b013e3180342087

Lisboa, P. J. G. (2002). A review of evidence of health benefit from artificial neural networks in medical intervention. *Neural Networks*, 15, 9–37. doi:10.1016/S0893-6080(01)00111-3

Lisboa, P. J. G., Vellido, A., Tagliaferri, R., Napolitano, F., Ceccarelli, M., Martin-Guerrero, J. D., & Biganzoli, E. (2004). Data mining in cancer research. *IEEE Computational Intelligence Magazine*, 5(1), 14–18. doi:10.1109/MCI.2009.935311

Liu, J. S., & Chen, R. (1998). Sequential Monte Carlo methods for dynamical systems. *Journal of the American Statistical Association*, 93, 1032–1044. doi:10.2307/2669847

Livingston, D. H., Mosenthal, A. C., & Deith, E. A. (1995). Sepsis and multiple organ dysfunction syndrome: A clinical-mechanistic overview. *New Horizons (Baltimore, Md.)*, 3, 257–266.

Lloyd, D. G., Buchanan, T. S., & Besier, T. F. (2005). Neuromuscular biomechanical modeling to understand knee ligament loading. *Medicine and Science in Sports and Exercise*, 37(11), 1939–1947. doi:10.1249/01.mss.0000176676.49584.ba

Logar, V., & Belič, A. (2011). Brain-computer interface analysis of a dynamic visuo-motor task. *Artificial Intelligence in Medicine*, 51(1), 43–51. doi:10.1016/j.artmed.2010.10.004

Logar, V., Belič, A., Koritnik, B., Brežan, S., Zidar, J., Karba, R., & Matko, D. (2008a). Using ANNs to predict a subject's response based on EEG traces. *Neural Networks*, 21(7), 881–887. doi:10.1016/j.neunet.2008.03.012

Logar, V., Škrjanc, I., Belič, A., Brežan, S., Koritnik, B., & Zidar, J. (2008b). Identification of the phase code in an EEG during gripping-force tasks: A possible alternative approach to the development of the brain-computer interfaces. *Artificial Intelligence in Medicine*, 44(1), 41–49. doi:10.1016/j.artmed.2008.06.003

López de Mántaras, R. (1991). A distance-based attribute selection measure for decision tree induction. *Machine Learning*, 6, 81–92. doi:10.1023/A:1022694001379

Lorich, D. G., Geller, D. S., & Nielson, J. H. (2004). Osteoporotic pertrochanteric hip fractures. *The Journal of Bone and Joint Surgery. American Volume*, 86, 398–410.

Lowe, D. G. (2004). Distinctive image features from scale-invariant keypoints. *International Journal of Computer Vision*, 60(2), 91–110. doi:10.1023/B:VISI.0000029664.99615.94

Lucas, P. J., de Bruijn, N. C., Schurink, K., & Hoepelman, A. (2000). A probabilistic and decision-theoretic approach to the management of infectious disease at the ICU. *Artificial Intelligence in Medicine*, 19(3), 251–279. doi:10.1016/S0933-3657(00)00048-8

Luce, J. (1987). Pathogenesis and management of septic shock. *Chest*, 91, 883–888. doi:10.1378/chest.91.6.883

Luts, J., Heerschap, A., Suykens, J. A. K., & Van Huffel, S. (2007). A combined MRI and MRSI based multiclass system for brain tumour recognition using LS-SVMs with class probabilities and feature selection. *Artificial Intelligence in Medicine, 40*(2), 87–102. doi:10.1016/j.artmed.2007.02.002

Mac Namee, B., Cunningham, P., Byrne, S., & Corrigan, O. (2002). The problem of bias in training data in regression problems in medical decision support. *Artificial Intelligence in Medicine, 24*(1), 51–70. doi:10.1016/S0933-3657(01)00092-6

MacDonald, D., & Fyfe, C. (2000). The kernel self organising map. In *Proceedings of the 4th International Conference on Knowledge-Based Intelligent Engineering Systems and Allied Technologies*, Vol. 1, (pp. 317-320).

MacKay, D. J. C. (1992). A practical Bayesian framework for back-propagation networks. *Neural Computation, 4*(3), 448–472. doi:10.1162/neco.1992.4.3.448

MacKay, D. J. C. (1992). The evidence framework applied to classification networks. *Neural Computation, 4*(5), 720–736. doi:10.1162/neco.1992.4.5.720

Manganotti, P., Gerloff, C., Toro, C., Katsuta, H., Sadato, N., & Zhuang, P. (1998). Task-related coherence and task-related spectral power changes during sequential finger movements. *Electroencephalography and Clinical Neurophysiology, 109*, 50–62. doi:10.1016/S0924-980X(97)00074-X

Manning, C., & Schutze, H. (1999). *Foundations of statistical natural language processing*. Cambridge, MA: MIT Press.

Marcos, M., Balser, M., ten Teije, A., & van Harmelen, F. (2002). From informal knowledge to formal logic: A realistic case study in medical protocols. In *Proceedings of the 13th International Conference on Knowledge Engineering and Knowledge Management*. New York, NY: Springer-Verlag.

Marcos, M., Berger, G., van Harmelem, F., & ten Teije, A. Roomans, H., & Miksch, S. (2001). Using critiquing for improving medical protocols: harder than it seems. *Proceedings of the Eighth European Conference on Artificial Intelligence in Medicine (AIME'01), LNAI, vol. 2101*, (pp. 431-441). New York, NY: Springer-Verlag.

Marcus, A. (2006). Dashboards in your future. *Interaction, 13*(1), 48–60. doi:10.1145/1109069.1109103

Marks, L. W., & Gardner, T. N. (1993). The use of strain energy as a convergence criterion in the finite element modeling of bone and the effect of model geometry on stress convergence. *Journal of Biomechanical Engineering-Transactions of the ASME, 15*, 474–476.

Martín, J. D., & Lisboa, P. J. G. (2010). Computational intelligence in biomedicine: Some contributions. *Proceedings of the 18th European Symposium on Artificial Neural Networks (ESANN)*, (pp. 429-438).

Martin, G. S., Mannino, D. M., Eaton, S., & Moss, M. (2003). The epidemiology of sepsis in the United States from 1979 to 2000. *The New England Journal of Medicine, 348*, 1546–1554. doi:10.1056/NEJMoa022139

Martín-Merino, M., & Blanco, A. (2009a). A local semi-supervised Sammon algorithm for textual data visualization. *Journal of Intelligent Information Systems, 33*(1), 23–40. doi:10.1007/s10844-008-0056-5

Martín-Merino, M., Blanco, A., & De Las Rivas, J. (2009b). Combining dissimilarities in a hyper reproducing kernel Hilbert space for complex human cancer prediction. *Journal of Biomedicine & Biotechnology, 2009*, 1–9. doi:10.1155/2009/906865

Matsumoto, H., & Seedhom, B. B. (1994). Treatment of the pivot-shift intraarticular versus extraarticular or combined reconstruction procedures. A biomechanical study. *Clinical Orthopaedics and Related Research, 299*, 298–304.

McNaught, K., Clifford, S., Vaughn, M., Fogg, A., & Foy, M. (2001). *A Bayesian belief network for lower back pain diagnosis*. Paper presented at the European Conference on Artificial Intelligence in Medicine.

Mencar, C., & Fanelli, A. M. (2008). Interpretability constraints for fuzzy information granulation. *Information Sciences, 178*, 4585–4618. doi:10.1016/j.ins.2008.08.015

Menetrey, J., Duthon, V. B., Laumonier, T., & Fritschy, D. (2008). "Biological failure" of the anterior cruciate ligament graft. *Knee Surgery, Sports Traumatology, Arthroscopy, 16*(3), 224–231. doi:10.1007/s00167-007-0474-x

Michalewicz, Z. (1992). *Genetic algorithms + Data structures = Evolution programs*. Berlin, Germany: Springer.

Michalski, R. S. (1983). A theory and methodology of inductive learning. In Michalski, R. S., Carbonell, T. J., & Mitchell, T. M. (Eds.), *Machine learning: An artificial intelligence approach* (pp. 111–161). Palo Alto, CA: TIOGA Publishing Co.doi:10.1016/0004-3702(83)90016-4

Miller, P. L. (1985). Goal-directed critiquing by computer: Ventilator management. *Computers and Biomedical Research, an International Journal, 18*, 422–438. doi:10.1016/0010-4809(85)90020-5

Miller, P. L. (1986). *Expert critiquing systems: Practice-based medical computing.* New York, NY: Springer Verlag.

Miller, R. A., Pople, H. E., & Myers, J. D. (1984). An experimental computer based diagnostic consultant for general internal medicine. In Clancey, W. J., & Shortliffe, E. H. (Eds.), *Readings in medical AI: The first decade.* Reading, MA: Addison-Wesley. doi:10.1056/NEJM198208193070803

Mitchell, M. (1996). *An introduction to genetic algorithms.* Cambridge, MA: Bradford.

Mitchell, T. M. (1997). *Machine learning. McGraw-Hill* (International Editions). Computer Science Series.

Mitchell, T. M., Keller, R. M., & Kedar-Cabelli, S. T. (1986). Explanation-based learning: A unifying view. *Machine Learning, 1*(1), 47–80. doi:10.1007/BF00116250

Mitsumori, T., Murata, M., Fukuda, Y., Doi, K., & Doi, H. (2006). Extracting protein-protein interaction information from biomedical text with SVM. *IEICE Transactions on Information and Systems. E (Norwalk, Conn.), 89D*(8), 244–246.

Mobley, B. A., Schechter, E., & Moore, W. E. (2000). Predictions of coronary artery stenosis by artificial neural network. *Artificial Intelligence in Medicine, 18*(3), 187–203. doi:10.1016/S0933-3657(99)00040-8

MOH. (2009). *Health facts 2009.* Retrieved from http://www.moh.gov.my/images/gallery/stats/heal_fact/healthfact-P_2009.pdf

Mohamed, N., Rubin, D. M., & Marwala, T. (2006) Detection of epileptiform activity in human EEG signals using Bayesian neural networks. In *Proceedings of the IEEE 3rd International Conference on Computational Cybernetics, ICCC 2005,* (pp. 231-237). IEEE.

Mondorf, W., Siegmund, B., Mahnel, R., Richter, H., Westfeld, M., & Galler, A. (2009). Haemoassist 'TM' - A hand-held electronic patient diary for haemophilia home care. *Haemophilia, 15*(2), 464–472. doi:10.1111/j.1365-2516.2008.01941.x

Monti, M. (2011). *Ostetricia e Ginecologia on line.* Retrieved April 5, 2011, from http://www.ginecolink.net/percorso_non_medici/ EsamiGrav.htm

Morris, A. (1987). Expert systems - Interface insight. In Diaper, D., & Winder, R. (Eds.), *People and Computers, 3* (pp. 307–324). Cambridge University Press.

Mukherjee, S., & Hill, S. M. (2011). Network clustering: probing biological heterogeneity by sparse graphical models. *Bioinformatics (Oxford, England), 27*(7), 994–1000. doi:10.1093/bioinformatics/btr070

Mukhi, S. N. (2007). *Integrated approach to real-time biosurveillance in a federated data source environment.* Winnipeg, Manitoba, Canada: University of Manitoba.

Nagl, S., Williams, M., & Williamson, J. (2006). Objective Bayesian nets for systems modelling and prognosis in breast cancer. In Holmes, D., & Jain, L. C. (Eds.), *Innovations in Bayesian networks: Theory and applications.* Springer Verlag. doi:10.1007/978-3-540-85066-3_6

Nauck, D., & Kruse, R. (1999). Obtaining interpretable fuzzy classification rules from medical data. *Artificial Intelligence in Medicine, 16*, 149–169. doi:10.1016/S0933-3657(98)00070-0

Neapolitan, R. (1990). *Probabilistic reasoning in expert systems.* New York, NY: Wiley & Sons Ltd.

Neapolitan, R. (2004). *Learning Bayesian networks.* New Jersey: Prentice Hall.

Neapolitan, R. E. (2003). *Learning Bayesian networks.* Prentice Hall.

Neill, D. B., Moore, A. W., Sabhnani, M., & Daniel, K. (2005). *Detection of emerging space-time clusters.*

Neill, D. B., Moore, A. W., Sabhnani, M. R., & Daniel, K. (2006). An expectation-based scan statistic for detection of space-time clusters. *Advances in Disease Surveillance, 1*(1), 56.

Neill, D., Moore, A., & Cooper, G. (2006). A Bayesian spatial scan statistic. *Advances in Neural Information Processing Systems, 18*, 1003.

NICE. (2003). *Antenatal care, routine care for the healthy pregnant woman.* National Collaborating Centre for Women's and Children's Health by NICE, Clinical Guidelines. RCOG Press, 2003.

Nikovski, D. (2000). Constructing Bayesian networks for medical diagnosis from incomplete and partially correct statistics. *IEEE Transactions on Knowledge and Data Engineering, 12*, 509–516. doi:10.1109/69.868904

Nixon, M., & Aguado, A. (2008). *Feature extraction and image processing* (2nd ed.). Amsterdam, The Netherlands: Elsevier.

Nugent, C., Doyle, D., & Cunningham, P. (2009). Gaining insight through case-based explanation. *Journal of Intelligent Information Systems, 32*(3), 267–295. doi:10.1007/s10844-008-0069-0

Nunez, P. L., & Srinivasan, R. (2006). *Electric fields of the brain.* New York, NY: Oxford University Press. doi:10.1093/acprof:oso/9780195050387.001.0001

Nyblom, H., Berggren, U., Balldin, J., & Olsson, R. (2004). High AST/ALT Ratio may indicate advanced alcoholic liver disease rather than heavy drinking. *Alcohol and Alcoholism (Oxford, Oxfordshire), 39*(4), 336–339. doi:10.1093/alcalc/agh074

Ohlsson, M. (2004). WeAidU–A decision support system for myocardial perfusion images using artificial neural networks. *Artificial Intelligence in Medicine, 30*, 49–60. doi:10.1016/S0933-3657(03)00050-2

Ojala, T., Mäenpää, T., Pietikäinen, M., Viertola, J., Kyllönen, J., & Huovinen, S. (2002). Outex - New framework for empirical evaluation of texture analysis algorithms. In *International Conference on Pattern Recognition,* Vol. 1, (p. 10701). Los Alamitos, CA: IEEE Computer Society.

Olarte Rodríguez, O. J., & Sierra Bueno, D. A. (2010) Determinación de los parámetros asociados al filtro wavelet por umbralización aplicado a filtrado de interferencias electrocardiográficas (in Spanish). *Revista UIS Ingenierías, 6*(2).

Olier, I., Vellido, A., & Giraldo, J. (2010). Kernel generative topographic mapping. In *Proceedings of the 18th European Symposium on Artificial Neural Networks* (ESANN 2010), (pp. 481-486).

Olona-Cabases, M. (1994). The probability of a correct diagnosis. In Candell-Riera, J., & Ortega-Alcalde, D. (Eds.), *Nuclear cardiology in everyday practice* (pp. 348–357). Dordrecht, The Netherlands: Kluwer Academic Publishers. doi:10.1007/978-94-011-1984-9_19

O'Neill, M., & Morris, A. (1989). Expert systems in the United Kingdom: An evaluation of development methodologies. *Expert Systems: International Journal of Knowledge Engineering and Neural Networks, 6*(2), 90–99. doi:10.1111/j.1468-0394.1989.tb00082.x

Opitz, D. W., & Maclin, R. (1999). Popular ensemble methods: An empirical study. *Journal of Artificial Intelligence Research, 11*, 169–198.

Oum, S., Chandramohan, D., & Cairncross, S. (2005). Community based surveillance: A pilot study from rural Cambodia. *Tropical Medicine & International Health, 10*(7), 689–697. doi:10.1111/j.1365-3156.2005.01445.x

Overington, J. P., Al-Lazikani, B., & Hopkins, A. L. (2006). How many drug targets are there? *Nature Reviews. Drug Discovery, 5*, 993–996. doi:10.1038/nrd2199

Paliwal, M., & Kumar, U. A. (2009). Neural networks and statistical techniques: A review of applications. *Expert Systems with Applications, 36*(1), 2–17. doi:10.1016/j.eswa.2007.10.005

Palniappan, S., & Ling, C. S. (2008). Clinical decision support using OLAP with data mining. *International Journal of Computer Science and Network Security, 8*(9).

Pandey, B., & Mishra, R. B. (2009). Knowledge and intelligent computing system in medicine. *Computers in Biology and Medicine, 39*(3), 215–230. doi:10.1016/j.compbiomed.2008.12.008

Pan, J., & Tomkins, W. (1985). A real-time QRS detection algorithm. *IEEE Transactions on Bio-Medical Engineering, BME-32*(3), 230–236. doi:10.1109/TBME.1985.325532

Park, K. W., Smaltz, D., McFadden, D., & Souba, W. (2009). The operating room dashboard. *Journal of Surgical Research, 164*(2), 294-300. doi: DOI: 10.1016/j.jss.2009.09.011

Parsian, M. (2006). *JDBC metadata, MySQL, & Oracle recipes: A problem-solution approach.* Apress Academic.

Patcha, A., & Park, J. M. (2007). An overview of anomaly detection techniques: Existing solutions and latest technological trends. *Computer Networks, 51*(12), 3448–3470. doi:10.1016/j.comnet.2007.02.001

Patrick, J., & Asgari, P. (2008). *A brief summary about the approach and explanation of the attributes of the developed system.* Paper presented at the i2b2 Workshop on Challenges in Natural Language Processing for Clinical Data, Washington, DC.

Pattacini, C., Rivolta, G. F., Perna, C. D., Riccardi, F., & Tagliaferri, A. (2009). A web-based clinical record 'xl'Emofilia^{®}' for outpatients with haemophilia and allied disorders in the Region of Emilia-Romagna: Features and pilot use. *Haemophilia, 15*(1), 150–158. doi:10.1111/j.1365-2516.2008.01921.x

Pearl, J. (1988). *Probabilistic reasoning in intelligent systems: Networks of plausible inference.* Morgan Kaufmann Publishers.

Pearson, K. (1901). Principal components analysis. *The London, Edinburgh, and Dublin Philosophical Magazine and Journal of Science*, 559.

Peek, N. (2001). *The notion of diagnosis in decision-theoretic planning.* Paper presented at the Eoropean Conference on Artificial Intelligence in Medicine Workshop on Bayesian Models in Medicine.

Pekalska, E., Paclick, P., & Duin, R. (2004). A generalized kernel approach to dissimilarity-based classification. *Journal of Machine Learning Research, 2*, 175-211, 2001.

Peña, J. M., Bjorkegren, J., & Tegner, J. (2005). Growing Bayesian network models of gene networks from seed genes. *Bioinformatics (Oxford, England), 21*(Suppl 2), ii224–ii229. doi:10.1093/bioinformatics/bti1137

Peng, Y., Yao, B., & Jiang, J. (2006). Knowledge-discovery incorporated evolutionary search for microcalcification detection in breast cancer diagnosis. *Artificial Intelligence in Medicine, 37*(1), 43–53. doi:10.1016/j.artmed.2005.09.001

Perkins, B. A., Olaleye, D., Zinman, B., & Bril, V. (2001). Simple screening tests for peripheral neuropathy in the diabetes clinic. *Diabetes Care, 24*(2), 250–256. doi:10.2337/diacare.24.2.250

Perrin, B. E., Ralaivola, L., Mazurie, A., Bottani, S., Mallet, J., & d'Alche-Buc, F. (2003). Gene networks inference using dynamic Bayesian networks. *Bioinformatics (Oxford, England), 19*(Suppl 2), ii138–ii148. doi:10.1093/bioinformatics/btg1071

Pervez, H., & Parker, M. J. (2001). Results of the long gamma nail for complex proximal femoral fractures. *Injury-International Journal of the Care of the Injured, 32*, 704–707.

Pevec, D., Štrumbelj, E., & Kononenko, I. (2011). Evaluating reliability of single classifications of neural networks. In Dobnikar, A., Lotrič, U., & Šter, B. (Eds.), *Adaptive and Natural Computing Algorithms* (*Vol. 5182*, pp. 22–30). Lecture Notes in Computer Science Berlin, Germany: Springer-Verlag. doi:10.1007/978-3-642-20282-7_3

Pfurtscheller, G., & Andrew, C. (1999). Event-related changes of band power and coherence: Methodology and interpretation. *Journal of Clinical Neurophysiology, 16*, 512–519. doi:10.1097/00004691-199911000-00003

Pierce, K. L., Premont, R. T., & Lefkowitz, R. J. (2002). Seven-transmembrane receptors. *Nature Reviews. Molecular Cell Biology, 3*, 639–650. doi:10.1038/nrm908

Pin, J. P., Galvez, T., & Prézeau, L. (2003). Evolution, structure and activation mechanism of family 3/C G-protein-coupled receptors. *Pharmacology & Therapeutics, 98*(3), 325–354. doi:10.1016/S0163-7258(03)00038-X

Piotrowski, Z., & Rozanowski, K. (2010). Robust algorithm for heart rate (HR) detection and heart rate variability (HRV) estimation. *Acta Physica Polonica A, 118*.

Pollock, B. H. (1983). Computer-assisted interpretation of noninvasive tests for diagnosis of coronary artery disease. *Cardiovascular Reviews & Reports, 4*, 367–375.

Pournara, I., & Wernisch, L. (2004). Reconstruction of gene networks using Bayesian learning and manipulation experiments. *Bioinformatics (Oxford, England)*, *20*(17), 2934–2942. doi:10.1093/bioinformatics/bth337

Powell, L. T., Diamond, G. A., Prediman, K. S., & Ferguson, J. G. (1989). CorSage: A critiquing system for coronary care. *Computer Applications in Medical Care: Proceedings of the Thirteenth Annual Symposium*, November 5-8, Washington, D.C., USA, (pp. 152-156).

Pryor, T. A., Gardner, R. M., Clayton, P. D., & Warner, H. R. (1983). The HELP system. *Journal of Medical Systems*, *7*(2), 87–102. doi:10.1007/BF00995116

Puig, S., Argenziano, G., Zalaudek, I., Ferrara, G., Palou, J., & Massi, D. (2007). Melanomas that failed dermoscopic detection: A combined clinicodermoscopic approach for not missing melanoma. *Dermatologic Surgery*, *33*(10), 1262–1273. doi:10.1111/j.1524-4725.2007.33264.x

Pu, P., & Chen, L. (2007). Trust-inspiring explanation interfaces for recommender systems. *Knowledge-Based Systems*, *20*, 542–556. doi:10.1016/j.knosys.2007.04.004

Quaglini, S. (2008). Compliance with clinical practice guidelines. In Lucas, P. (Ed.), *Computer-based Medical Guidelines and Protocols: A Primer and current Research Trends* (pp. 160–179). Amsterdam, The Netherlands: IOS Press.

Quinlan, R. (1986). Induction of decision trees. *Machine Learning*, *1*(1), 81–106. doi:10.1007/BF00116251

Quinlan, R. (1993). *C4.5: Programs for machine learning*. San Mateo, CA: Morgan Kaufmann Publishers.

Radović, M., & Filipović, N. (2010). Mining data from hemodynamic simulations via multilayer perceptron neural network. *Journal of Serbian Society for Computational Mechanics*, *4*(1), 31–42. Retrieved from http://www.singipedia.com/attachment.php?attachmentid=2381

Rankin, I. (1989). Deep generation of a critique. *Second European Natural Language Generation Workshop*, Edinburgh, April, (pp. 39-44).

Rennals, G. R., Shortliffe, E. H., Stockdale, F. E., & Miller, P. L. (1989). Reasoning from the clinical literature: The Roundsman system. In Salmon, R., Blum, B., & Jorgenson, M. (Eds.), *MEDINFO 86*. New York, NY: Elsevier Science.

Rigau-Pérez, J. G., Clark, G. G., Gubler, D. J., Reiter, P., Sanders, E. J., & Vance Vorndam, A. (1998). Dengue and dengue haemorrhagic fever. *Lancet*, *352*(9132), 971–977. doi:10.1016/S0140-6736(97)12483-7

Rivas, E., Burgos, J. C., & García-Prada, J. C. (2009). Condition assessment of power OLTC by vibration analysis using wavelet transform. *IEEE Transactions on Power Delivery*, *24*(2), 687–694. doi:10.1109/TPWRD.2009.2014268

Roberts, K., Rink, B., & Harabagiu, S. (2010). *Extraction of medical concepts, assertions, and relations from discharge summaries for the fourth i2b2/VA shared task*. Paper presented at the i2b2 Workshop on Challenges in Natural Language Processing for Clinical Data, Washington, DC.

Robnik-Šikonja, M., & Kononenko, I. (2003). Theoretical and empirical analysis of ReliefF and RReliefF. *Machine Learning*, *53*, 23–69. doi:10.1023/A:1025667309714

Rogers, Y., & Leiser, B. (1987). *What do you mean by that? Designing user requirements for expert system explanation. Colloquium on Man-Machine Interfaces for Intelligent Knowledge-Based Systems, 27 November*. London: IEEE Computer and Control Division.

Romero, E., Vellido, A., Julià-Sapé, M., & Arús, C. (2009). Discriminating glioblastomas from metastases in a SV ^{1}H-MRS brain tumour database. In *Proceedings of the 26th Annual Meeting of the European Society for Magnetic Resonance in Medicine and Biology, ESMRMB 2009*, (p. 18). Antalya, Turkey.

Rondard, P., Goudet, C., Kniazeff, J., Pin, J.-P., & Prézeau, L. (2011). The complexity of their activation mechanism opens new possibilities for the modulation of mGlu and GABAB class C G protein-coupled receptors. *Neuropharmacology*, *60*, 82–92. doi:10.1016/j.neuropharm.2010.08.009

Rosario, B., & Hearst, M. A. (2004). Classifying semantic relations in bioscience text. *In Proceedings of the 42nd Annual Meeting on Association for Computational Linguistics.*

Rosenblum, M. G., Cimponeriu, L., Bezerianos, A., Patzak, A., & Mrowka, R. (2002). Identification of coupling direction: Application to cardiorespiratory interaction. *Physical Review E: Statistical, Nonlinear, and Soft Matter Physics, 65*(4), 041909. doi:10.1103/PhysRevE.65.041909

Rosow, E., Adam, J., Coulombe, K., Race, K., & Anderson, R. (2003). Virtual instrumentation and real-time executive dashboards: Solutions for health care systems. *Nursing Administration Quarterly, 27*(1), 58–76.

Rossille, D., Cuggia, M., Arnault, A., Bouget, J., & Le Beux, P. (2008). Managing an emergency department by analysing HIS medical data: A focus on elderly patient clinical pathways. *Health Care Management Science, 11*, 139–146. doi:10.1007/s10729-008-9059-6

Ruha, A., Sallinen, S., & Nissila, S. (1997). A real-time microprocessor QRS detector system with a 1-ms timing accuracy for the measurement of ambulatory HRV. *IEEE Transactions on Bio-Medical Engineering, 44*(3). doi:10.1109/10.554762

Runge-Ranzinger, S., Horstick, O., Marx, M., & Kroeger, A. (2008). What does dengue disease surveillance contribute to predicting and detecting outbreaks and describing trends? *Tropical Medicine & International Health, 13*(8), 1022–1041. doi:10.1111/j.1365-3156.2008.02112.x

Sahami, M. (1996). Learning limited dependence Bayesian classifiers. In *KDD-96: Proceedings of the Second International Conference on Knowledge Discovery and Data Mining*, (pp. 335–338). AAAI Press.

Šajn, L., & Kononenko, I. (2008). Multiresolution image parametrization for improving texture classification. *EURASIP Journal on Advances in Signal Processing*, (1): 1–13. doi:10.1155/2008/617457

Šajn, L., & Kononenko, I. (2009). Image segmentation and parametrization for automatic diagnostics of whole-body scintigrams. In *Computational intelligence in medical imaging: Techniques & applications* (pp. 347–377). Boca Raton, FL: CRC Press. doi:10.1201/9781420060614.ch12

Sá, R. C., & Verbandt, Y. (2002). Automated breath detection on long-duration signals using feedforward backpropagation artificial neural networks. *IEEE Transactions on Bio-Medical Engineering, 49*(10), 1130–1141. doi:10.1109/TBME.2002.803514

Schipper, I. B., Steyerberg, E. W., & Castelein, R. M. (2004). Treatment of unstable trochanteric fractures: Randomized comparison of the gamma nail and the proximal femoral nail. *The Journal of Bone and Joint Surgery. British Volume, 86*, 86–94.

Schmid, F., Hirschen, K., Meynen, S., & Schäfer, M. (2005). An enhanced approach for shape optimization using an adaptive algorithm. *Finite Elements in Analysis and Design, 41*, 521–543. doi:10.1016/j.finel.2004.07.005

Schneider, P., Schneider, A., & Schwarz, P. (2002). A modular approach for simulation-based optimization of MEMS. *Microelectronics Journal, 33*, 29–38. doi:10.1016/S0026-2692(01)00101-X

Schnitzler, A., & Gross, J. (2005). Normal and pathological oscillatory communication in the brain. *Nature Reviews. Neuroscience, 6*, 285–296. doi:10.1038/nrn1650

Schölkopf, B., Smola, A., & Müller, K. R. (1997). Kernel principal component analysis. In *Proceedings of the 7th International Conference on Artificial Neural Networks* (ICANN 1997), (pp. 583-588).

Schölkopf, B., & Smola, A. (2002). *Learning with kernels.* Cambridge, MA: The MIT Press.

Schölkopf, B., Tsuda, K., & Vert, J.-P. (2004). *Kernel methods in computational biology.* Cambridge, MA: The MIT Press.

Schöllhorn, W. I. (2004). Applications of artificial neural nets in clinical biomechanics. *Clinical Biomechanics (Bristol, Avon), 19*, 876–898. doi:10.1016/j.clinbiomech.2004.04.005

Schulz, U. G. R., & Rothwell, P. M. (2001). Sex differences in carotid bifurcation anatomy and the distribution of atherosclerotic plaque. *Stroke, 32*(7), 1525–1531. Retrieved from http://stroke.ahajournals.org/cgi/content/abstract/32/7/1525doi:10.1161/01.STR.32.7.1525

Seng, S. B., Chong, A. K., & Moore, A. (2005). *Geostatistical modelling, analysis and mapping of epidemiology of Dengue fever in Johor State.* Malaysia.

Shawe-Taylor, J., & Cristianini, N. (2004). *Kernel methods for pattern analysis*. Cambridge University Press. doi:10.1017/CBO9780511809682

Shen, Y., & Cooper, G. F. (2007). A Bayesian biosurveillance method that models unknown outbreak diseases. *Lecture Notes in Computer Science, 4506*, 209. doi:10.1007/978-3-540-72608-1_21

Shinzawa, H., Morita, S., Ozaki, Y., & Tsenkova, R. (2006). New method for spectral data classification: Two-way moving window principal component analysis. *Applied Spectroscopy, 60*(8), 884–891. doi:10.1366/000370206778062020

Shokrieh, M. M., & Rezaei, D. (2003). Analysis and optimization of a composite leaf spring. *Composite Structures, 60*, 317–325. doi:10.1016/S0263-8223(02)00349-5

Shortliffe, E. H. (1976). *Computer-based medical consultations: MYCIN*. New York, NY: North Holland.

Siddiq, J., Akhgar, B., Gruzdz, A., Zaefarian, G., & Ihnatowicz, A. (2009). *Automated diagnosis system to support colon cancer treatment: MATCH*. Fifth International Conference on Information Technology: New Generations.

Silverman, B. G. (1992). Survey of expert critiquing systems: practical and theoretical frontiers. *Communications of the ACM, 35*(4), 107–127. doi:10.1145/129852.129861

Singer, W., & Gray, C. M. (1995). Visual feature integration and the temporal correlation hypothesis. *Annual Review of Neuroscience, 18*, 555–586. doi:10.1146/annurev.ne.18.030195.003011

Sips, R. J., Braun, L. M. M., & Roos, N. (2006). Medical expert critiquing using a BDI approach. In P-Y. Schobbens, W. Vanhoof, & G. Schwanen (Eds.), *Proceedings of the 18th Belgium-Netherlands Conference on Artificial Intelligence* (BNAIC 06) (pp. 283-290). Namur, Belgium.

Sips, R. J., Braun, L., & Roos, N. (2008). *Enabling medical expert critiquing using a BDI approach*.

Slender, G. (2009). *Overview of Ext GWT and GWT*. Springer. doi:10.1007/978-1-4302-1941-5

Slomka, P. J., Nishina, H., Berman, D. S., Akincioglu, C., Abidov, A., & Friedman, J. D. (2005). Automated quantification of myocardial perfusion spect using simplified normal limits. *Journal of Nuclear Cardiology, 12*(1), 66–77. doi:10.1016/j.nuclcard.2004.10.006

Solt, I., Tikk, D., Gal, V., & Kardkovacs, Z. T. (2009). Semantic classification of diseases in discharge summaries using a context-aware rule-based classifier. *Journal of the American Medical Informatics Association, 16*(4), 580–584. doi:10.1197/jamia.M3087

Soon Ong, C., Smola, A., & Williamson, R. (2005). Learning the kernel with hyperkernels. *Journal of Machine Learning Research, 6*, 1043–1071.

Spirtes, P., Glymour, C., & Scheines, R. (2000b). *Constructing Bayesian network models of gene expression networks from microarray data*. Paper presented at the The Atlantic Symposium on Computational Biology, Genome Information Systems & Technology.

Spirtes, P., Glymour, C., & Scheines, R. (2000a). *Causation, prediction, and search*. The MIT Press.

Stapley, B. J., & Benoit, G. (2000). Bibliometrics: Information retrieval visualization from co-occurrences of gene names in MEDLINE Abstracts. *In Proceedings of the Pacific Symposium on Biocomputing*: Vol. 5. (pp. 526–537).

Stegle, O., Fallert, V., MacKay, D., & Brage, S. (2008). Gaussian process robust regression for noisy heart rate data. *IEEE Transactions on Bio-Medical Engineering, 55*(9), 2143–2151. doi:10.1109/TBME.2008.923118

Stempfel, G., & Ralaivola, L. (2009). Learning SVMs from sloppily labeled data. *International Conference on Artificial Neural Networks*, Vol. 1, (pp. 884-893).

Stewart, B. W., & Kleihues, P. (2003). *World cancer report*. IARC Press.

Stolba, N., & Tjoa, A. M. (2007). The relevance of data warehousing and data mining in the field of evidence based medicine to support healthcare decision-making. *International Journal of Computer Systems Science and Engineering, 3*(3), 143–149.

Stoto, M. A., Schonlau, M., & Mariano, L. T. (2004). Syndromic surveillance: Is it worth the effort. *Chance, 17*(1), 19–24.

Szathmary, L. (2006). *Symbolic data mining methods with the Coron Platform*. University Henri Poincaré, Nancy 1, laboratory of LORIA - INRIA Lorraine, France.

Talarmin, A., Peneau, C., Dussart, P., Pfaff, F., Courcier, M., & de Rocca-Serra, B. (2000). Surveillance of dengue fever in French Guiana by monitoring the results of negative malaria diagnoses. *Epidemiology and Infection, 125*(1), 189–193. doi:10.1017/S0950268899004239

Taylor, D. M., Tillery, S. I. H., & Schwartz, A. B. (2002). Direct cortical control of 3D neuroprosthetic devices. *Science, 296*, 1829–1832. doi:10.1126/science.1070291

Teach, R. L., & Shortliffe, E. H. (1981). An analysis of physician's attitudes regarding computer-based medical consultation systems. *Computers and Biomedical Research, an International Journal, 14*, 542–558. doi:10.1016/0010-4809(81)90012-4

Thayer, D. T., &. R. (1982). EM algorithms for ML Factor analysis. *Psychometrica, 47*, 69–76. doi:10.1007/BF02293851

Thomas, J., Milward, D., Ouzounis, C., Pulman, S., & Carroll, M. (2000). Automatic extraction of protein interactions from scientific abstracts. *In Proceedings of the Pacific Symposium on Biocomputing*: Vol. 5. (pp. 538–549).

Uysal, H., Gul, R., & Uzman, U. (2007). Optimum shape design of shell structures. *Engineering Structures, 29*, 80–87. doi:10.1016/j.engstruct.2006.04.007

Uzuner, O., Zhang, X., & Sibanda, T. (2009). Machine learning and rule-based approaches to assertion classification. *Journal of the American Medical Informatics Association, 16*(1), 109–115. doi:10.1197/jamia.M2950

van Harmelen, F., Lifschitz, V., & Porter, B. (2008). *Handbook of knowledge representation*. Amsterdam, The Netherlands: Elsevier.

Van Melle, W. (1979). A domain-independent production rule system for consultation programs. *Proceedings of the Sixth International Joint Conference on Artificial Intelligence*, Tokyo, (pp. 923 -925).

Vapnik, V. (1998). *Statistical learning theory*. New York, NY: John Wiley & Sons.

Verma, T., & Pearl, J. (1991). Equivalence and synthesis of causal models. In P. Bonissone & M. Henrion (Eds.), *Proceedings of Seventh Conference Uncertainty in Artificial Intelligence*. Amsterdam, The Netherlands: North Holland.

Vestergaard, M. E., & Menzies, S. W. (2008). Automated diagnostic instruments for cutaneous melanoma. *Seminars in Cutaneous Medicine and Surgery, 27*(1), 32–36. doi:10.1016/j.sder.2008.01.001

Viceconti, M., Casali, M., Massari, B., Cristofolini, L., Bassini, S., & Toni, A. (1996). The 'Standardized femur program' proposal for a reference geometry to be used for the creation of finite element models of the femur. *Journal of Biomechanics*, (9): 1241. doi:10.1016/0021-9290(95)00164-6

Vilalta, R., Giraud-Carrier, C., & Brazdil, P. (2010). Meta-learning: Concepts and techniques. In Maimon, O., & Rokach, L. (Eds.), *The data mining and knowledge discovery handbook* (pp. 717–731). Springer.

Vincent, J. L. (1996). Definition and pathogenesis of septic shock. *Current Topics in Microbiology and Immunology, 216*, 1–13. doi:10.1007/978-3-642-80186-0_1

Vincent, J. L., de Mendoça, A., Cantraine, F., Moreno, R., Takala, J., & Suter, P. M. (1998). Use of the SOFA score to assess the incidence of organ dysfunction/failure in intensive care units: Results of a multicenter, prospective study. *Critical Care Medicine, 26*, 1793–1800. doi:10.1097/00003246-199811000-00016

Vincent, J. L., Moreno, R., Takala, J., Willats, S., De Mendoca, A., & Burining, H. (1996). The SOFA (Sepsis-related organ failure assessment) score to describe organ dysfunction/failure. *Critical Care Medicine, 22*, 707–710.

von der Malsburg, C. (1985). Nervous structures with dynamical links. *Berichte der Bunsengeselschaft Physical Chemistry, 89*, 703–710.

von der Malsburg, C., & Schneider, W. (1986). A neural coctail-party processor. *Biological Cybernetics, 54*, 29–40. doi:10.1007/BF00337113

Walker, I., Sigouin, C., Sek, J., Almonte, T., Carruthers, J., & Chan, A. (2004). Comparing hand-held computers and paper diaries for haemophilia home therapy: A randomized trial. *Haemophilia, 10*(6), 698–704. doi:10.1111/j.1365-2516.2004.01046.x

Wang, C. J., Brown, C. J., Yettram, A. L., & Procter, P. (2000). Intramedullary femoral nails: One or two lag screws? A preliminary study. *Medical Engineering & Physics, 22*, 613–624. doi:10.1016/S1350-4533(00)00081-3

Ware, H., Mullet, C. J., & Jagannathan, V. (2009). Natural language processing framework to assess clinical conditions. *Journal of the American Medical Informatics Association, 16*(4), 585–589. doi:10.1197/jamia.M3091

Wessberg, J., Stambaugh, C. R., Kralik, J. D., Beck, P. D., Laubach, M., & Chapin, J. K. (2000). Real-time prediction of hand trajectory by ensembles of cortical neurons in primates. *Nature, 408*(6810), 361–365. doi:10.1038/35042582

Williamson, J. (2005). Objective Bayesian nets. In Artemov, S. (Eds.), *We will show them! Essays in honour of Dov Gabbay* (pp. 713–730). College Publications.

Willoughby, R. (2005). Dynamic hip screw in the management of reverse obliquity intertrochanteric neck of femur fractures. *Injury-International Journal of the Care of the Injured, 36*, 105–109.

Witten, I. H., & Frank, E. (2005). *Data mining: Practical machine learning tools and techniques* (2nd ed.). San Francisco, CA: Morgan Kaufmann.

Wolpaw, J. R., & McFarland, D. J. (2004). Control of a two-dimensional movement signal by a noninvasive brain-computer interface in humans. *Proceedings of the National Academy of Sciences of the United States of America, 101*(51), 17849–17854. doi:10.1073/pnas.0403504101

Wong, W. K., Moore, A., Cooper, G., & Wagner, M. (2002). *Rule-based anomaly pattern detection for detecting disease outbreaks.*

Wong, W. K., Moore, A., Cooper, G., & Wagner, M. (2003). WSARE: What's strange about recent events? *Journal of Urban Health: Bulletin of the New York Academy of Medicine, 80*(2 Supplement 1).

Wong, W., Moore, A., Cooper, G., & Wagner, M. (2003). *Bayesian network anomaly pattern detection for disease outbreaks.*

Wong, D. T., Crofts, S. L., McGuire, G. P., & Byrick, R. J. (1995). Evaluation of predictive ability of APACHE II system and hospital outcome in Canadian intensive care unit patients. *Critical Care Medicine, 23*(7), 1177–1183. doi:10.1097/00003246-199507000-00005

Wong, W. K. (2004). *Data mining for early disease outbreak detection.* Pittsburgh, PA: Carnegie Mellon University.

Woods, W. A. (1970). Transition network grammars for natural language analysis. *Communications of the ACM, 13*, 591–606. doi:10.1145/355598.362773

Woznica, A., Kalousis, A., & Hilario, M. (2007). Learning to combine distances for complex representations. In *Proceedings of the 24th International Conference on Machine Learning*, (pp. 1031-1038). Corvallis, USA.

Wright, A., & Sittig, D. F. (2008). A four-phase model of the evolution of clinical decision support architectures. *International Journal of Medical Informatics, 77*, 641–649. doi:10.1016/j.ijmedinf.2008.01.004

Wu, G., Chang, E. Y., & Panda, N. (2005). *Formulating distance functions via the kernel trick* (pp. 703–709). Chicago: ACM SIGKDD.

Xing, E., Ng, A., Jordan, M., & Russell, S. (2003). Distance metric learning, with application to clustering with side-information. *Advances in Neural Information Processing Systems, 15*, 505–512.

Xiong, H., & Chen, X.-W. (2006). Kernel-based distance metric learning for microarray data classification. *BMC Bioinformatics, 7*(299), 1–11.

Yakushiji, A., Tateisi, Y., Miyao, Y., & Tsujii, J. (2001). Event extraction from biomedical papers using a full parser. *In Proceedings of the Pacific Symposium on Biocomputing*: Vol. 6. (pp. 408–419).

Yamada, T., & Meng, E. (Eds.). (2010). *Practical guide for clinical neurophysiologic testing: EEG*. Philadelphia, PA: Lippincott Williams & Wilkins.

Yang, J., & Honavar, V. (1998). Feature subset selection using a genetic algorithm. In *IEEE Intelligent Systems*, (pp. 380–385).

Yang, H., Spasic, I., Keane, J. A., & Nenadic, G. (2009). A text mining approach to the prediction of a disease status from clinical discharge summaries. *Journal of the American Medical Informatics Association, 16*(4), 596–600. doi:10.1197/jamia.M3096

Young, D. W. (1984). What makes doctors use computers? *Journal of the Royal Society of Medicine, 77*, 663.

Zadeh, L. A. (1973). Outline of a new approach to the analysis of complex systems and decision processes. *IEEE Transactions on Systems, Man, and Cybernetics, 3*, 28–44. doi:10.1109/TSMC.1973.5408575

Zadeh, L. A. (1975). The concept of a linguistic variable and its application to approximate reasoning. *Information Sciences, Part I - 8*, 199-249, *Part II - 8*, 301-357. *Part III, 9*, 43–80.

Zalizah, A. L., Abu Bakar, A., Hamdan, A. R., & Sahani, M. (2010). Multiple attribute frequent mining-based for dengue outbreak. *Proceedings of the 6th International Conference on Advanced Data Mining and Applications, Part 1*.

Zalizah, A. L., Hamdan, A. R., & Azuraliza, A. B. (2009 5-6 Jun 2009). *Framework on outlier sequential patterns for outbreak detection*. Paper presented at the International Conference Knowledge Discovery (ICKD) Manila

Zalizah, A. L., Hamdan, A. R., & Norsuhaili, S. (2008). *Outbreak detection techniques for public health surveillance: A preliminary study* Paper presented at the 2nd International Conference on Science & Technology (ICSTIE 2008).

Zhang, Y., Meratnia, N., & Havinga, P. J. M. (2007). *A taxonomy framework for unsupervised outlier detection techniques for multi-type data sets*.

Zhao, B., Kwok, J. T., & Zhang, C. (2009). Multiple kernel clustering. *Proceedings of the Ninth SIAM International Conference on Data Mining*, (pp. 638-649). Nevada.

Zhao, Q., & Bhowmick, S. S. (2006). *Association rule mining: A survey*. Singapore: Nanyang Technological University.

Zheng, Z., Wu, X., & Srihari, R. (2004). Feature selection for text categorization on imbalanced data. *SIGKDD Explorations Newsletter, 6*(1), 80–89. doi:10.1145/1007730.1007741

Zhou, Z. H. (2003). Three perspectives of data mining. *Artificial Intelligence, 143*(1), 139–146. doi:10.1016/S0004-3702(02)00357-0

Ziegler, D. (2005). Validation of a novel screening device (Neuroquick) for quantitative assessment of small nerve fiber dysfunction as an early feature of diabetic polyneuropathy. *Diabetes Care, 28*(5), 1169–1174. doi:10.2337/diacare.28.5.1169

Zou, M., & Conzen, S. D. (2005). A new dynamic Bayesian network (DBN) approach for identifying gene regulatory networks from time course microarray data. *Bioinformatics (Oxford, England), 21*(1), 71–79. doi:10.1093/bioinformatics/bth463

Zurada, J. M. (1992). Applications of neural algorithms and systems. In *Artificial neural systems*. St. Paul, MN: West Publishing.

About the Contributors

Rafael Magdalena-Benedito was born in 1968 in Segovia (Castellón). Between 1986 and 1991, he studied a degree in Physics at the University of Valencia, Computer and Electronic specialty. In 1993 he worked in the company of electro DextroMédica as dictafonía technician in cardiology and medical physics. In 1998 he joined the Group Processing Digital Signal Department, where he currently works on research projects, is an Assistant Professor. His areas of work are data security, multimedia networks, standardization in biomedical engineering, and telemedicine.

Emilio Soria received an MS degree in Physics (1992) and a PhD degree (1997) in Electronics Engineering from the Universitat de Valencia (Spain). He has been an Assistant Professor at the University of Valencia since 1997. His research is centered mainly in the analysis and applications of adaptive and neural systems.

Juan Guerrero Martínez earned his degree in Physics, specializing in Electrical Engineering and Electronics and Computer Science in 1984 and PhD in Physics from the University of Valencia in 1988. He has been Associate Professor at the University of Valencia since 1985 and Associate Professor in the area of Electronics since 1992. He has participated in several research projects and R & D contracts with companies on issues related to the development of control systems based on microprocessors, as well as biomedical instrumentation and processing of biosignals. He has written several papers published in conferences and national and international journals. He is currently coordinating a research group Digital Signal Processing (GPDS) on Digital Processing, with applications in various fields but preferably oriented biosignals, which is developing research projects. His main interests are the development of biomedical instrumentation systems based on microprocessor or PC and the digital processing of biosignals, including real-time applications.

Juan Gómez-Sanchis received a B.Sc. degree in Physics (2000) and a B.Sc. degree in Electronics Engineering from the University of Valencia (2003). He joined at the Public Research Institute IVIA in 2004, developing is Ph.D. in hyperspectral computer vision systems applied to the agriculture. He joined to the Department of Electronics Engineering at University of Valencia in 2008, where he currently works as Assistant Professor in Pattern Recognition using Neural Networks.

Antonio Jose Serrano-López received a BS degree in Physics in 1996, a MS degree in Physics in 1998, and a Ph.D. degree in Electronics Engineering in 2002, from the University of Valencia. He is currently an Associate Professor in the Electronics Engineering Department at this same university. His research interest is machine learning methods for biomedical signal processing. Currently, he teaches courses of Analog Electronic Design and Digital Signal Processing.

* * *

Jose M. Alonso received his M.S. degree (2003) and the Ph.D. degree (2007) in Telecommunication Engineering, both from the Technical University of Madrid, Spain. From 2003-2005, he was involved in the ADVOCATE2 project, funded by European Union. Between 2005-2007, he enjoyed as visiting researcher at Cemagref (Montpellier, France), an agricultural and environmental engineering research centre; and ECSC, European Centre for Soft Computing (Mieres, Spain). Since November 2007, he is postdoctoral researcher in the Fundamentals of Soft Computing Unit at the ECSC. His main research line is related to knowledge extraction and representation in fuzzy modeling. Two kinds of knowledge, expert and induced knowledge, are considered paying attention to their integration and final model interpretability-accuracy trade-off. He has published more than 40 peer-reviewed papers in international journals and conference proceedings.

Juan I. Alonso-Barba received the B.E and M.S. in Information Technology from the University of Castilla-La Mancha, Spain, in 2007 and 2008, respectively. He joined the Intelligent Systems and Data Mining research group in 2006 and he is currently a granted Ph.D. student by the Junta de Comunidades de Castilla-La Mancha. He has been working on several projects related with the applications of metaheuristics in the field of data mining. Currently, his research work focuses on automatic learning of probabilistic graphical models, mainly Bayesian Networks and Chain Graphs.

Dario Antonelli holds a M.S. degree in Mechanical Engineering from the Politecnico di Torino, 1990. He is currently Associate Professor at the Department of Production Systems and Economics of Politecnico di Torino. His scientific activity is mainly related to finite element simulation of metalworking processes, to experimental identification of process parameters and to collaborative networks management. He is member of COVE, IFIP-WG5.5.

Carlos Julio Arizmendi received his degree in Electronic Engineering from the Industrial University of Santander (Bucaramanga-Colombia), is a currently postgraduate student of the Artificial Intelligence program adscript to the Department of Computer Languages and Systems at Technical University (Catalonia-Barcelona). Also, he is a Professor of the Autonomous University (Bucaramanga-Colombia) in the Mechatronics Department. His currently interest areas are: pattern recognition, machine learning, data mining, neural networks, biomedical engineering and signal treatment, and processing in general.

Azuraliza Abu Bakar is a Professor at the School of Computer Science, Faculty of Technology and Information Science, UKM. She was awarded PhD in Artificial Intelligence from UPM. Currently she is the head of the Center for Artificial Intelligence Technology, a research center in the faculty. Her research interests include data mining, artificial intelligence, rough sets, outlier detection, and knowledge-based technology.

Elena Baralis received the Master's degree in Electrical Engineering and the Ph.D. degree in Computer Engineering from the Politecnico di Torino, Italy. She is full Professor at the Dipartimento di Automatica e Informatica of the Politecnico di Torino since January 2005. Her current research interests are in the field of databases, in particular data mining, sensor databases, and bioinformatics. She is the author or coauthor of numerous papers on journal and conference proceedings, and she has managed several Italian and EU research projects.

Aleš Belič is an Associate Professor at the Faculty of Electrical Engineering, University of Ljubljana where he is involved in modelling and analysis of biological and pharmaceutical systems with major stress on the analysis of EEG signals, systems biology, pharmacokinetics, and modelling in pharmaceutical technology. He received his BSc and PhD degrees from the Faculty of Electrical Engineering, University of Ljubljana in 1994 and 2000, respectively. He has been involved in several industrial projects as well as national and international research activities (6th and 7th European Framework Projects: STEROLTALK, FightingDrugFailure). His professional bibliography consists of more than 150 contributions in international and domestic journals, international conferences, and book chapters.

Radoslav Bortel received the M.S. and Ph.D. degrees in Electrical Engineering from the Faculty of Electrical Engineering of the Czech Technical University (FEE CTU), Prague, Czech Republic, in 2005 and 2010, respectively. He is currently an Assistant Professor at FEE CTU. His research interests include statistical signal analysis, EEG coherence analysis and spatial filtering, ECG signal processing, and electronic circuits for the measurement of biological signals with dry electrodes.

Zoran Bosnić obtained his Master and Doctor degrees in Computer Science at University of Ljubljana, Slovenia in 2003 and 2007, respectively. Since 2006 he has been employed at Faculty of Computer and Information Science and currently works as an Assistant Professor in the Laboratory of Cognitive Modeling. He teaches courses on computer networks, communication protocols, and web programming. His research interests include artificial intelligence, machine learning, regression, and reliability estimation for individual predictions, as well as medical and other applications in these areas. He is a (co)author of about 20 research papers and a textbook in international journals and conference proceedings.

Giulia Bruno holds a Master degree and a Ph.D. in Computer Engineering from Politecnico di Torino, Italy. She is currently working in the field of data mining and bioinformatics. Her activity is focused on anomaly detection in temporal and biological databases and on microarray data analysis to select genes relevant for tumor classification. She is also investigating data mining techniques for clinical analysis, particularly the extraction of medical pathways from electronic patients' records.

Martha Ivón Cárdenas received his degree in Mathematics from the Department of Mathematics and Computer, University of Havana (Cuba) in 1996. She received his MSc in Artificial Intelligence from the Technical University of Catalonia (UPC) in 2011 under careful supervision of Dr. Alfredo Vellido and Dr. Jesús Giraldo. Her research interests cover machine learning and pattern recognition applied to proteomics area, specifically in G protein-coupled receptors (GPCR) where a protein sequences comparison approach is developed.

Ciro Castiello is an Assistant Professor at the Department of Informatics of the University of Bari since 2009. He graduated (cum laude) in Informatics at the University of Bari and received from the same university also his PhD in Informatics in 2005. His research activity mainly concerns the fields of Artificial Intelligence and Machine Learning. Particularly, his research is focused on: the development of Knowledge-Based Neurocomputing methodologies and their application for solving different problems; the study of inductive learning mechanisms for assessing the theoretical basis of meta-learning approaches; the application of Soft Computing techniques in the contexts of image processing and Semantic Web; and the definition of interpretability evaluation techniques for fuzzy rule based classifiers. Dr. Castiello is author of more than fifty scientific papers, he took part as a speaker in several national and international conferences, and he is involved in different national research projects. Dr. Castiello regularly participates in the didactic activity of the II Science Faculty of the University of Bari, where he acts as a member.

Silvia Chiusano is an Assistant Professor at the Dipartimento di Automatica e Informatica of the Politecnico di Torino since January 2004. She holds a Master degree and a Ph.D. in Computer Engineering, both from Politecnico di Torino. Her current research interests are in the areas of data mining and database systems, in particular integration of data mining techniques into relational DBMSs, and classification of structured and sequential data.

Luis de la Ossa received the MSc. and PhD degrees in Computer Science in 2002 and 2007, respectively, from the University of Castilla-La Mancha, Spain. He is currently working as Associate Professor in the Computing Systems Department of this university, and he is also member of the Intelligent Systems and Data Mining research group in the Albacete Research Institute of Informatics I3A. Most of his former research was related to evolutionary computation, and he is currently working on evolutionary fuzzy systems, Bayesian network learning, and data mining.

Claudia Diamantini is associate professor at the Università Politecnica delle Marche, Department of Information Engineering, where she leads the Knowledge Discovery & Management research group. She received the Laurea degree in Computer Science with honors in 1990 from the University of Milan, and the PhD degree in Artificial Intelligent Systems from the University of Ancona in 1995. Her research interests are in the areas of business intelligence (in particular data mining and data warehousing) and semantic interoperability, with special attention to interdisciplinary relationships among them. On these topics she has published more than 70 technical papers in refereed journals and conferences. She is a member of the IEEE and ACM.

Ian Douglas, Ph.D., is an Associate Program Director at the Learning Systems Institute at Florida State University and an Associate Professor in the university's College of Communications and Information. His research interests focus on improving human performance, particularly through knowledge management and user-centered design of technology. Dr. Douglas has a multidisciplinary background, with an M.A. (hons) in Psychology, an M.S. in Computing and Cognition, and a Ph.D. in Computing. He began his career in medical AI and has worked as an educator in the USA, UK, and Singapore. He has also been a visiting Professor at the University of the Philippines, Dalian Maritime University, China, and the Informatics Institute of the Russian Academy of Sciences.

Sandro Fioretti graduated in 1979 in Electronic Engineering at Ancona University and presently is Associate Professor in Bioengineering at the Department of Information Engineering – Università Politecnica delle Marche - Ancona. He teaches Movement Biomechanics and Bioengineering of Motor Rehabilitation at the Biomedical Engineering course of the same university. His main research interests are in the field of human movement analysis and its related fields such as: stereophotogrammetry, linear and nonlinear filtering, joint kinematics, analysis and identification of postural control, static and perturbed posturography, gait analysis, and dynamic electromyography. He participated in various European and National research projects in the field of movement analysis for motor rehabilitation. He is author of numerous scientific publications in international journals, books, and congress proceedings.

Oana Frunza is a Ph.D. candidate at the SEECS (School of Electrical Engineering and Computer Science), University of Ottawa, Canada. She holds an M.C.S. degree from the same university and a B.C.S. in Computer Science from Babes-Bolyai University, Romania. Her research interests include different areas of artificial intelligence, natural language processing and text analysis, machine learning, and medical informatics. Affiliated with several renowned associations such as CAIAC (Canadian Artificial Intelligence Association) she is an active reviewer for prestigious journals and conferences. She is the author of the book: "Cognates, False Friends, and Partial Cognates" and more than 20 publications including: a book chapter, 6 journal articles, and 14 conference papers.

Jesús Giraldo received his PhD in Chemistry from Universitat Autònoma de Barcelona (UAB), Spain. He is currently based at the Institut de Neurociències and Unitat de Bioestadística (UAB) where he works mainly in the molecular and mathematical modeling of G protein-coupled receptor (GPCR) structure and function. The complexity of GPCR signaling requires collaborative efforts between researchers from all the disciplines involved-both experimental and theoretical. Because of this, his research is conducted in an integrative way, combining methods and techniques from computational chemistry, statistics, and bioinformatics, with the general aim of providing a mechanistic interpretation of biological function.

Ciril Grošelj, MD, PhD is internal medicine specialist, working at Nuclear medicine Department in University Medical Center Ljubljana, Slovenia and member of research group of the institution. He is also an Assistant Professor of Internal Medicine at Medical Faculty Ljubljana. His research interest include coronary artery disease, lung diseases, myocardial and lung nuclear medicine diagnostics, machine learning, data mining, and their applications in medicine. He is co-author of a few chapters in Slovenian medical books and of more than 60 scientific publications.

Abdul Razak Hamdan is a Professor in Intelligent System, Faculty of Information Science and Technology, Universiti Kebangsaan Malaysia (UKM).Currently he is the dean of the faculty, and also a head of Data Mining & Optimization Research Group. He received his BSc degree from UKM (1975), MSc degree from University of Newcastle Upon Tyne, UK (1977) and PhD in Artificial Intelligence from Loughborough University of Technology, United Kingdom in 1987. His research interests include data mining & optimization, ICT strategic & policy, and intelligent decision support.

Ching-Chi Hsu was born in Hsinchu, Taiwan, Republic of China, on September 24th, 1977. He received his Ph.D. degree in Mechanical Engineering from National Taiwan University of Science and Technology (NTUST) in December 2005. In August 2007, he joined in the Department of Mechanical Engineering of NTUST as a Project-Appointed Assistant Professor. In August 2009, he moved to the Graduate Institute of Engineering of NTUST as an Assistant Professor. In August 2011, The Graduate Institute of Engineering is renamed as the Graduate Institute of Applied Science and Technology. Dr. Hsu has taught and published in the field of biomechanics. His main research interests are in analyses and improvements of the orthopaedic implants, applications of engineering algorithms and artificial intelligence in biomedicine, and applications of nonlinear finite element analyses for biomechanical problems.

Diana Inkpen is an Associate Professor the School of Electrical Engineering and Computer Science at the University of Ottawa. She obtained her PhD in 2003 from the University of Toronto, Department of Computer Science. She obtained her M.Sc. from the Department of Computer Science, Technical University of Cluj-Napoca, Romania, in 1999, and a B.Eng. from the same university, in 1994. Her research interests are in the areas of Computational Linguistics and Artificial Intelligence, more specifically: Natural Language Understanding, Natural Language Generation, Lexical Semantics, and Information Retrieval. She has many research grants from NSERC, SSHRC, and OCE, including industrial collaborations. She is a reviewer for several journals and a program committee member for many conferences (ACL, NAACL. EMNLP, RANLP, CICLing, TANL, AI, etc.). She published 6 book chapters, 20 journal papers, and 61 conference and workshop papers. She organized 4 international workshops. She is member of the Association for Computational Linguistics (ACL).

Igor Kononenko received his PhD in Computer Science in 1990 from University of Ljubljana, Slovenia. He is the Professor at the Faculty of Computer and Information Science in Ljubljana and the head of Laboratory for Cognitive Modeling. His research interests include artificial intelligence, machine learning, and data mining. He is the (co)author of about 200 papers and 13 textbooks (two in English). His papers were cited over 1000 times by other authors. Igor Kononenko was actively involved in research in 20 national and international research projects. He is the member of the editorial board of *Applied Intelligence Journal* and *Informatica Journal*. He was a chair and the proceedings editor of three international scientific conferences.

Domen Košir received his Bachelor's degree in Computer Science from University of Ljubljana in 2010. He is currently a PhD student and a junior researcher in the Laboratory of Cognitive Modeling at the Faculty of Computer and Information Science. He is employed at Httpool Online Advertising Limited as a senior software architect where he works mostly on web content analysis and contextual advertising. His research is partly financed by the European Union, European Social Fund. His interests include artificial intelligence, machine learning, and data mining with focus on natural language processing, online advertising, and web user profiling.

Matjaž Kukar is an Assistant Professor at the Faculty of Computer and Information Science in Ljubljana, Slovenia, and a member of Laboratory for Cognitive Modeling as well as of Artificial Intelligence Department at the same Faculty. His research interests include machine learning, data mining and their applications in medicine, ROC analysis, cost-sensitive learning, combinations of classifiers, classification reliability in machine learning, and spatial learning. He is the co-author of the book Machine Learning and Data Mining: Introduction to Principles and Algorithms (with Igor Kononenko) and of more than 70 scientific publications.

Vito Logar received his B.Sc. and Ph.D. degrees from the Faculty of Electrical Engineering, University of Ljubljana, Slovenia in 2004 and 2009, respectively. He is currently working as a researcher/assistant at the same institution. At the time his main research interests are modeling of the industrial systems, namely modeling of the electric-arc processes. Furthermore, modelling and identification of the neurophysiological systems based on the EEG measurements and development of the web-based applications regarding e-learning solutions are also a part of his research work. His professional bibliography consists of more than 50 contributions in international and domestic journals, international conferences, and book chapters.

Zalizah Awang Long is currently a Senior Lecturer at the Malaysia Institute Information Technology (MIIT), Universiti Kuala Lumpur. She is currently pursuing PhD at Universiti Kebangsaan Malaysia. Her research interests in data mining for public health applications. She has taught for more than 10 years, consisting mainly of courses in Information Systems.

Marco Lucarelli is currently a PhD student at the Department of Informatics of the University of Bari (since 2011) with a grant by the same university. In 2007 he received his B.Sc. degree in Informatics and Digital Communications at the University of Bari. In 2010, at the same University, he received his M.Sc. degree in Informatics (summa cum laude) defending the thesis "Interpretable Fuzzy Knowledge Discovery for IgA Nephropathy." Currently, his research field is soft computing, in particular with focus on granular computing, human centric information processing, and interpretable fuzzy modelling. He is co-author of three peer-reviewed scientific papers.

Naeem A. Mahoto received the Master's degree in Computer Engineering from Mehran University of Engineering and Technology Jamshoro, Pakistan. He is PhD student at Politecnico di Torino, Italy since January 2010. He works in the field of data mining and bioinformatics with the Databases and Data Mining Group of Politecnico di Torino, Italy. His activity is focused on pattern extraction and classification of electronic records in the medical domain.

Manuel Martín-Merino received the B. S. degree in Physics from the University of Salamanca (Spain) in 1996 and the PhD. degree in Applied Physics from the same university in 2003. He is currently an Associate Professor in the Computer Science school at the University Pontificia of Salamanca. His research interests include visualization and clustering algorithms for the analysis of high dimensional data, pattern recognition techniques, and particularly kernel methods and Support Vector Machines. Currently he is focusing on practical problems related to Bioinformatics (gene expression data analysis and proteomics), data mining, and text mining. He is a member of the IEEE.

Corrado Mencar is currently Assistant Professor at the University of Bari, Faculty of Sciences, Department of Informatics, in Bari (Italy). He got a "laurea" (Ms.Sci) degree in Informatics in 2000 and a PhD degree in Informatics in 2005, both at the University of Bari. In 2001 he was employed as software analyst and designer for some Italian software firms. From 2005, he started his academic career as Assistant Professor by actively doing research in Computational Intelligence and Soft Computing. In his research activities, he joined several research projects and published more than 50 peer-reviewed international publications. He also acts as a reviewer for several international journals and conferences, as well as for the *ACM Computing Reviews*. His current research topics include fuzzy logic, granular computing, neuro-fuzzy systems, computational web intelligence, and intelligent data analysis.

Jens Dalgaard Nielsen received the MS degree in Software Engineering in 2002, and the PhD degree in Computer Science in 2007, both from the Department of Computer Science at the University of Aalborg, Denmark. From 2007 to 2008 he was a research assistant at the Department of Statistics and Applied Mathematics at the University of Almerìa, Spain. From 2008 to 2011 he was a researcher at the Department of Computer Systems, University of Castilla-La Mancha, Spain. He has been working of various research projects on the development of learning algorithms for probabilistic graphical models, and his research interests include machine learning and graphical models and the application of these techniques in genetics and bioinformatics. Since 2011 he has been a Postdoctoral Research Associate at the Department of Cardiovascular Science and the University of Sheffield (UK).

Iván Olier is currently a Marie Curie research fellow at the School of Psychological Sciences, The University of Manchester, UK. Previously, he was a postdoctoral fellow at the Institute of Neurosciences, Universitat Autdnoma de Barcelona, Spain, during the period 2009–2010. He received his Ph.D. in Computer Science from the Universitat Politècnica de Catalunya, Barcelona, Spain, in 2008. His research interests include Bayesian modeling of cognitive processes, statistical machine learning, and biomedicine.

Caterina Petrigni received the Master degree in Biomedical Engineering at Politecnico di Torino (2007). She was a research assistant at the Department of Production Systems and Business Economics of Politecnico di Torino. She is currently Ph.D. student at Universita` degli Studi di Torino and grant researcher at Istituto Superiore di Sanità. Her main research activity is focused on the transferability of industrial management concepts to healthcare networks. She actively collaborates with the AIIC (The Italian Association of Clinical Engineers).

Domenico Potena received the MSc degree in Electronic Engineering from the University of Ancona, Italy, in 2001, and the Ph.D. in Information Systems Engineering from the Università Politecnica delle Marche, Italy, in 2004. From June 2005 to October 2008, he was post-doctoral fellow at the Dipartimento di Ingegneria Informatica, Gestionale e dell'Automazione - Università Politecnica delle Marche. Since 2008 he is an Assistant Professor at the the Department of Information Engineering of the same University. His research interests include knowledge discovery in databases, data mining, data warehousing, information systems, and service oriented architectures.

Jose M. Puerta received a M.S. degree in Computer Science in 1991, and a Ph.D. degree in Computer Science in 2001, both from the University of Granada, Spain. He joined the Department of Computer Systems at the University of Castilla-La Mancha (UCLM) in 1991, where he is currently an Associate Professor. He currently serves as Vice-Dean of the Escuela Superior de Ingeniería Informática (UCLM) and is the co-leader of the Intelligent Systems and Data Mining research group. He carries out his research at the Laboratory of Intelligent Systems and Data Mining (SIMD) and his main research interest include probabilistic graphical models, Bayesian networks, evolutionary algorithms, machine learning, and data mining. Dr. Puerta has published more than 50 papers on these topics. Dr. Puerta has served in the organization of International Conferences and Workshops as Program Co-Chair and Technical Program Committee Member.

Vicent Ribas received an MSc in Telecommunications Engineering from the Royal Institute of Technology in Stockholm (Sweden) from Universitat Politècnica de Catalunya (Spain) with majors in Digital Signal Processing and Radiocommunications Technology in 2000. At UPC, he also followed the studies of Mathematical Engineering focusing on the mathematical modelling of physiological processes. He is currently pursuing a PhD degree at the Department of Languages and Information Systems of UPC. Vicent Ribas has extensive experience as a technology specialist (10+ years). He worked as a Project Manager at T-Systems Spain and as Management Consultant at Accenture Technology Labs in Sophia Antipolis, France. His research interests include, pattern recognition, machine learning, signal processing, and mathematical modelling applied to medicine. He has authored and co-authored more than 5 patents and papers on these topics.

Enrique Romero received a B.Sc. degree in Mathematics in 1989 from the *Universitat Autònoma de Barcelona* (UAB). In 1994, he received a B.Sc. degree in Computer Science from the *Universitat Politècnica de Catalunya* (UPC). In 1996, he joined the Department of *Llenguatges i Sistemes Informátics* at UPC, as an Assistant Professor. In 2004, he received the Ph.D. degree in Computer Science from the UPC. His research interests include pattern recognition, neural networks, support vector machines, and feature selection.

X. Rovira graduated with a degree in Biology at the University of Girona (Spain) in 2003. He received his PhD from the Universitat Autònoma de Barcelona (Spain) in 2010 at the Laboratory of Systems Pharmacology and Bioinformatics lead by Dr Jesús Giraldo. Currently, Dr. Rovira held a Federation of European Biochemical Societies (FEBS) long-term fellowship at the Institute of Functional Genomics (IGF) in Montpellier under the supervision of Dr Jean-Philippe Pin. His research is focussed on the study of the functional significance of the oligomerization phenomenon in G protein-coupled receptors (GPCRs). To that aim, he develops mathematical and computational theoretical models which can shed light on some apparent pharmacological abnormalities that can be explained in the context of a receptor dimer. These hypotheses are then used to design new experimental assays.

Juan Carlos Ruiz-Rodriguez graduated in Medicine and Surgery (University of Barcelona) and specialized in Intensive Care Medicine (Vall d' Hebron University Hospital, Barcelona). Medical staff of the Critical Care Department, Vall d' Hebron University Hospital and member of the Research Group for Shock, Organ Disfunction and Resuscitation (SODIR Research Group), Vall d' Hebron Institut de Recerca,

Universitat Autònoma de Barcelona. His research interests include sepsis and technological innovation projects. Active member of Scientific Committee of the Catalan Society of Critical Care Medicine. He was a member of Extended Scientific Committee of the Spanish Society of Intensive Care Medicine, Critical and Coronary Units (SEMICYUC) and he was national coordinator of the Working Group on Blood Products and Transfusion Alternatives SEMICYUC. Is also a member of the European Society of Intensive Care Medicine and the Spanish Society of Transplantation. He is author and coauthor of several articles, book chapters, and books.

Vasco Saavedra graduated in Information Systems (2002, Oporto University). Currently he teaches several subjects in the Computer Science domain in University of Aveiro. His main research areas are Computer Science, also including the Healthcare Information System domain. He has several articles published in journals, book chapters, and proceedings in several national and international conferences. He also works since 2003 with Portugal Telecom Inovação, a major telecommunication company, as software analyst and developer.

Mazrura Sahani is a senior medical fellow at the Faculty of Health Sciences, UKM. Her domain specialization is Environmental and Occupational Epidemiology. She obtained a medical degree from Catholic University of Leuven Belgium. She was awarded a Master degree on Public health in 1997 from UKM and PhD on Environmental Management for Health in 2004 from University of Western Sydney, Richmond, Australia. Her research interests include environmental and occupational health sciences, public health, and not limited to artificial intelligence.

João Pedro Simões received his MSc in Computer Science in 2009 from the University of Coimbra, Portugal. At this moment he is a Software Developer consultant at Accenture. Before joining Accenture, he worked on PT Inovação, Aveiro, where he was a Software Developer for two years. In this period he had the opportunity to publish in some conferences.

Pavel Sovka received the M.S. and Ph.D. degrees in Electrical Engineering from the Faculty of Electrical Engineering of the Czech Technical University (FEE CTU), Prague, Czech Republic, in 1981 and 1986, respectively. From 1985 to 1991, he was with the Institute of Radioengineering and Electronics of the Czech Academy of Sciences, Prague. In 1991, he joined the Department of Circuit Theory, FEE CTU. Since 2000, he has been a Full Professor. His research interests include the application of adaptive systems to noise and echo cancellation, speech analysis, changepoint detection, and signal separation. He is a member of the International Speech Communication Association (ISCA).

Leonor Teixeira graduated in Management and Industrial Engineering, received an MSc degree in Information Management and a PhD in Health Information Systems area. She is currently an Assistant Professor with the Department of Economics, Management and Industrial Engineering at the University of Aveiro and teaching in Technology and Information Systems areas. She has published in several conferences and journals, and currently she is researcher at the Governance, Competitiveness and Public Politics (GOVCOPP) and of the Institute of Electronics and Telematics Engineering (IEETA) of Aveiro research units.

Alfredo Vellido received his degree in Physics from the Department of Electronics and Automatic Control of the University of the Basque Country (Spain) in 1996. He completed his PhD at Liverpool John Moores University (UK) in 2000. After a few years of experience in the private sector, he briefly joined Liverpool John Moores University again as senior research officer. Following a Ramón y Cajal research fellowship, he is currently Assistant Professor at Technical University of Catalonia in Barcelona, Spain. Research interests include, but are not limited to, pattern recognition, machine learning, and data mining, as well as their applications in medicine, market analysis, ecology, and e-learning, subjects on which he has published widely.

Index

A

ABCD rule 291
Acute Physiology and Chronic Health Evaluation II (APACHE II) 4
Algebraic Statistical Models (ASM) 14
Anterior Cruciate Ligament injury (ACL) 190
anterior-posterior (AP) 23
anti-unification (AU) 291, 293, 296-297
area under the ROC curve (AUC) 43, 302
ArTex with resolutions (ARes) 95
arthrokinetics restrictions 190
artificial intelligence (AI) 175
Artificial Neural Networks (ANN) 30
Association rules for Textures (ArTex) 95
Attending system 214

B

Bag-of-Words (BOW) 242
balanced error rate (BER) 43
basal neck fractures 139
baseline wander 69
Bayesian Network (BN) 225
Bayes Vector Quantizer (BVQ) 18
Best Matching Unit (BMU) 188
Body Mass Index (BMI) 244
Brain Computer Interface (BCI) 186

C

CaMML 233, 236
care guidelines 274
carotid artery bifurcation 114
carotid artery stenosis 114, 124
Case-based reasoning (CBR) 293
Center for Disease Control (CDC) 2
central nervous system (CNS) 6, 31, 198
centre-of-pressure (COP) 18-19

CFC Stock Data Management (CFCSDM) 163
Chain Graphs (CG) 225
chemtherapeutic agents 197
chronic diseases 162
chunklets 54
classification performance 115
clippy 213
clustering 51
Coagulation Factor Concentrate (CFC) 162
Complement Naive Bayes (CNB) 249
Complete Blood Count (CBC) 275
comprehensibility postulate (CP) 257
comprehensive yeast genome database (CYGD) 59
Computerized Tomography (CT) 31
conditional probability tables (CPT) 230
conflict strategy 215
Confusion Matrix 21
constraint-based learning 228
control subjects (CNTR) 23
co-occurrences analysis 239
coronary artery disease (CAD) 92
CORSAGE 215
CuSUM 126
cysteine-rich domain (CRD) 198

D

data collection and segmentation phase 276-277, 279
data mining 274
decision-making process 161
decision trees (DT) 302-303
de-fuzzyfication 179
DENDRAL 210
Dermoscopy 291
diabetic neuropathy 18
Directed Acyclic Graph (DAG) 71, 224
Discrete Wavelet Transform (DWT) 30

Dissimilarity Index Matrix (DIM) 34
dynamic hip screw 139
    lag screw 139
    locking screws 139
    metal plate 139

E

Electrocardiogram (ECG) 88, 93, 105
electromyography 18, 26
electronic medical records 273-274
Elvira 233, 236
end-diastolic volume (EDV) 98
end-stage renal disease (ESRD) 255-256, 262
Essential-Attending (E-Attending) 215
European Society of Intensive Care Medicine (ES-ICM) 4
exam log data 276
Expectation-Maximization (EM) 200
explanation-based learning (EBL) 292
eyes closed (EC) 23
eyes open (EO) 23

F

Factor Analysis 7
femoral shaft fractures 139
Fisher's Linear Discriminant Analysis (FLDA) 22
follow-ups (FU) 263
frequent mining 127
frequent outlier 128
functional magnetic resonance imaging (fMRI) 173
Fuzzy Decision Tree (FDT) 265
fuzzy models 179
    Mamdani 179
    Takagi-Sugeno (TS) 179
fuzzy rule-based classifiers (FRBCs) 255-256
Fuzzy Set Theory (FST) 258
Fuzzy toolbox 180

G

gamma nails 139
    proximal lag screw 139
    set screw 139
Gaussian process (GP) 71
Generative Topographic Mapping (GTM) 199
genetic algorithms (GAs) 147
GeNIe&SMILE 233, 236
Google Web Toolkit (GWT) 165
G protein-coupled receptors (GPCRs) 196
grid-based filter 72
guanosine triphosphate (GTP) 197

H

Haematology Service of Coimbra Hospital Centre (SH_CHC) 161
healthcare professional (HCPs) 160
Health Information Systems (HISs) 161
heart rate (HR) 67-68, 87
HELP 216
hemo@care_dashboard 163
Hepatitis B antibody test (HBV) 275
Hepatitis C antibody test (HCV) 275
heptahelical domain (HD) 198
Highly Interpretable Linguistic Knowledge (HILK) 255-256, 260
HT-Advisor 215
Hugin Expert 233, 235
human immune-deficiency virus (HIV) 275

I

ICON 215
ILIAD 216, 220
I-map 229
imbalanced datasets 116
Immunoglobin A Nephropathy (IgAN) 255-256
Independent Component Analysis (ICA) 43, 175, 186
inference engine 210
information and communications technologies (ICTs) 160
input vector 188
Intelligent Data Analysis (IDA) 257
Intensive Care Unit (ICU) 1-2
INTERNIST consultant system 215
INTERPRET database 34
intertrochanteric fractures 139
in vitro 30
in vivo 31

K

kernel-GTM (KGTM) 201
Kernel PCA (KPCA) 201
Kernel SOM (KSOM) 201
Key Performance Indicators (KPIs) 160-161
k-Nearest Neighbour (kNN) 21
knowledge base 210, 212, 255, 257-258, 260-261, 265, 267, 271
knowledge discovery (KD) 292
Kullback-Leibler (KL) 227

L

Labeled Vector Quantizer (LVQ) 22
Lazy Induction of Descriptions (LID) 291, 297
Least-Squares Support Vector Machine (LS-SVM) 43
left anterior descending (LAD) 98
Left bundle branch block (lbbb) 105
left cirumflex (LCx) 98
Left-Down Corner 189
left ventricular ejection fraction (LVEF) 98
Linear Discriminant Analysis (LDA) 18-19, 21, 43
logistic regression (LR) 14

M

machine learning (ML) 237
    domain specific knowledge 239
    lexical knowledge 239, 249
    semantic knowledge 239, 241
machine learning techniques 241
    distribution of data 57, 162, 200, 241
    labeling cost 242
    misclassification cost 26-27, 242
    noise 7, 30, 34-35, 39, 54, 59-60, 63, 69-70, 78, 81-82, 86, 127, 188, 200, 241-242
    representation 11, 14, 22, 30, 34, 55, 88, 91, 95-96, 103, 105, 169, 189, 191, 194, 200-201, 204-205, 210-211, 213, 215, 222-225, 240-247, 249-251, 256, 258-259, 266, 268, 279, 302, 307
Magnetic Resonance Spectroscopy(MRS) 30
Malignant melanoma (MM) 290
maximal wall shear stress (MWSS) 113
maximum a posteriori probability (MAP rule) 20
Maximum Frequent Itemsets (MFI) 275
maximum likelihood (ML) 7
mean square error (MSE) 38
medial-lateral (ML) 23
medical decision support systems (MDSS) 30
memorize (M) 175
memorize-reorder (M-R) 175
Mercer Kernel 65
metabotropic glutamate receptors (mGluRs) 197
metric learning 51, 58-59, 61-62
Microarrays 50
missed QRS detection 79
Model-View-Controller (MVC) 166
modus ponens 259
monitoring systems 161
mortality prediction 10
Moving Average (MA) 125, 132

Moving Window and Variance Analysis (MWVA) 30
Moving Window (MW) 33
Multi-Layer Perceptron (MLP) 255, 267
Multiple Attribute Value (MAV) 125
Multiple linear regressions (MLRs) 145
MYCIN 210

N

National Health Service (NHS) 162
National Institute of Health (NIH) 258
natural language processing (NLP) 237
nerve conduction studies 17-18
Netica 233, 236
Neural networks toolbox 180
no answer (NA) 299
Non-Negative Matrix Factorization (NMF) 6
not-enough-information strategy 216
Nuclear Magnetic Resonance (NMR) 31
number of decomposition coefficients (NDC) 38

O

ONCOCIN 216
oscillatory motions 18
outbreak 126
outbreak detection 128
    field investigation 128
    forensic stage 128
    outbreak detection stage 128
    pre-processing stage 21, 24-25, 34, 38, 45, 97-98, 124, 128, 130, 263
outlier mining 127-128

P

particle filters 75
part-of-speech (POS) 240
pathway evaluation phase 277, 279
pathway mining phase 276, 278
Patient Clinical Data Management (PCDM) 163
Peak Integration (PI) 43
penalized likeihood-scores 228
perfect-map 229
Peripheral Neuropathy (PN) 17
pharmacology 198
phase demodulation (PD) 175
Pointwise Mutual Information (PMI) 240
posturography 18-19
Principal Component Analysis (PCA) 6, 175, 186
Probabilistic Graphical Models (PGM) 223

prognostic reasoning 231
protein sequence 195
pursue strategy 215

Q

QRD complex 68
QRS detector 68

R

RaPiD 216
Receiver Operating Characteristic (ROC) 301
receptor 197
reflectance confocal microscopy 291
relational databases (RDB) 166
Relevance Vector Machines 5
Relevant Component Analysis algorithm (RCA) 54
renal biopsy (RB) 263
reorder (R) 175
Research Patient Data Repository (RPDR) 244
Rich Internet Applications (RIA) 165
right coronary artery (RCA) 98
Risk-of-Death (ROD) 12
Roundsman 216
R-R intervals 70
rule-based approaches 239
rule-in-rule-out strategy 216

S

SamIam 233, 236
Scale Invariant Feature Transform (SIFT) 95
scintigraphic images 98
score-and-search-based learning 227
Self-Organizing Map (SOM) 188
Sepsis 2
    Sepsis Induced Hypotension 3
    Severe Sepsis 2-3, 5-6, 14-15
Septic Shock and Multiorganic Dysfunction Syndrome (MODS) 2
sequence extraction 275
Sequential Organ Failure Assessment (SOFA) 4, 14
signal-to-noise ratio (SNR) 30, 38

Single Prediction Reliability Estimate 124
statistical approach 240
Statistical Pattern Recognition 17-20, 25, 27, 196
stenosis 114, 124
Strong Fuzzy Partitions (SFPs) 260
structured query language (SQL) 169
subtrochanteric fractures 139
Support Vector Machine (SVM) 1, 267
surveillance system 128
Surviving Sepsis Campaign (SSC) 6
symptomatic ones (SN) 23
synthetic examples 114
Synthetic Minority Oversampling Technique (SMOTE) 113

T

TETRAD 233, 236
time of echo (TE) 32
time repetition (TR) 33
Treatment Data Management (TDM) 163
true positive rate (TPR) 302

U

Undirected Graph (UG) 224
universe of discourse (UD) 260
Up-Right Corner 189
user interface 210

V

Vector Quantizer (VQ) 22
Venus flytrap domain (VFT) 198
visual data mining 188
visuo-motor task (VM) 175

W

wait (W) 175
weight vector 188
within-groups variance (WGV) 33, 49
World Health Organization (WHO) 32